New Insights into Cardiothoracic Surgery

New Insights into Cardiothoracic Surgery

Editor: Daniel Willson

AMERICAN
MEDICAL PUBLISHERS
www.americanmedicalpublishers.com

AMERICAN
MEDICAL PUBLISHERS
www.americanmedicalpublishers.com

Cataloging-in-Publication Data

New insights into cardiothoracic surgery / edited by Daniel Willson.
p. cm.
Includes bibliographical references and index.
ISBN 979-8-88740-329-8
1. Heart--Surgery. 2. Chest--Surgery. 3. Cardiovascular system--Surgery.
4. Heart--Surgery--Technological innovations. I. Willson, Daniel.
RD598 .N49 2023
617.412--dc23

American Medical Publishers,
41 Flatbush Avenue,
1st Floor, New York,
NY 11217, USA

ISBN 979-8-88740-329-8 (Hardback)

Contents

Preface

Cardiothoracic surgery is the medical specialty involved with the surgical treatment of organs within the thorax, principally, the heart, lungs, chest wall, esophagus and diaphragm. There are three major subspecialties of cardiothoracic surgery, namely, cardiac, thoracic and congenital. There are a variety of cardiothoracic surgeries and procedures. Angioplasty is a commonly used surgical procedure, which helps in the restoration of healthy blood flow to the heart. This is done by reopening the arteries that are narrowed by the accumulation of fatty plaque. Stent placement is another cardiothoracic surgical method that involves the placement of a small metal coil or tube to hold open the narrowed arteries. Some other surgical procedures and device implantations under cardiothoracic surgery are coronary artery bypass grafting (CABG), heart valve repair or replacement, ventricular assist devices, heart transplant, carotid surgery, pacemakers and implantable cardioverter defibrillators (ICDs). This book is a valuable compilation of topics, ranging from the basic to the most complex advancements in the field of cardiothoracic surgery. It consists of contributions made by international experts. The book will serve as a valuable source of reference for graduate and post graduate students.

All of the data presented henceforth, was collaborated in the wake of recent advancements in the field. The aim of this book is to present the diversified developments from across the globe in a comprehensible manner. The opinions expressed in each chapter belong solely to the contributing authors. Their interpretations of the topics are the integral part of this book, which I have carefully compiled for a better understanding of the readers.

At the end, I would like to thank all those who dedicated their time and efforts for the successful completion of this book. I also wish to convey my gratitude towards my friends and family who supported me at every step.

Editor

1

Predictors of acute kidney insufficiency post isolated coronary artery bypass grafting surgery

Waleed Aty[1,2*], Eric Lo[1], Wei Xuan[3], Rebecca J. Dignan[1,3], Bruce French[1] and Rebecca Verchin[1]

Abstract

Background: Despite the advances of cardiac surgery in the last decades, the incidence of acute kidney insufficiency (AKI) post isolated coronary artery bypass grafting surgery (iCABG) is increasing. The purpose of this study was to identify the potential predictors of postoperative AKI in iCABG in order to implement measures to reduce its incidence.

Results: We reviewed the data of 1914 patients who had on-pump iCABG from January 2008 to December 2015, using the cardiothoracic surgery unit database of Liverpool Hospital, Sydney, New South Wales, Australia. Patients were divided into two groups according to the occurrence of postoperative AKI. The incidence of postoperative AKI was 5.3% in 8 years ($n = 101/1914$ patients). Multivariable analysis has identified the following independent predictors of postoperative AKI; age older than 80 years (OR 4.27; 95% CI 1.6–11.81) ($p < 0.005$), diabetes mellitus (OR 1.96; 95% CI 1.073–3.65) ($p = 0.034$), peripheral vascular disease (OR 2.55; 95% CI 1.16–5.59) ($p < 0.01$), severe congestive cardiac symptoms (i.e., NYHA III & IV) (OR 1.9; 95% CI 1.26–2.92) ($p = 0.002$), surgical re-exploration (OR 2.49; 95% CI 1.07–5.76) ($p = 0.04$), postoperative red blood cell (RBC) transfusion (OR 4.93; 95% CI 2.25–10.80) ($p < 0.0001$), and postoperative low cardiac output syndrome (OR 2.85; 95% CI 1.49–5.46) ($p < 0.0001$).

Conclusion: Postoperative AKI after iCABG is a complex problem. Predictors of postoperative AKI can be mitigated by accurate risk-based assessment and intraoperative proper surgical hemostasis.

Keywords: Acute kidney insufficiency, Isolated coronary artery bypass grafting surgery, Postoperative blood transfusion

Background

Acute kidney insufficiency (AKI) post isolated coronary artery bypass grafting surgery (iCABG) is a serious complication associated with increased morbidity and mortality [1–6]. Despite the advancements achieved in cardiac surgery and postoperative care, the incidence of AKI is increasing [6]. The reported incidence of AKI after cardiac surgery ranged between 2.4 and 40%; this variability is attributed to different AKI definitions and patients' characteristics among studies [7–10]. AKI increased hospital mortality by 10–30%, and it can be as high as 40–60% if continuous renal replacement therapy (CRRT) was required [11, 12].

The aim of this study was to identify the potential risk factors of postoperative AKI in patients undergoing iCABG in order to implement measures to reduce its incidence in high-risk patients.

Methods

Study design and data collection

This is a retrospective cohort study performed at the Cardiothoracic Surgery Unit - Liverpool Hospital, Sydney, New South Wales, Australia. Data were retrieved from the prospectively maintained database collected at the time of surgery using the questionnaire of the Australian and New Zealand Society of Cardiac and Thoracic Surgeons (ANZSCTS) database. An "opt- out" consent and information sheet were utilized. This study was approved by the Sydney South West Area Health Service Human Research Ethics Committee (Western Zone, HREC reference number: HE17/015)

* Correspondence: waleedaty@yahoo.com.au
[1]Department of Cardiac Surgery, Liverpool Hospital, Level 1, New Clinical Building, Elizabeth St, Liverpool, Sydney, New South Wales, Australia
[2]Department of Cardiac Surgery, Faculty of Medicine, Suez Canal University, Ismailia, Egypt
Full list of author information is available at the end of the article

The definition of new AKI and grouping

The last serum creatinine prior to cardiac surgery and the highest postoperative serum creatinine prior to discharge were used to define the stage of AKI. AKI stages were defined by Acute Kidney Injury Network (AKIN) definitions as follows: stage 1: 50% increase in serum creatinine from baseline, stage 2: a 2-fold increase in serum creatinine, and stage 3: a 3-fold increase in serum creatinine or a new dialysis-dependent renal failure.

Because of the small proportion of patients with new AKI, we merged stages 1, 2, and 3 in one group (AKI group), and patients with normal postoperative serum creatinine were designated as No AKI group.

Patients

All iCABG patients operated between January 2008 to December 2015 were included in the study ($n = 1914$). Patients with new AKI ($n = 101$) were compared to patients with No AKI ($n = 1813$). Patients who had off-pump CABG or concomitant valve surgery with CABG were excluded to create homogenous cohort of patients. Factors investigated included age; gender; comorbidities; perioperative baseline data including the clinical status; operative data including cardiopulmonary bypass, aortic cross clamp times; and need for intra-aortic balloon pump (IABP); and postoperative data which could be associated with the development of postoperative AKI.

Statistical analysis

Continuous variables were presented as mean ± standard deviation (SD) and categorical data as frequencies and percent. A chi-square test was used to investigate the association between the presence of AKI and the categorical risk factors. Student's t test and the Wilcoxon rank-sum test were used to compare continuous variables between AKI and No AKI groups. For the dichotomized outcome variable (AKI presence/absence), multivariable logistic regression analysis was implemented to investigate the independent predictors of postoperative AKI. All analyses were performed using SAS statistical software (SAS v9.4; SAS Institute, Cary, North Carolina, USA), and p value < 0.05 was considered statistically significant.

Table 1 Comparisons of demographic and clinical variables in patients with and without postoperative AKI in isolated CABG cohort

Variables	No AKI group (*N* 1813)	AKI group (*N* 101)	*p* value
Age, years			
≤ 65	925 (51.02)	30 (29.7)	
65–80	788 (43.5)	56 (55.5)	
> 80	100 (5.5)	15 (14.9)	< 0.0001
Gender (male)	1490 (77.9)	80 (79.2)	0.44
Body mass index (kg/m^2)	30.2 ± 17.3	30.1 ± 14.9	0.99
Positive smoking history	1231 (67.9)	59 (58.4)	0.04
Family history of IHD	803 (44.4)	45 (44.6)	0.96
Hypertension	1488 (82.1)	96 (95.1)	0.0008
Dyslipidemia	1529 (84.4)	88 (87.1)	0.45
Respiratory disease	323 (16.9)	21 (20.8)	0.67
Diabetes mellitus	770 (42.5)	65 (64.4)	< 0.0001
Cerebrovascular disease	152 (8.4)	14 (13.9)	0.057
Peripheral vascular disease	149 (8.2)	19 (18.8)	0.0003
Acute myocardial infarction < 30 days	1133 (62.5)	75 (74.3)	0.017
Moderate to severe LVD	304 (16.8)	24 (24.1)	0.06
Congestive heart failure	232 (12.8)	31 (30.7)	< 0.0001
Cardiogenic shock	39 (2.2)	10 (9.9)	< 0.0001
NYHA grade III & IV	137 (7.6)	23 (22.8)	< 0.0001
Urgency of surgery			
Elective	1225 (67.6)	65 (64.4)	
Urgent	507 (28.0)	25 (24.8)	
Emergent	80 (4.4)	8 (7.9)	< 0.0001
CPB time (min)	100.76 ± 47.39	106 ± 56.8	0.23
Aortic cross clamp time (min)	71.3 ± 31.2	69.3 (39.3)	0.54
Intra-aortic balloon pump	100 (5.5)	20 (19.8)	< 0.0001

Categorical variables are presented as number (%) and continuous variables as mean (SD)

AKI acute kidney insufficiency, *CABG* coronary artery bypass grafting, *IHD* ischemic heart disease, *LVD* left ventricular dysfunction, *NYHA* New York Heart Association, *CPB* cardiopulmonary bypass

Results

Patients' characteristics and operative data

Incidence of AKI post iCABG was 5.3% ($n = 101/1914$ patients) during the study period. Comparison of the patients' demographic and perioperative characteristics between patients with and without postoperative AKI is shown in Table 1.

Patients who had postoperative AKI were significantly older ($p < 0.0001$), smoker ($p = 0.04$), hypertensives ($p = 0.0008$), and diabetics ($p < 0.0001$) and had more peripheral vascular disease ($p = 0.0003$), had recent MI ($p < 0.0001$), had congestive heart failure symptoms (NYHA III & IV) ($p < 0.0001$), had severe left ventricular dysfunction ($p < 0.0001$), and had cardiogenic shock ($p < 0.0001$).

Postoperative data

Postoperatively, the patients in the AKI group had more cardiac support with IABP ($p < 0.0001$), inotropic support, blood transfusion ($p < 0.0001$), and more frequent surgical re-exploration ($p < 0.0001$) (Table 2).

Predictors of AKI

A multivariable logistic regression analysis model was constructed using variables presented in Table 3, and it

Table 2 Comparison of postoperative variables between the AKI group and No AKI group

Variable	No AKI group	AKI group	*p* value
Return for exploration	70 (3.9)	22 (21. 8)	< 0.0001
Low cardiac out put	370 (20.4)	53 (52.5)	< 0.0001
Vasoplegic shock	387 (21.4)	40 (39.6)	< 0.0001
Blood product transfusion			
Red blood cell	605 (33.4)	76 (75.3)	< 0.0001
Other blood product	449 (24.8)	52 (51.5)	< 0.0001

Categorical variables are presented as *n* (%) and continuous variables as mean ± SD
AKI acute kidney insufficiency

identified the following risk factors as predictors of postoperative AKI after iCABG (Table 3): age above 80 years (OR 4.27; 95% CI 1.6–11.81), diabetes mellitus (OR 1.96; 95% CI 1.073–3.65), peripheral vascular disease (OR 2.55; 95% CI 1.16–5.59), severe congestive cardiac symptoms (NYHA III & IV) (OR 1.9; 95% CI 1.26–2.92), surgical re-exploration (OR 2.49; 95% CI 1.07–5.76), postoperative red blood cell (RBC) transfusion (OR 4.93; 95% CI 2.25–10.80), and postoperative low cardiac output syndrome (OR 2.85; 95% CI 1.49–5.46).

Table 3 Multivariable analysis of predictors of postoperative acute kidney insufficiency (AKI) in isolated coronary artery bypass grafting

Variables	Adjusted OR (95%CI)	*p* value
Age, years		
≤ 65	Reference value	
65–80	1.4 (0.7–3.1)	0.39
> 80	4.27 (1.6–11.8)	0.005
Smoking	0.64 (0.3–1.2)	0.17
Diabetes mellitus	1.96 (1.1–3.7)	0.04
Cerebrovascular disease	0.94 (0.4–2.4)	0.94
Peripheral vascular disease	2.55 (1.2–5.6)	0.02
Acute myocardial infarction < 30 days	1.48 (0.7–2.9)	0.27
History of congestive heart failure	0.80 (0.4–1.9)	0.64
NYHA III & IV	1.90 (1.3–2.9)	0.002
Cardiogenic shock	0.34 (0.3–2.9)	0.16
Urgency		
Elective	Reference value	
Urgent	0.56 (0.3–1.2)	0.12
Emergency	0.70 (0.2–2.4)	0.56
Use intra-aortic balloon pump	0.98 (0.3–2.9)	0.97
Surgical re-exploration	2.49 (1.1–5.8)	0.04
Postoperative atrial fibrillation	1.54 (0.8–2.9)	0.19
Postoperative low cardiac output syndrome	2.85 (1.5–5.5)	< 0.0001
Blood product transfusion		
Red blood cells	4.93 (2.3–10.8)	< 0.0001
Other blood products	0.65 (0.1–1.3)	0.24

CI confidence interval, *OR* odds ratio, *NYHA* New York Heart Association

Discussion

In this study, the incidence of AKI was 5.2% which is higher than the expected for the isolated CABG but lies within the reported range (2.4–40%) of AKI after cardiac surgery [1, 5, 6, 8, 10, 13–16]. The higher incidence of AKI in our study could be explained by merging patients with different AKIN stages into one stage. The variation in the incidence of AKI in literature is likely due to two reasons: a lack of universal definition for postoperative AKI and difference in patient population among studies. Warren and colleagues defined AKI as the rise in creatinine 25% from baseline or an absolute increase of > 0.5 mg/dL [6]. Other studies used different equations to calculate the effective glomerular filtration rate (EGFR) and then defined the AKI according to the change in the pre- and postoperative EGFR [10]. AKI definition in other studies was based on the calculated creatinine clearance [8]. In a large cohort, Chertow and associates defined AKI as the deterioration of the renal function sufficient to require dialysis within 30 days after surgery [13]. The difference in the demographics and operative variations of the studied populations affected the occurrence of postoperative AKI; previous studies included the results of valvular and combined cardiac surgeries which are more complex than iCABG [5, 7–13, 17]. Despite the advances in cardiac surgery and postoperative care in the last decades, the incidence of postoperative AKI is increasing which may be explained by the increased number of high-risk patients undergoing iCABG in recent decades making them vulnerable to postoperative AKI [1, 6].

The pathogenesis of AKI after iCABG is still not fully understood and likely multifactorial. In general, it requires combinations of risk factors as well as several intraoperative or postoperative insults. The independent risk factors for AKI identified in this cohort were age above 80 years, diabetes mellitus, peripheral vascular disease, and the presence of congestive heart failure symptoms. Similar findings were reported in our previous study and other studies [18–20]. Unsurprisingly, the combination of elderly, diabetics, and patients with vascular disease predisposed patient to AKI with minimal insult. These are non-modifiable multi-systemic risk factors which affected both heart, kidney and neurovascular systems. In our institute, we did not use any preoperative risk stratification algorithms [9, 21, 22] to predict and identify high-risk patients who were vulnerable to have AKI and could benefit from peri- or intraoperative renal protective strategies. Huen and their colleagues concluded in their reviews that these scoring systems require more validation across huge cohorts in different centers before being adopted [9].

Operative factor predicting AKI in this cohort was emergency surgery. Patients who suffer from inadequate renal perfusion due to acute coronary syndrome and cardiogenic shock are often associated with postoperative low cardiac output syndrome which causes renal hypoperfusion especially to vulnerable kidneys. Additionally, operating urgently on a patient just loaded by coronary angiogram contrast dye adds more insult to those vulnerable kidneys. In recent series [4, 23, 24], prolonged cardiopulmonary bypass was associated with postoperative AKI, a finding which was not confirmed in our study as the univariable analysis revealed no difference in CPB and ischemic time between AKI and No AKI groups.

We found that surgical re-exploration due to postoperative bleeding or cardiac tamponade were the most significant postoperative predictors of AKI post iCABG; this result was also reported by others [10, 25]. We assumed that postoperative surgical re-exploration exacerbated other risk factors that add more insult to the renal perfusion as hemodynamic instability, anemia, blood transfusion, and the use of vasopressors. Postoperative bleeding may also initiate multiple episodes of renal hypoperfusion due to either hypotension or cardiac tamponade. Loor and Ranucci and their colleagues found anemia to be independent predictor of postoperative AKI [26, 27]. Anemia decreases renal oxygen delivery, impairs hemostasis and enhances oxidative stress contributing to the risk of renal insult. Anemia and blood transfusion had a synergistic effect on postoperative AKI, as there is an increasing risk of postoperative AKI in transfused anemic patient compared to non-transfuse anemic patient which was attributed to the increased risk of post-transfusion oxidative injury in anemic patients with abnormal iron metabolism [28, 29].

This study found that the transfusion of RBCs postoperatively was an independent predictor of AKI. We believed that blood transfusion was a consequence of postoperative bleeding and many studies reported that stored RBC transfusions contributed to organ dysfunction in borderline patients. Stored RBCs have no ability to generate nitric osxide, increasing its adhesive power to the vascular endothelium which may result in impairment of tissue oxygen delivery, increasing oxygen oxidative stress and coagulation cascade which may contribute to the establishment of postoperative AKI [28–30].

Study limitations

This study was a retrospective and observational study, and therefore, the conclusion drawn should be considered according to these constraints. Because of the inclusion of on-pump isolated CABG only, our results cannot be generalized to other populations; additionally, the small number of events compared to the variables included in the logistic regression model added more limitation to this study. The effect of unknown confounders on the observed associations between the risk factors and AKI, such as contrast used in coronary angiogram and CT scan, perioperative and postoperative use of nephrotoxic medication, hydration state or perioperative anemia, intraoperative hypotension, the effect of CPB, and intraoperative hematocrit level, cannot be ruled out. It is difficult to implicate or conclude a temporal relationship between AKI and iCABG and whether all AKI events in iCABG were due to correlation and not a causation

Conclusion

This study identified the predictors of acute kidney insufficiency after isolated CABG. Older patients with non-modifiable comorbidities such as diabetes mellitus, peripheral vascular disease, and symptomatic heart failure could be identified preoperatively and should have accurate risk-based assessments to give the patients and their families accurate risk prediction; moreover, measures can be put in place by the heart team to decrease the risk of postoperative AKI. Postoperative predictors can be mitigated by preoperative optimization of hemoglobin levels, coagulation profiles, and proper surgical hemostasis.

Abbreviations

AKI: Acute kidney insufficiency; CABG: Coronary artery bypass grafting; iCABG: Isolated coronary artery bypass grafting; IHD: Ischemic heart disease; LVD: Left ventricular dysfunction; NYHA: New York Heart Association; IABP: Intra-aortic balloon pump; AKIN: Acute Kidney Injury Network; CPB: Cardiopulmonary bypass; M ± SD: Mean and standard deviation; CI: Confidence interval; OR: Odds ratio; ANZSCTS: Australian and New Zealand Society of Cardiac and Thoracic Surgeons; CRRT: Continuous renal replacement therapy

Acknowledgements

Not applicable

Authors' contributions

WA wrote the study protocol. RD and BF reviewed the protocol before it was submitted to the ethics committee. WA and RV reviewed and collected the missing data. WA and XW did the statistical analysis. WA and ER wrote the manuscript. All authors read and approved the manuscript for submission and publications.

Author details

[1]Department of Cardiac Surgery, Liverpool Hospital, Level 1, New Clinical Building, Elizabeth St, Liverpool, Sydney, New South Wales, Australia. [2]Department of Cardiac Surgery, Faculty of Medicine, Suez Canal University, Ismailia, Egypt. [3]Sydney Southwest Clinical School, University of New South Wales, Liverpool, New South Wales, Australia.

References

1. ElBardissi AW, Aranki SF, Sheng S, O'Brien SM, Greenberg CC, Gammie JS (2012) Trends in isolated coronary artery bypass grafting: an analysis of the Society of Thoracic Surgeons adult cardiac surgery database. J Thorac Cardiovasc Surg 143(2):273–281
2. Gelsomino S, Del Pace S, Parise O, Caciolli S, Matteucci F, Fradella G et al (2017) Impact of renal function impairment assessed by CKDEPI estimated glomerular filtration rate on early and late outcomes after coronary artery bypass grafting. Int J Cardiol 227:778–787
3. Liotta M, Olsson D, Sartipy U, Holzmann MJ (2014) Minimal changes in postoperative creatinine values and early and late mortality and cardiovascular events after coronary artery bypass grafting. Am J Cardiol 113(1):70–75
4. Pickering JW, James MT, Palmer SC (2015) Acute kidney injury and prognosis after cardiopulmonary bypass: a meta-analysis of cohort studies. Am J Kidney Dis 65(2):283–293
5. Thakar CV, Worley S, Arrigain S, Yared JP, Paganini EP (2005) Influence of renal dysfunction on mortality after cardiac surgery: modifying effect of preoperative renal function. Kidney Int 67(3):1112–1119
6. Warren J, Mehran R, Baber U, Xu K, Giacoppo D, Gersh BJ et al (2016) Incidence and impact of acute kidney injury in patients with acute coronary syndromes treated with coronary artery bypass grafting: insights from the Harmonizing Outcomes With Revascularization and Stents in Acute Myocardial Infarction (HORIZONS-AMI) and Acute Catheterization and Urgent Intervention Triage Strategy (ACUITY) trials. Am Heart J 171(1):40–47
7. Coca SG, Yusuf B, Shlipak MG, Garg AX, Parikh CR (2009) Long-term risk of mortality and other adverse outcomes after acute kidney injury: a systematic review and meta-analysis. Am J Kidney Dis 53(6):961–973
8. Doddakula K, Al-Sarraf N, Gately K, Hughes A, Tolan M, Young V et al (2007) Predictors of acute renal failure requiring renal replacement therapy post cardiac surgery in patients with preoperatively normal renal function. Interact Cardiovasc Thorac Surg 6(3):314–318
9. Huen SC, Parikh CR (2012) Predicting acute kidney injury after cardiac surgery: a systematic review. Ann Thorac Surg 93(1):337–347
10. Karkouti K, Wijeysundera DN, Yau TM, Callum JL, Cheng DC, Crowther M et al (2009) Acute kidney injury after cardiac surgery: focus on modifiable risk factors. Circulation 119(4):495–502
11. Mangano CM, Diamondstone LS, Ramsay JG, Aggarwal A, Herskowitz A, Mangano DT (1998) Renal dysfunction after myocardial revascularization: risk factors, adverse outcomes, and hospital resource utilization. The Multicenter Study of Perioperative Ischemia Research Group. Ann Intern Med 128(3):194–203
12. Ryden L, Sartipy U, Evans M, Holzmann MJ (2014) Acute kidney injury after coronary artery bypass grafting and long-term risk of end-stage renal disease. Circulation 130(23):2005–2011
13. Chertow GM, Levy EM, Hammermeister KE, Grover F, Daley J (1998) Independent association between acute renal failure and mortality following cardiac surgery. Am J Med 104(4):343–348
14. Cooper WA, O'Brien SM, Thourani VH, Guyton RA, Bridges CR, Szczech LA et al (2006) Impact of renal dysfunction on outcomes of coronary artery bypass surgery: results from the Society of Thoracic Surgeons National Adult Cardiac Database. Circulation 113(8):1063–1070
15. Lagny MG, Jouret F, Koch JN, Blaffart F, Donneau AF, Albert A et al (2015) Incidence and outcomes of acute kidney injury after cardiac surgery using either criteria of the RIFLE classification. BMC Nephrology 16:76
16. Rosner MH, Okusa MD (2006) Acute kidney injury associated with cardiac surgery. Clin J Am Soc Nephrol 1(1):19–32
17. O'Neal JB, Shaw AD, FTt B (2016) Acute kidney injury following cardiac surgery: current understanding and future directions. Crit Care (London, England). 20(1):187
18. Ahmed WA, Tully PJ, Baker RA, Knight JL (2009) Survival after isolated coronary artery bypass grafting in patients with severe left ventricular dysfunction. Ann Thorac Surg 87(4):1106–1112
19. Chertow GM, Lazarus JM, Christiansen CL, Cook EF, Hammermeister KE, Grover F et al (1997) Preoperative renal risk stratification. Circulation 95(4): 878–884
20. Fortescue EB, Bates DW, Chertow GM (2000) Predicting acute renal failure after coronary bypass surgery: cross-validation of two risk-stratification algorithms. Kidney Int 57(6):2594–2602
21. Eriksen BO, Hoff KR, Solberg S (2003) Prediction of acute renal failure after cardiac surgery: retrospective cross-validation of a clinical algorithm. Nephrol Dial Transplant 18(1):77–81
22. Thakar CV, Arrigain S, Worley S, Yared JP, Paganini EP (2005) A clinical score to predict acute renal failure after cardiac surgery. J Am Soc Nephrol 16(1): 162–168
23. Axtell AL, Fiedler AG, Melnitchouk S, D'Alessandro DA, Villavicencio MA, Jassar AS et al Correlation of Cardiopulmonary Bypass Duration with Acute Renal Failure after Cardiac Surgery. J Thorac Cardiovasc Surg
24. Li Z, Fan G, Zheng X, Gong X, Chen T, Liu X et al (2019) Risk factors and clinical significance of acute kidney injury after on-pump or off-pump coronary artery bypass grafting: a propensity score-matched study. Interact Cardiovasc Thorac Surg
25. Moulton MJ, Creswell LL, Mackey ME, Cox JL, Rosenbloom M (1996) Reexploration for bleeding is a risk factor for adverse outcomes after cardiac operations. J Thorac Cardiovasc Surg 111(5):1037–1046
26. Loor G, Li L, Sabik JF 3rd, Rajeswaran J, Blackstone EH, Koch CG (2012) Nadir hematocrit during cardiopulmonary bypass: end-organ dysfunction and mortality. J Thorac Cardiovasc Surg 144(3):654–662 e4
27. Ranucci M, Conti D, Castelvecchio S, Menicanti L, Frigiola A, Ballotta A et al (2010) Hematocrit on cardiopulmonary bypass and outcome after coronary surgery in nontransfused patients. Ann Thorac Surg 89(1):11–17
28. Karkouti K (2012) Transfusion and risk of acute kidney injury in cardiac surgery. Br J Anaesth 109 Suppl 1:i29–i38
29. Karkouti K, Wijeysundera DN, Yau TM, McCluskey SA, Chan CT, Wong PY et al (2011) Influence of erythrocyte transfusion on the risk of acute kidney injury after cardiac surgery differs in anemic and nonanemic patients. Anesthesiology 115(3):523–530
30. Cardo LJ, Hmel P, Wilder D (2008) Stored packed red blood cells contain a procoagulant phospholipid reducible by leukodepletion filters and washing. Transfus Apher Sci 38(2):141–147

2

Coronary artery bypass surgery in type 2 diabetic patients: predictors of mortality and morbidity

Younes Moutakiallah[1,2*], Abdelatif Boulahya[1,2], Aniss Seghrouchni[1,2], Reda Mounir[1,2], Noureddine Atmani[1,2], Mohammed Drissi[1,3], El Ghadbane Abdedaim Hatim[1,3], Zouhair Lakhal[1,4], Iliyasse Asfalou[1,4], Youssef El Bekkali[1,2], Redouane Abouqal[1,5] and Mahdi Aithoussa[1,2]

Abstract

Background: Coronary artery bypass grafting has been widely admitted in the therapeutic arsenal of coronary artery disease in diabetics with low morbi-mortality. However, it requires special management which may be challenging in low-volume centers especially in African countries. We aimed to analyze the outcome of coronary artery bypass graft in our diabetic population and define predictors of adverse events.

Patients and methods: We retrospectively enrolled 529 consecutive diabetic patients (type 2) who underwent on-pump coronary artery bypass grafting at our institution between January 2000 and June 2018. The mean age was 61.1 ± 8.3 years with 4.04 as sex ratio (M/F) and 2.95 as mean EuroSCORE II. History of acute myocardial infarction, left main coronary artery stenosis, and three-vessel disease was present in respectively 58%, 26.1%, and 72.2% of patients. The average number of bypass was 2.4 ± 0.8. Duration of cardiopulmonary bypass and aortic cross-clamping were respectively 124.8 ± 43.5 and 79.7 ± 32.9 min.

Results: In-hospital mortality was 5.9% (n = 31) and the late mortality was 6.9% (n = 32). Duration of artificial ventilation, ICU stay, and postoperative stay were respectively 7 h, 44 h, and 13 days. Postoperative complications were myocardial infarction, superficial wound infection, mediastinitis, and low cardiac output syndrome in respectively 9.1%, 25.5%, 3.8%, and 12.7% of patients. Multivariable logistic regression analysis revealed that left ventricular ejection fraction < 40% (OR = 1.88; 95% CI 1.30–2.47; p = 0.03), poor perioperative glycemic control (OR = 1.53; 95% CI 1.12–2.38; p = 0.014), intra-aortic balloon pump insertion (OR = 2.29; 95% CI 1.47–3.10; p < 0.001), and postoperative cardiac complications (OR = 2.01; 95% CI 1.23–2.78; p < 0.001) were predictors of in-hospital mortality. Predictors of mediastinitis were obesity (OR = 5.86; 95% CI 1.43–23.95; p = 0.014), inotropic drugs use (OR = 8.14; 95% CI 1.57–42.34; p = 0.013), chest reopening for bleeding (OR = 4.01; 95% CI 0.62–25.85; p = 0.014), and blood transfusion (OR = 7.56; 95% CI 1.09–52.76; p = 0.041). Follow-up was 86.1% complete, with a mean follow-up of 63.5 ± 48.3 months (1–192 months), and cumulative survival at 5, 10, and 15 years was respectively 95.5 ± 1.1%, 86.3 ± 2.9%, and 76.9 ± 6.9%.

Conclusion: Even in low-volume centers in developing areas, coronary artery bypass surgery is an effective therapy for coronary artery disease in diabetic patients despite a relative high morbidity and mortality.

Keywords: Diabetes mellitus, Coronary artery bypass grafting surgery, Low-volume center, Low-income countries, Africa

* Correspondence: dryouns@hotmail.com
[1]Faculty of Medicine and Pharmacy, Mohammed V University, Rabat, Morocco
[2]Cardiac Surgery Department, Mohammed V Teaching Military Hospital, Hay Riyad, PB 10100 Rabat, Morocco
Full list of author information is available at the end of the article

Background

Diabetes mellitus (DM), an important risk factor of coronary artery disease (CAD) [1, 2], is a rapidly progressing public health problem in our country, with a prevalence in adult population varying from 6.6% in 2000 to 12.4% in 2016 [3–5]. This unrestrained evolution of DM and CAD among our population has drastically modified our surgical activity formerly dominated by rheumatic valve disease and now balanced by coronary artery bypass grafting (CABG) which has been largely described by the most internationally accepted studies as the standard of care for CAD [6–8].

DM is constantly increasing throughout the world [9, 10], especially in developing countries, because of rapid changes in lifestyles and dietary habits [11]. However, these radical changes have not been followed, as is the case in developed countries, with adequate care. Therefore, diabetics in developing countries had more complications because of delayed diagnosis and treatment which might have a negative impact on surgical results [11].

Traditionally, DM has been associated with poor results and adverse outcomes after CABG for both the short term and long term [12–14]. However, several recent series conducted mainly in developed countries have shown that DM is not in itself an additional risk in CABG with almost similar results in diabetic and non-diabetic patients [12, 15–17]. However, can these results obtained in high-volume and experienced centers in high socio-economic countries be replicated in low-volume centers in developing areas such as Africa? This concern is largely justified by the frequency of co-morbidities and degenerative disorders which require special management and may be challenging in low-income African countries. The aim of the current study was to analyze the outcome of CABG in diabetic population and to define predictors of adverse events.

Methods

Study design

After approval of our institutional review board and registered in ISRCTN registry, we conducted an observational retrospective cohort study about outcomes of CABG in diabetic patients. We collected and analyzed the data of 529 consecutive type 2 diabetic patients who underwent on-pump CABG at our institution between January 2000 and June 2018. Data were extracted from preoperative and postoperative clinical notes, anesthesia and operating data records, intensive care unit (ICU) progress notes, and laboratory data. Patients were divided into two groups: insulin-treated group (IT group) (n = 322) and non-insulin-treated group (NIT group) (n = 207).

Inclusion and exclusion criteria

The inclusion criteria were all type 2 diabetic patients with diagnostic coronary artery disease and who underwent on-pump CABG. The exclusion criteria were type 1 diabetes and off-pump CABG.

Definitions

DM type 2 is defined according to the American Diabetes Association as fasting plasma glucose (FPG) ≥ 126 mg/dl or 2-h plasma glucose ≥ 200 mg/dl during oral glucose tolerance test and A1c hemoglobin (HbA1c) ≥ 6.5% [2]. All patients underwent a systematic arterial ultrasound examination of the abdominal aorta, the supra-aortic trunks, and the lower extremity arteries for peripheral atherosclerosis. In case of significant stenosis, a CT scan was performed. Polyvascular atherosclerotic disease (PVAD) was defined as follows a history of vascular reconstruction; bypass surgery or percutaneous intervention on carotid, abdominal aorta, or any peripheral artery for atherosclerotic lesion; documented aortic aneurysm; or significant atherosclerotic arterial stenosis. Anemia was defined as hemoglobin level below 11 g/dl for women and 13 g/dl for men.

Diabetes management

Anti-diabetic treatment was substituted 2 days before surgery by a standard sliding scale subcutaneous insulin injection. In the operating room and ICU, blood glucose level (BGL) was routinely measured and controlled by intermittent intravenous injection of insulin or by continuous intravenous insulin (50 IU of insulin in 50 ml 0.9% normal saline) adjusted to target intraoperative BGL between 120 and 180 mg/dl. In the ward, patients were switched back to subcutaneous insulin injection and then resumption of the preoperative anti-diabetic regimen usually on the fifth postoperative day.

Operative protocol

All patients were operated according to the same protocol by the same team. General anesthesia was made by cisatracurium besylate, midazolam, thiopental, and propofol. After sternotomy, the pericardium space was opened and the internal thoracic arteries (ITA) and the saphenous vein graft (SVG) were harvested. Initially, for almost all diabetic patients, only the left internal thoracic artery (LITA) was harvested in addition to the SVG until 2010, when we started to harvest both skeletonized ITA. Bilateral internal thoracic artery (BITA) was avoided in patients with one of the following criteria: age > 70 years, obesity, and chronic obstructive pulmonary disease.

Cardiopulmonary bypass (CPB) conventionally performed by standard aortic and venous cannulation was conducted under moderate systemic hypothermia (32 °C). Myocardial protection was achieved with antegrade cold (4 °C) crystalloid St. Thomas cardioplegia and/or antegrade cold blood cardioplegia. We carried on by the right coronary artery anastomosis, then the left marginal arteries, and finally the left anterior descending artery. After aortic clamp release and heart defibrillation, proximal anastomoses to the ascending aorta were performed by partial aortic clamping.

Postoperative management and follow-up

Postoperative events and results are described as follows: in-hospital mortality indicates death occurring during the hospitalization in which CABG was performed, an early complication was defined as an event occurring during hospitalization, and a late complication was defined as an event occurring after discharge. A bleeding event is any episode of major internal or external bleeding that causes death, hospitalization, or permanent injury or required blood transfusion. A neurologic event includes any new, temporary, or permanent focal or global neurologic deficit. Cardiac complication was defined by one of the following: inotropic drug ≥ 72 h, acute myocardial infarction (AMI), low cardiac output syndrome (LCOS), insertion of intra-aortic pump balloon (IABP), return to operating room for bleeding or tamponade, new onset of atrial fibrillation (A. Fib), permanent pacemaker placement, or in-hospital cardiac arrest. Respiratory complication was defined by one of the following: lung collapse, atelectasis, acute respiratory distress syndrome, respiratory failure and pleural effusions, duration of mechanical ventilation ≥ 24 h, re-intubation, or tracheostomy. Infective complication was defined by one of the following: pneumonia, sternum or leg wound infection, mediastinitis, or sepsis. Renal complication was defined by new-onset renal failure (serum creatinine elevation > 2 times) or new-onset renal replacement therapy.

Follow-up data were obtained from our local database. After discharge, all patients were included in our scheduled follow-up protocol with routine clinical controls at 1, 3, 6, and 12 months and annually afterwards. Follow-up data were provided either routinely by our outpatient clinic evaluation (medical visits of the systematic and programmed controls) or by telephone interviews with patients, relatives or referring physicians. The control was based on clinical examination, electrocardiogram, chest X-ray, and echocardiography. In case of residual angina, exertional dyspnea, and electrical or echocardiographic signs of myocardial ischemia, patients were explored by stress test and coronary angiogram.

Statistical analysis

The statistical analysis was performed by IBM statistical package software for social sciences 19.0 (SPSS, Chicago, IL, USA). Data were presented as mean ± standard deviation (SD), median (range), and n (%). For comparisons, chi-square test or Fisher's test were used for categorical variables and Student's t test or non-parametric Wilcoxon rank-sums test for continuous variables. Survival curves were made with Kaplan-Meier method with group comparisons by log-rank test. Independent predictors of in-hospital mortality and adverse outcomes with a p value of less than 0.2 on univariate analysis were considered in the multivariate analysis using stepwise selection. Results are expressed using odds ratio (OR). For all analyses, p values < 0.05 were considered statistically significant.

Results

Total population: See Table 1.

Baseline characteristics

The mean age of patients was 61.1 ± 8.3 years with 4.04 as sex ratio (M/F). More than three cardiovascular risk factors were found in 32.9% of patients, and mean body mass index was 26.5 ± 3.4 kg/m^2. Previous percutaneous coronary intervention and vascular surgery were respectively noticed in 10% and 1.9% of patients. Angina was present in 93.8% of patients, and 42% had Canadian Cardiovascular Society class 3–4. New York Heart Association (NYHA) class 3–4 was found in 23.6% of patients. A. Fib and chest X-ray cardiomegaly were detected respectively in 1.7% and 34.6% of patients. Left ventricular (LV) ejection fraction and systolic pulmonary arterial pressure were respectively 55% (range 20–80%) and 25 mmHg (range 12–96 mmHg). More than mild mitral regurgitation was found in 12.7% of patients. EuroSCORE II and HbA_1c were respectively 1.68 (range 0.7–47) and 8% (range 5.3–14.9%).

Operative data

CPB and aortic cross-clamping times were respectively 124.8 ± 43.5 min and 79.7 ± 32.9 min. Cardioplegia protocol consisted of three categories: cold blood cardioplegia (45.7%), cold crystalloid (39.5%), and mixed cardioplegia (14.7%), and 10% of patients had hot reperfusion just before aortic clamp release. The used grafts were LITA, SVG, and RITA in respectively 97.2%, 78.4%, and 17.4% of patients with 20.6% as rate of all arterial revascularization. Complete revascularization was achieved in 50.5% of patients, and the main reason of the incomplete revascularization, as mentioned on individual surgical reports, was the complexity of lesions and the poor quality of coronary arteries which were of small caliber and unsuitable for bypass. CABG was associated to other procedures in 53 patients (10%) and consisted of 24 aortic valve replacements (4.5%), 10 carotid surgeries, 9 mitral valve replacements, 3 mitral and aortic valve replacements, 1 mitral valve replacement with tricuspid repair, 1 LV aneurysm repair, 1 postinfarction ventricular septal defect (VSD) closure, 1 LV aneurysm repair with VSD closure, 1 abdominal aortic aneurysm repair, and 1 peripheral vascular surgery. Those associated procedures were significantly associated with high rate of mortality

Table 1 Baseline and operative characteristics and outcomes of all patients. Data are expressed as *n* (%) for categorical variables, mean ± standard deviations, or median (range) for continuous variables

Variable	
Age > 70 years	86 (16.3%)
Female, *n* (%)	105 (19.9%)
Cardiovascular risk factor	
Hypertension, *n* (%)	267 (50.5%)
Hyperlipidemia, *n* (%)	206 (38.9%)
Smoking, *n* (%)	288 (54.4%)
Comorbidities	
Renal failure (severe or more), *n* (%)	31 (5.9%)
Stroke, *n* (%)	15 (2.8%)
Chronic obstructive pulmonary disease, *n* (%)	94 (17.8%)
Anemia, *n* (%)	117 (22.1%)
Polyvascular atherosclerotic disease, *n* (%)	97 (18.3%)
Acute myocardial infarction < 3 months, *n* (%)	193 (36.5%)
Echocardiographical and coronary angiogram finding	
Left ventricular ejection fraction < 40%, *n* (%)	66 (12.5%)
Pulmonary hypertension, *n* (%)	183 (34.6%)
Tri-vessels disease, *n* (%)	382 (72.2%)
Left main coronary artery stenosis, *n* (%)	138 (26.1%)
Operative parameters	
Urgency-emergency, *n* (%)	66 (12.5%)
Distal anastomosis per patient	2.3 ± 0.8
Bilateral internal thoracic artery use, *n* (%)	88 (16.6%)
"Y" anastomosis, *n* (%)	43 (8.1%)
Associated procedures, *n* (%)	53 (10%)
Postoperative course	
In-hospital deaths, *n* (%)	31 (5.9%)
Ventilator support, (hours)	7 (2–1560)
Intensive care unit stay, (hours)	44 (18–1560)
Hospital stay (days)	13 (2–106)
Cardiac complications, *n* (%)	117 (22.1%)
Infective complications, *n* (%)	142 (26.8%)
Respiratory complications, *n* (%)	92 (17.4%)
Renal failure, *n* (%)	68 (12.9%)
Cerebro-vascular accident, *n* (%)	11 (2.1%)

($p < 0.001$) and all cardiac complications ($p < 0.001$). The weaning of CPB was difficult in 48 patients (9.1%) and needed inotropic drug use and intra-aortic balloon pump insertion in 40 patients (7.6%).

Postoperative course

The postoperative course was marked by complications in 44% of patients; half was benign in nature (paroxystic A. Fib, transient hypoxemia, and poor glycemic control). Cardiac complications were present in 22.1% of patients and were as follows: inotropic drugs use ≥ 72 h (19.5%), LCOS (12.7%), IABP insertion (9.3%), and AMI (9.1%). However, infections were the most frequent complications (26.8%); the rate of mediastinitis was 3.8% while wound infection and pneumonia rates were respectively 25.5% and 8.7%. Glucose level was poorly controlled in 34.6% of patients. Univariate and multivariate binary logistic regression analysis identified several independent predictors of in-hospital and late mortality and major adverse cardiac and cerebral event (MACCE) (Tables 2 and 3).

Intergroup comparison

We compared IT and NIT group data and found that preoperative parameters were quite similar except for some variables such as diabetes duration, anemia, PVAD, degenerative retinopathy and nephropathy, EuroSCORE II, fasting plasma glucose, HbA_1c, and C reactive protein which were worse in the IT group. However, gastro-duodenal ulcer was more frequent in the NIT group (6.3% vs. 1.9%, $p = 0.01$). There were no significant differences in echocardiography and coronary angiogram findings.

Operative data showed an almost complete similarity between the two groups with no significant difference in surgical techniques, number of distal anastomoses, and grafts used except for complete revascularization which was significantly more reached in the NIT group.

In contrast, outcomes were clearly different, since the IT group showed significantly higher morbidity and mortality. All cardiac complications were significantly more frequent in the IT group except for the rate of AMI which was higher in the IT group without crossing the threshold of significance (10.6% vs. 6.8%, $p = 0.163$). Pneumonia and superficial wound infection rates were also significantly higher in the IT group (29.5% vs. 19.3%, $p = 0.01$; and 11.2% vs. 4.9%, $p = 0.011$ respectively), but the difference was not significant for mediastinitis (4.3% vs. 2.9%, $p = 0.49$) (Table 4).

Follow-up and long-term outcomes

Follow-up was closed on June 1, 2019, and was 86.1% complete, with a cumulative duration of follow-up of 30, 692 patient-years and a mean follow-up period of 63.5 ± 48.3 months (1–192 months). Mortality rate was 6.9% (n = 32), and cumulative survival calculated by Kaplan-Meier method at 5, 10, and 15 years was respectively 95.5 ± 1.1%, 86.3 ± 2.9%, and 76.9 ± 6.9% (Fig. 1), with no significant difference at 15 years between the IT and NIT groups (respectively 72.2 ± 13.5% vs. 79.5 ± 7.8%; $p = 0.311$) (Fig. 2). Similarly, there was no significant difference between complete and incomplete revascularization (respectively 74.9 ± 9.8% vs. 80.1 ± 8.2%; $p = 0.69$) (Figs. 3 and 4).

Table 2 Independent predictors of in-hospital mortality on binary logistic regression analysis (all patients)

Characteristics	Univariate analysis			Multivariate analysis		
	OR	95% CI	*p* value	OR	95% CI	*p* value
Left ventricular ejection fraction < 40%	1.06	0.46–1.66	< 0.001	1.88	1.30–2.47	0.003
Left ventricular diastolic dysfunction	1.17	0.68–1.66	< 0.001	1.28	0.14–9.20	0.008
Right ventricular dysfunction	2.83	1.64–4.01	< 0.001	1.28	0.34–2.23	0.008
Poor glycemic control	3.27	2.95–4.63	0.001	1.53	1.12–2.38	0.014
Low cardiac output syndrome	4.29	3.80–4.77	< 0.001	1.58	0.87–2.29	< 0.001
Intra-aortic balloon pump insertion	4.53	3.95–5.10	< 0.001	2.29	1.47–3.10	< 0.001
Cardiac complications	5.76	5.15–6.38	< 0.001	2.01	1.23–2.78	< 0.001
Postoperative renal failure	3.88	3.38–4.38	< 0.001	1.47	0.93–2.02	< 0.001
Postoperative stroke	3.12	1.73–4.50	< 0.001	1.96	1.05–2.88	< 0.001
Tracheal re-intubation	5.20	4.11–6.28	< 0.001	2.46	1.44–3.49	< 0.001
Respiratory complications	2.58	2.10–3.06	< 0.001	1.04	0.98–1.75	0.035

OR odds ratio, *CI* confidence interval

Exertional angina and NYHA class 3–4 were respectively observed in 6.1% and 5.6% of patients. Rehospitalization for MACCE was observed in 26.8% of patients (27.2% of cardiac events and 1.8% of stroke). Myocardial revascularization was needed in 6.9% of patients (1 redo CABG because of graft failure and 30 percutaneous coronary interventions). There was no significant difference between IT and NIT groups except for hospitalizations for heart failure (8.6% vs. 1.7%; $p = 0.002$).

In contrast, some variables were identified in univariate analysis as having a protector effect on late outcome such as BITA use (OR 1.53, 95% CI 1.01–2.5; $p < 0.001$), complete revascularization (OR 1.31, 95% CI 0.48–1.71; $p = 0.03$), all-arterial revascularization (OR 1.62, 95% CI 0.87–1.93; $p = 0.008$), and hot blood reperfusion (OR 1.42, 95% CI 1.10–1.83; $p = 0.08$), but on multivariate analysis, only complete revascularization (OR 1.70, 95% CI 1.12–2.31; $p = 0.04$) and hot blood reperfusion (OR 1.22, 95% CI 1.06–1.80; $p = 0.02$) were statistically significant predictors of better outcome.

Discussion

As the main finding of our study, CABG can provide relatively good results in diabetic patients with acceptable morbidity and mortality even in low-volume centers in low-middle-income countries. In addition, we have identified several parameters as independent predictors of in-hospital mortality (Table 3). Indeed, our in-hospital mortality rate was relatively high in comparison with large series in developed countries [13, 16, 18, 19], with also a high incidence of postoperative complications.

Surely, the literature had widely debated and treated the outcome and results of CABG in DM in all its aspects, but unfortunately, it is largely dominated by

Table 3 Independent predictors of late mortality and major adverse cardiovascular and cerebral events on binary logistic regression analysis (all patients)

Characteristics	Univariate analysis			Multivariate analysis		
	OR	95% CI	*p* value	OR	95% CI	*p* value
Age > 70 years	2.01	1.18–3.41	0.010	2.93	1.47–5.83	0.002
Female sex	1.21	0.37–1.40	0.048	1.40	1.20–1.80	0.009
Chronic obstructive pulmonary disease	1.97	1.19–3.28	0.009	2.07	1.01–4.23	0.047
Anemia	2.40	1.48–3.91	< 0.001	1.97	1.03–3.80	0.042
Left atrium dilation	1.94	1.27–2.95	0.002	2.16	1.01–4.61	0.046
Lower extremity arterial disease	1.80	1.41–2.32	< 0.001	1.68	1.09–2.59	0.018
Electrical heart defibrillation	1.92	1.27–2.92	0.002	2.25	1.23–3.89	0.004
Postoperative acute myocardial infarction	5.07	2.32–11.07	< 0.001	5.72	1.87–17.46	0.002
Chest reopening for bleeding	4.61	1.48–14.36	0.008	7.72	1.30–45.85	0.025
Prolonged ventilator support	1.02	1.01–1.04	0.001	1.02	1.00–1.04	0.046
Prolonged postoperative stay	1.04	1.02–1.07	< 0.001	1.04	1.00–1.08	0.043

OR odds ratio, *CI* confidence interval

Table 4 Baseline characteristics, operative data, and outcome: comparison between insulin-treated and non-insulin-treated groups. Data are expressed as mean ± SD, median (range), and *n* (%)

Variable	IT group, *n* = 322	NIT group, *n* = 207	*p* value
Baseline characteristics			
Diabetes duration (months)	120 (1–648)	84 (0–468)	< 0.001
Peripheral vascular surgery, *n* (%)	9 (1.7)	1 (0.2)	0.009
Renal failure (severe or more), *n* (%)	22 (6.8)	9 (4.3)	0.27
Chronic obstructive pulmonary disease, *n* (%)	62 (19.3)	32 (15.5)	0.29
Anemia, *n* (%)	81 (25.2)	36 (17.4)	0.04
Polyvascular atherosclerotic disease, *n* (%)	70 (21.7)	27 (13)	0.01
Retinopathy and/or nephropathy, *n* (%)	36 (11.6)	8 (3.9)	0.015
EuroSCORE II	1.9 (0.7–47)	1.4 (0.7–32.8)	0.001
A1c hemoglobin (%)	8.5 (5.8–14.9)	7.3 (5.3–13.8)	< 0.001
Operative data			
Urgency-emergency, *n* (%)	43 (13.4)	23 (11.1)	0.58
Distal anastomosis per patient	2.3 ± 0.8	2.4 ± 0.8	0.1
Complete revascularization, *n* (%)	151 (46.9)	116 (56)	0.04
All arterial revascularization, *n* (%)	65 (20.2)	44 (21.3)	0.84
Difficult weaning of cardio-pulmonary bypass, *n* (%)	36 (11.2)	12 (5.8)	0.04
Intra-aortic balloon pump insertion, *n* (%)	31 (9.6)	9 (4.3)	0.03
Postoperative course			
In-hospital deaths, *n* (%)	24 (7.5)	7 (3.4)	0.036
Ventilator support (hours)	8 (3–1560)	6 (2–524)	< 0.001
Intensive care unit stay (hours)	44 (18–1560)	44 (18–528)	0.001
Postoperative stay (days)	13 (2–106)	13 (2–53)	0.09
Cardiac complications, *n* (%)	82 (25.5)	35 (16.9)	0.024
Infective complications, *n* (%)	102 (31.7)	40 (19.3)	0.002
Respiratory complications, *n* (%)	68 (21.1)	24 (11.6)	0.005
Renal failure, *n* (%)	50 (15.5)	18 (8.7)	0.024
Cerebro-vascular accident, *n* (%)	8 (2.5)	3 (1.5)	0.541
Poor glycemic control, *n* (%)	134 (41.6)	49 (23.7)	< 0.001

IT insulin-treated group, *NIT* non-insulin-treated

series of high-volume centers in developed countries endowed with important logistics, modern hospitals with sophisticated medical equipment, good organization of the health care systems, and a high expertise of the practitioners. However, what about the situation in small centers in developing countries? In our daily practice, we are always extrapolating data from experiences of centers which share few things with our realities. Our study has the advantage to reflect as closely as possible the real-life situation in centers like ours and put the spotlight on the difficulties faced daily to perform CABG in "our" diabetic patients who present a high prevalence of chronic diabetic complications with microvascular lesions which were mainly due to non-compliance with diet, medications, lack of therapeutic education, and delay between the onset of diabetes and diagnosis time. Chadli et al. found in an epidemiologic study that the majority of diabetic patients in our country had at least one diabetes-associated complication and did not achieve the recommended triple target of glycemic, blood pressure and lipid control, suggesting that there is a huge gap between evidence-based diabetes management and real-life practice [20]. Bos et al. stipulated that most diabetic patients in northern Africa were unaware of their complications, and a high percentage of patients with severe complications had never been consulted by a specialist before [11]. Similarly, our patients referred for CABG often had severe diabetic complications and comorbidities such as micro- and macroangiopathy, renal failure, PVAD, and anemia, and frequently, they have never had an

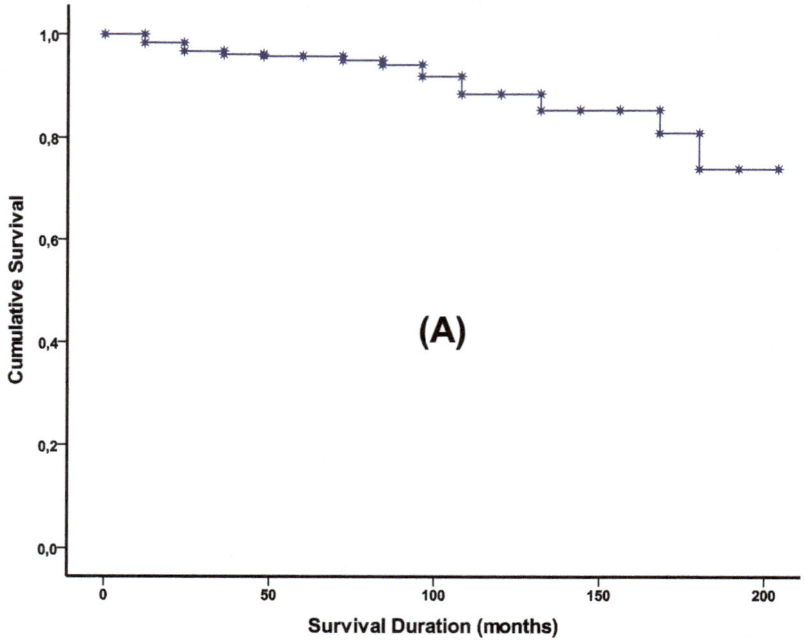

Number of patients at risk

429 263 108 27 1

Fig. 1 Kaplan-Meier survival curve (A) for the whole cohort with all patients enrolled in the study

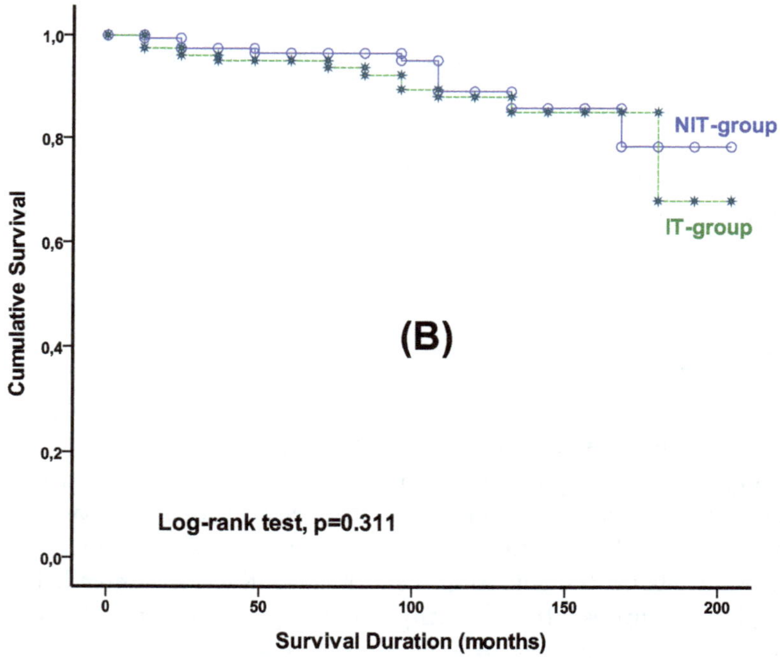

Number of patients at risk

IT-group	180	105	47	14	1
NIT-group	249	158	61	12	1

IT: Insulin-treated
NIT: Non-insulin-treated

Fig. 2 Kaplan-Meier survival curve (B) for the whole cohort with all patients enrolled in the study with comparison between insulin-treated (*n* = 322) and non-insulin-treated (*n* = 207) patients. IT: insulin-treated, NIT: non-insulin-treated

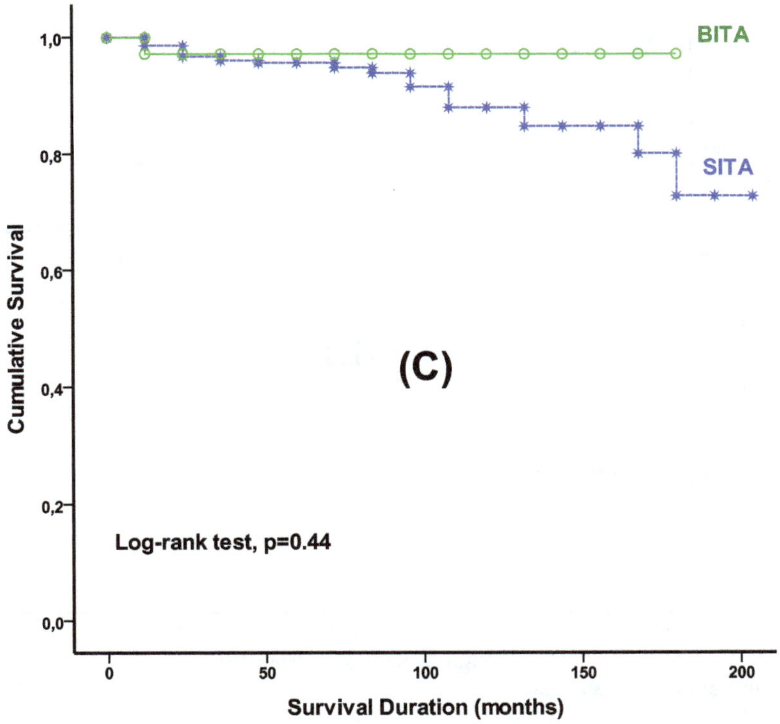

Number of patients at risk

SITA	357	239	103	25	2
BITA	72	23	5	1	/

SITA: Single Internal Thoracic Artery
BITA: Bilateral Internal Thoracic Artery

Fig. 3 Kaplan-Meier survival curve (C) for the whole cohort with comparison between patients who received bilateral internal thoracic artery use (n = 88, 16.6%) and single internal thoracic artery (n = 441, 83.4%). SITA: single internal thoracic artery. BITA: bilateral internal thoracic artery

evaluation of their cardiovascular system until after the declaration of complications such as inaugural AMI whose rate in our series remains very high.

We experienced that perioperative management of diabetes is one of the key of safe, secure, and efficient CABG. Poor perioperative glycemic control was clearly identified in our study as an independent predictor of in-hospital mortality, MACCE, and mediastinitis. That has been shared by most investigators who have focused on the association between perioperative hyperglycemia and mortality after CABG [21–23]. Ujueta et al. mentioned that peri-procedural BGL is associated with adverse clinical outcomes, by the bias of mechanisms of harm including increased inflammation, platelet reactivity, and endothelial dysfunction [24]. Magaji et al. showed the clear benefit of maintaining BGL between 110 and 140 mg/dl in immediate postoperative cardiac surgery by adopting a continuous insulin injection protocol for both glycemic control and hypoglycemia prevention [25].

Several studies had shown that insulin therapy was associated with higher mortality and morbidity [12–14, 18, 26, 27]. In our study, it has been associated in univariate analysis to higher in-hospital mortality and all adverse postoperative events, but it has not been identified in multivariate analysis as an independent predictor. That association might be explained by the fact that insulin therapy in our practice was usually indicated to more severe patients or after failure of conventional diet-oral hypoglycemic drugs; IT group had significantly older diabetes and more diabetes-related comorbidities (PVAD, anemia, higher EuroSCORE II, micro-angiopathy, and poor glycemic control). However, this needs more investigations to be proven.

Certainly, infection of incision sites is one of the most common complications after CABG in diabetic patients. Slightly more than a quarter of our patients presented infection which dominated by superficial and deep wound infection while mediastinitis rate was lesser. The incidence of infective complications was strongly associated with perioperative poor glycemic control. Several independent predictors of mediastinitis were identified in multivariate analysis: age, diabetes duration, obesity, poor perioperative glycemic control, prolonged ICU stay, inotropic support, chest reopening for bleeding, and

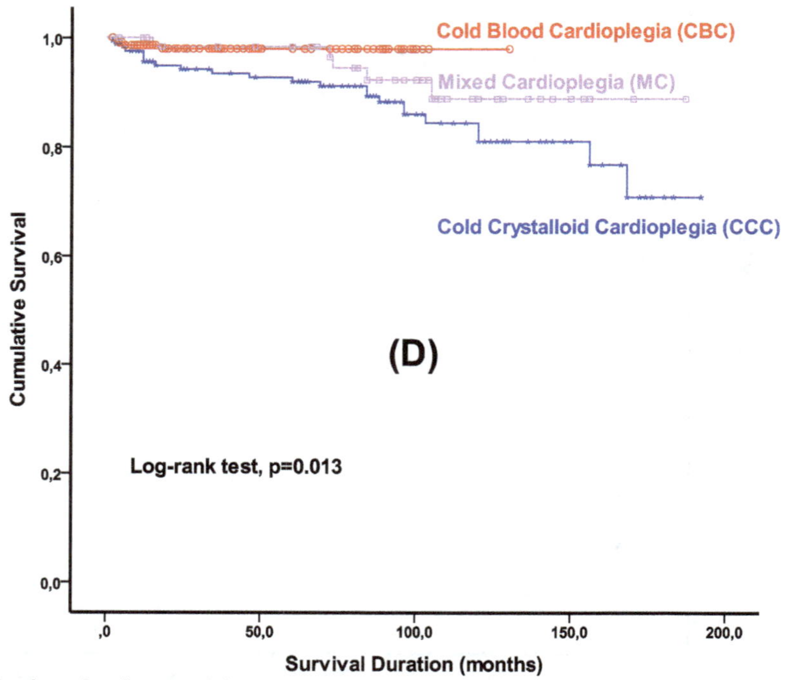

Number of patients at risk

CCC	169	123	57	19	1
MC	66	57	30	4	/
CBC	217	77	9	/	/

CCC: Cold Crystalloid Cardioplegia
MC: Mixed Cardioplegia
CBC: Cold Blood Cardioplegia

Fig. 4 Kaplan-Meier survival curve (D) for the whole cohort with comparison between cardioplegia protocols: cold blood cardioplegia (n = 242, 45.7%), mixed cardioplegia (n = 78, 14.7%), and cold crystalloid cardioplegia (n = 209, 39.5%). CCC: cold crystalloid cardioplegia, MC: mixed cardioplegia, CBC: cold blood cardioplegia

blood transfusion. However, BITA was indicated in the univariate analysis but was not significant in multivariate analysis as an independent predictor of mediastinitis. Even if several recent publications [28, 29] claimed that BITA use has not been associated with an increased risk of mediastinitis compared to SITA, the debate remains; Taggart et al. [30] had published the 5-year results of ART investigation and found that BITA was significantly associated with higher rate of both sternal wound complications and sternal reconstructions without benefit of survival or freedom from adverse events at 5 years. However, it seems that the risk can be lowered if graft harvesting was made by skeletonized fashion with meticulous attention to preserve sternal blood flow [31, 32].

Several studies have shown the superiority of arterial grafts over venous grafts in terms of long-term survival, need of repeated revascularization, and graft failure [28, 29, 31, 32] without impact on in-hospital mortality [33]. But in our practice, and for a long time, we considered diabetes as an absolute contraindication to BITA harvesting because of the "inevitable and frightening" mediastinitis. This situation has been a real obstacle to the development of all arterial revascularization strategies even in case of young and low-risk patients. Lately, since 2010, we have changed this paradigm and adopted a cautious and progressive strategy towards using skeletonized BITA [5]. There was no significant difference of mediastinitis rate between BITA and SITA use (6.8% vs. 3.2%, p = 0.121) (see Additional file 1: Table S1). Moreover, BITA was associated in univariate analysis with a protective effect on survival as well as complete revascularization. That concept was confirmed by many studies which have suggested a survival benefit for CABG versus percutaneous coronary intervention in DM, which can be due to the completeness of revascularization and to the good long-term patency of ITA over SVG [33–35].

Limitations of the study

Several important limitations exist in the current study. Mainly, it is limited by its mono-centric observational retrospective nature. The period of recruitment is too long, and the population is too small, which is an obstacle to draw strong conclusions. Some detailed data was not always available in our registry such as SYNTAX score and HbA1c measurement which was not a routine practice before 2015. The follow-up was only 86.1% completed and does not include a systematic angiographic control of the patency of grafts and anastomoses. Information about the main cause of death was not always available. The multivariable analysis of in-hospital mortality may be underpowered because of the relatively small number of deaths.

Conclusion

Even in low-volume centers in developing areas, CABG is an effective therapy for CAD in diabetic patients despite a relatively higher morbidity and mortality. We recommend strict perioperative glycemic control, complete revascularization, and BITA use. The authorities must apply a policy to improve early detection of diabetic patients who are at high risk of CAD, establish primary and secondary prevention protocols, and prepare appropriate structures with multi-disciplinary teams. As for practitioners, they have to improve their therapeutic protocols, which must be more aggressive for early management and better diabetic control.

Additional file

Additional file 1: Table S1. Independent predictors of mediastinitis by binary logistic regression analysis.

Abbreviations

A. Fib: Atrial fibrillation; AMI: Acute myocardial infarction; BGL: Blood glucose level; BITA: Bilateral internal thoracic artery; CABG: Coronary artery bypass grafting; CAD: Coronary artery disease; CPB: Cardiopulmonary bypass; DM: Diabetes mellitus; FPG: Fasting plasma glucose; HbA_1c: A_1c hemoglobin; IABP: Intra-aortic balloon pump; ICU: Intensive care unit; IT: Insulin-treated; ITA: Internal thoracic arteries; LCOS: Low cardiac output syndrome; LV: Left ventricular; MACCE: Major adverse cardiac and cerebral event; NIT: Non-insulin-treated; NYHA: New York Heart Association; PVAD: Polyvascular atherosclerotic disease; SITA: Single internal thoracic artery; SVG: Saphenous vein graft; VSD: Ventricular septal defect

Acknowledgements

We would like to appreciate the technical assistance of Mr. A. El Fadl for the English writing of the manuscript.

Authors' contributions

YM, RM, and MA collected the data. YM, AS, and NA performed the statistical analysis and analyzed the data. YM, MD, AHG, and IA designed, drafted, and corrected the manuscript. ZL, AM, YB, and AB revised the paper. All authors have read and approved the final manuscript.

Author details

[1]Faculty of Medicine and Pharmacy, Mohammed V University, Rabat, Morocco. [2]Cardiac Surgery Department, Mohammed V Teaching Military Hospital, Hay Riyad, PB 10100 Rabat, Morocco. [3]Intensive Care of Cardiac Surgery, Mohammed V Teaching Military Hospital, Rabat, Morocco. [4]Cardiology Department, Mohammed V Teaching Military Hospital, Rabat, Morocco. [5]Laboratory of Biostatistics, Clinical and Epidemiological Research (LBRCE), Faculty of Medicine and Pharmacy, Mohammed V University, Rabat, Morocco.

References

1. McGinn JT Jr, Shariff MA, Bhat TM, Azab B, Molloy WJ, Quattrocchi E, Farid M, Eichorn AM, Dlugacz YD, Silverman RA (2011) Prevalence of dysglycemia among coronary artery bypass surgery patients with no previous diabetic history. J Cardiothorac Surg. 6:104. https://doi.org/10.1186/1749-8090-6-104
2. American diabetes association (2017) Standards of medical care in diabetes – 2017. 2. Classification and Diagnosis of Diabetes. Diabetes Care 40(Suppl. 1):S11–S24
3. Tazi MA, Abir-Khalil S, Chaouki N, Cherqaoui S, Lahmouz F, Sraïri JE et al (2003) Prevalence of the main cardiovascular risk factors in Morocco: results of a National Survey, 2000. J Hypertens. 21(5):897–903
4. World Health Organization. Country profiles for diabetes 2016. Available at: http://www.who.int/diabetes/country-profiles/mar_en.pdf.
5. Moutakiallah Y, Benzaghmout K, Aithoussa M, Atmani N, Amahzoune B, Hatim A et al (2014) Coronary surgery under cardiopulmonary bypass in patients with diabetes. Pan Afr Med J. 17:199
6. Serruys PW, Morice MC, Kappetein AP, Colombo A, Holmes DR, Mack MJ, Ståhle E, Feldman TE, van den Brand M, Bass EJ, Dyck NV, Leadley K, Dawkins KD, Mohr FW, for the SYNTAX Investigators (2009) Percutaneous coronary intervention versus coronary-artery bypass grafting for severe coronary artery disease. N Engl J Med. 360(10):961–972
7. Mohr FW, Morice MC, Kappetein AP, Feldman TE, Ståhle E, Colombo A, Mack MJ, Holmes DR Jr, Morel MA, Dyck NV, Houle VM, Dawkins KD, Serruys PW (2013) Coronary artery bypass graft surgery versus percutaneous coronary intervention in patients with three-vessel disease and left main coronary disease: 5-year follow-up of the randomised, clinical SYNTAX trial. Lancet. 381(9867):629–638
8. Farkouh ME, Domanski M, Dangas GD, Godoy LC, Mack MJ, Siami FS, Hamza TH, Shah B, Stefanini GG, Sidhu MS, Tanguay JF, Ramanathan K, Sharma SK, French J, Hueb W, Cohen DJ, Fuster V (2019) for the FREEDOM Follow-On Study Investigators. Long-term survival following multivessel revascularization in patients with diabetes: the FREEDOM follow-on study. J Am Coll Cardiol. 73(6):629–638
9. Lam DW, LeRoith D (2012) The worldwide diabetes epidemic. Curr Opin Endocrinol Diabetes Obes. 19(2):93–96
10. Engoren M, Habib RH, Zacharias A, Schwann TA, Riordan CJ, Durham SJ, Shah A (2008) The prevalence of elevated hemoglobin A1c in patients undergoing coronary artery bypass surgery. J Cardiothorac Surg. 3:63. https://doi.org/10.1186/1749-8090-3-63
11. Bos M, Agyemang C (2013) Prevalence and complications of diabetes mellitus in Northern Africa, a systematic review. BMC Public Health. 13:387
12. Kogan A, Ram E, Levin S, Fisman EZ, Tenenbaum A, Raanani E et al (2018) Impact of type 2 diabetes mellitus on short- and long-term mortality after coronary artery bypass surgery. Cardiovasc Diabetol. 17(1):151
13. Carson JL, Scholz PM, Chen AY, Peterson ED, Gold J, Schneider SH (2002) Diabetes mellitus increases short-term mortality and morbidity in patients undergoing coronary artery bypass graft surgery. J Am Coll Cardiol. 40(3): 418–423
14. Mohammadi S, Dagenais F, Mathieu P, Kingma JG, Doyle D, Lopez S et al (2007) Long-term impact of diabetes and its comorbidities in patients undergoing isolated primary coronary artery bypass graft surgery. Circulation. 116(11 Suppl):I220–I225
15. Rawshani A, Rawshani A, Franzén S, Eliasson B, Svensson AM, Miftaraj M et al (2017) Mortality and cardiovascular disease in type 1 and type 2 diabetes. N Engl J Med. 376(15):1407–1418
16. Marui A, Kimura T, Nishiwaki N, Mitsudo K, Komiya T, Hanyu M et al (2015) Five-year outcomes of percutaneous versus surgical coronary revascularization in patients with diabetes mellitus (from the CREDO-Kyoto PCI/CABG Registry Cohort-2). Am J Cardiol. 115(8):1063–1072
17. Zalewska-Adamiec M, Bachorzewska-Gajewska H, Malyszko J, Tomaszuk-Kazberuk A, Nowak K, Hirnle T et al (2014) Impact of diabetes on mortality and complications after coronary artery by-pass graft operation in patients with left main coronary artery disease. Adv Med Sci. 59(2):250–255

18. Li Z, Amsterdam EA, Young JN, Hoegh H, Armstrong EJ (2015) Contemporary outcomes of coronary artery bypass grafting among patients with insulin-treated and non-insulin-treated diabetes. Ann Thorac Surg. 100(6):2262–2269
19. Wit MA, de Mulder M, Jansen EK, Umans VA (2013) Diabetes mellitus and its impact on long-term outcomes after coronary artery bypass graft surgery. Acta Diabetol. 50(2):123–128
20. Chadli A, El Aziz S, El Ansari N, Ajdi F, Seqat M, Latrech H et al (2016) Management of diabetes in Morocco: results of the International Diabetes Management Practices Study (IDMPS) – wave 5. Ther Adv Endocrinol Metab. 7(3):101–109
21. Thiele RH, Hucklenbruch C, Ma JZ, Colquhoun D, Zuo Z, Nemergut EC et al (2015) Admission hyperglycemia is associated with poor outcome after emergent coronary bypass grafting surgery. J Crit Care. 30(6):1210–1216
22. Doenst T, Wijeysundera D, Karkouti K, Zechner C, Maganti M, Rao V et al (2005) Hyperglycemia during cardiopulmonary bypass is an independent risk factor for mortality in patients undergoing cardiac surgery. J Thorac Cardiovasc Surg. 130(4):1144
23. Furnary AP, Wu Y (2006) Clinical effects of hyperglycemia in the cardiac surgery population: the Portland Diabetic Project. Endocrine practice. Endocr Pract 12(Suppl 3):22–26
24. Ujueta F, Weiss EN, Sedlis SP, Shah B (2016) Glycemic control in coronary revascularization. Curr Treat Options Cardiovasc Med. 18(2):12
25. Magaji V, Nayak S, Donihi AC, Willard L, Jampana S, Nivedita P et al (2012) Comparison of insulin infusion protocols targeting 110–140 mg/dl in patients after cardiac surgery. Diabetes Technol Ther. 14(11):1013–1017
26. Mohammadi S, Dagenais F, Voisine P, Dumont E, Baillot R, Doyle D, Charbonneau E, Kalavrouziotis D (2014) Lessons learned from the use of 1,977 in-situ bilateral internal mammary arteries: a retrospective study. J Cardiothorac Surg. 9:158. https://doi.org/10.1186/s13019-014-0158-9
27. Koshizaka M, Lopes RD, Reyes EM, Gibson CM, Schulte PJ, Hafley GE et al (2015) Long-term clinical and angiographic outcomes in patients with diabetes undergoing coronary artery bypass graft surgery: results from the Project of Ex-vivo Vein Graft Engineering via Transfection IV trial. Am Heart J. 169(1):175–184
28. Iribarne A, Westbrook BM, Malenka DJ, Schmoker JD, McCullough JN, Leavitt BJ et al (2018) Should diabetes be a contraindication to bilateral internal mammary artery grafting? Ann Thorac Surg. 105(3):709–714
29. Vrancic JM, Piccinini F, Camporrotondo M, Espinoza JC, Camou JI, Nacinovich F et al (2017) Bilateral internal thoracic artery grafting increases mediastinitis: myth or fact? Ann Thorac Surg. 103(3):834–839
30. Taggart DP, Altman DG, Gray AM, Lees B, Gerry S, Benedetto U, Flather M, for the ART Investigators (2016) Randomized trial of bilateral versus single internal-thoracic-artery grafts. N Engl J Med. 375(26):2540–2549
31. Deo SV, Shah IK, Dunlay SM, Erwin PJ, Locker C, Altarabsheh SE et al (2013) Bilateral internal thoracic artery harvest and deep sternal wound infection in diabetic patients. Ann Thorac Surg. 95(3):862–869
32. Toumpoulis IK, Theakos N, Dunning J (2007) Does bilateral internal thoracic artery harvest increase the risk of mediastinitis? Interact Cardiovasc Thorac Surg. 6(6):787–791
33. Dorman MJ, Kurlansky PA, Traad EA, Galbut DL, Zucker M, Ebra G (2012) Bilateral internal mammary artery grafting enhances survival in diabetic patients. A 30-year follow-up of propensity score–matched cohorts. Circulation. 126(25):2935–2942
34. Schwartz L, Bertolet M, Feit F, Fuentes F, Sako EY, Toosi MS, Davidson CJ, Ikeno F, King SB (2012) Impact of completeness of revascularization on long-term cardiovascular outcomes in patients with type 2 diabetes mellitus results from the Bypass Angioplasty Revascularization Investigation 2 Diabetes (BARI 2D). Circ Cardiovasc Interv. 5(2):166–173
35. Hlatky MA, Boothroyd DB, Bravata DM, Boersma E, Booth J, Brooks MM et al (2009) Coronary artery bypass surgery compared with percutaneous coronary interventions for multivessel disease: a collaborative analysis of individual patient data from ten randomized trials. Lancet. 373(9670):1190–1197

3

Are neonatal age and small weight predictive of in-hospital death and prolonged hospital stay in children undergoing heart surgery?

Osman O. Al-Radi

Abstract

Background: The effect of young age and low weight on outcomes of congenital heart disease surgery is controversial. It is still widely believed both by parents and referring cardiologists that they do have a significant deleterious effect and may prohibit surgical care. This study was intended to determine the independent predictors of in-hospital death and prolonged hospital stay in pediatric patients undergoing cardiac surgery. The effects of age and weight were the focus of analysis. To adjust for heterogeneity and complexity, the Risk Adjustment in Congenital Heart Surgery (RACHS-1) system and other factors were used.

Results: All patients between birth and 18 years of age who underwent cardiac surgery with or without the use of cardiopulmonary bypass from April 1, 2011, to September 30, 2019, were included. Patients undergoing isolated patent ductus ligation were excluded. For the analysis of in-hospital death, a multivariable logistic regression model was used. For the analysis of length of stay, a generalized linear regression model with Poisson distribution and a multivariable logistic regression model were used. The RACHS-1 categories were used to adjust for complexity.
The study included 934 index operations. Neonates (age < 28 days) accounted for 11% of the operations. After adjusting for complexity and other operative variables, we found that age and weight were not significant predictors of in-hospital death or prolonged hospital stay. RACHS category and cardio-pulmonary bypass time were, however, significant predictors of in-hospital mortality, p value 0.009, and 0.002, respectively. The complexity of the operation was also predictive of prolonged hospital stay.

Conclusion: Age and weight are not significant predictors of in-hospital death or prolonged hospital stay. Except for severe prematurity and prohibitive genetic or metabolic disease, patients with CHD should get appropriate and expeditious surgical care regardless of age and weight.

Keywords: Age, Bodyweight, Congenital cardiac surgery

Background

The outcomes of surgery for congenital heart disease (CHD) have markedly improved in the last 20 years [1, 2]. It is difficult to pinpoint a singular event or strategy that lead to this improvement. However, it is widely believed that improvements in surgical strategy, timing, and techniques, as well as postoperative care, additively led to this improvement. It is also still widely believed that neonates and very young infants, as well as low weight for age children, have worse outcomes [3]. This belief leads to delaying corrective or palliative surgical care in many children who are born with low weight or who fail to grow to satisfy arbitrary age or weight limits [4, 5]. In this study, we sought to investigate whether age or weight was independent predictors of surgical outcomes in a wide array of surgical procedures for CHD.

Methods

All children from age 0 to18 years who underwent surgery for CHD at our pediatric cardiac center between

Correspondence: oradi@kau.edu.sa
Department of Surgery, Faculty of Medicine, King Abdulaziz University, PO Box 80215, Jeddah 21589, Saudi Arabia

April 1, 2011, and September 30, 2019, were included. Only the first operation of the index admission was included. Patients who underwent isolated patent ductus ligation were excluded, as the length of stay and mortality in those patients were dependent on other factors not related to the cardiac pathology. We have also excluded patients with significant prematurity (< 28 weeks of gestation) and extreme small weight. Those patients may indeed be at higher risk due to technical and technological limitations of the current state of surgical and technological methods and tools.

The data was harvested from our prospective electronic database. The primary outcome of interest was operative mortality defined as death in the index admission at any time. The secondary outcomes were prolonged hospital stay more than 14 days and length of stay in hospital. Age and weight at the time of operation were the main predictors of interest. Other variables included to account for heterogeneity were gender, preoperative hospital stay, redo operation, cardiopulmonary bypass (CPB) time, aortic cross-clamp time, deep hypothermic circulatory arrest (DHCA) time, and the Risk Adjustment in Congenital Cardiac Surgery (RACHS) classification, version 1 [6]. Prematurity, birth weight, and the presence of extra-cardiac or chromosomal anomalies were not included as these variables were not reliably recorded in the prospective database. In patients who underwent surgery without CPB, CPB time was recorded as zero. Similarly, if the patient did not require aortic clamping or DHCA, the respective time variable was recorded as zero.

The surgical methods may vary as two surgeons contributed to the data; however, 98% of the operations were performed by a single surgeon (the author). In general, patients who required CPB were placed on bypass by aortic and bicaval or atrial cannulation as needed. Before June 2015, cold intermittent antegrade blood cardioplegia was used, and cold antegrade DelNido cardioplegia was used thereafter [7]. If DHCA was needed, it was established at 18°. Antegrade cerebral perfusion was applied at 30 ml/kg/min. Delayed sternal closure was used as needed.

All patients after September 2016 were cared for in a dedicated pediatric cardiac intensive care unit. Before that date, patients were cared for in a general pediatric intensive care unit.

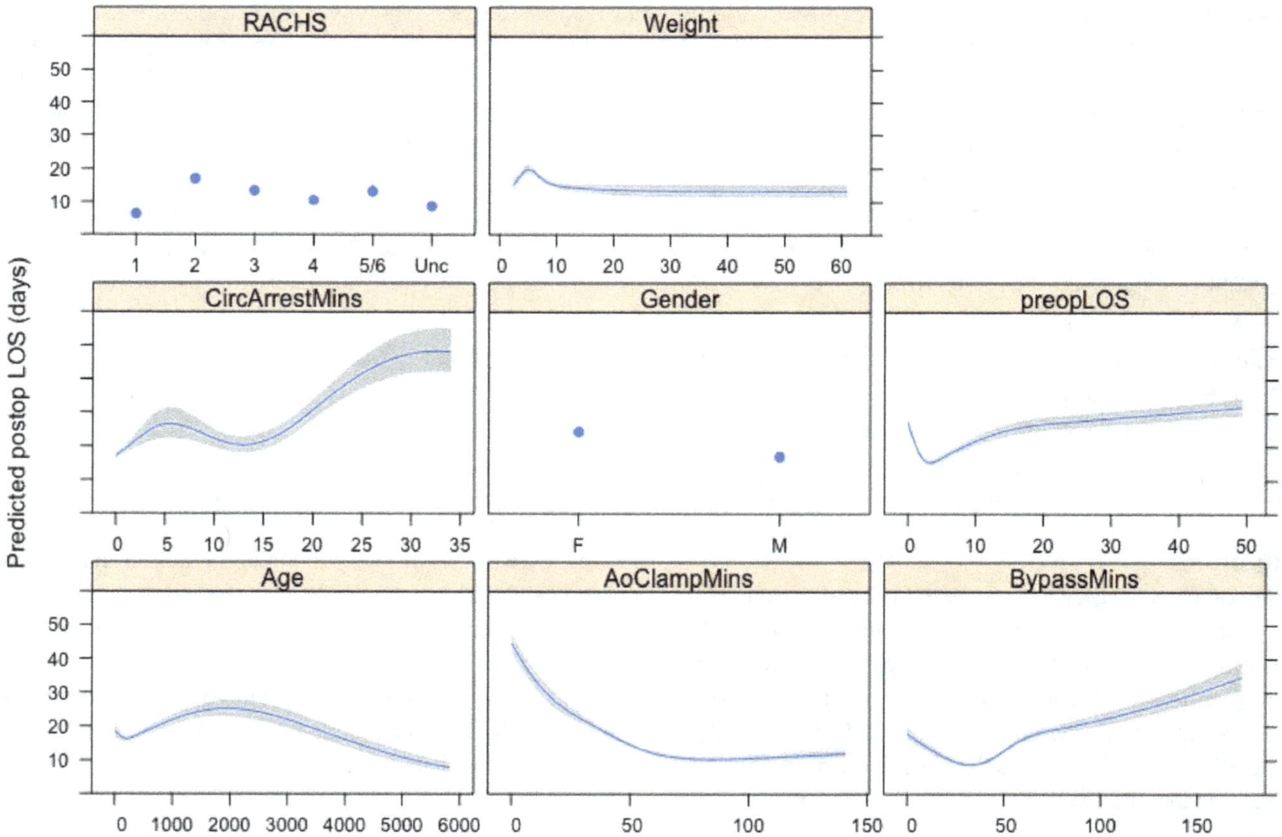

Fig. 1 Graphical description of the relationship between postoperative length of stay in days (y-axis) and age at operation in days, aortic clamp time in minutes (AoClampMins), CPB time in minutes (BypassMins), DHCA time in minutes (CircArrestMins), gender, preoperative length of stay in days (preopLOS), RACHS category, and weight in kg as predicted by a generalized linear model with Poisson distribution and 95% confidence bands for continuous variables

Statistical analysis

The data which was imported from the prospective electronic database into the R statistical system with the following packages was used for analysis: rms, Hmisc, and survival [8–11]. Categorical variables were described as frequency and percent. Continuous variables were described as median and upper and lower quartiles. For descriptive purposes, the data was divided into neonates, defined as age less than 28 days, and post-neonatal children age 29 days to 18 years. For statistical modeling, age was used as a continuous variable and the neonatal status was included as a separate variable as appropriate. The normality and linearity of continuous variables were tested, and the appropriate transformation was used. A restricted cubic spline function was used where non-linear association was identified. For the primary outcome of in-hospital mortality, logistic linear regression was used. For the postoperative length of stay, the analysis was restricted to survivors and a generalized linear regression model with Poisson distribution was used due to the skewed nature of the length of stay (Fig. 1). This model was used to graphically study the association between length of stay and the predictive variables. For ease of interpretation and clinical relevance, prolonged hospital stay was defined as a total postoperative length of stay of greater than 14 days. A logistic regression model was used to study factors associated with a prolonged hospital stay. A p value of 0.05 was accepted as significant.

The study was approved by the local Hospital board of research ethics.

Table 1 Descriptive statistics (N = 934)

	N	Neonate N = 103 a, b, c	Post neonate N = 831 a, b, c	Combined N = 934 a, b, c	p value
Age, days	934	8.00, 15.00, 20.50	202.50, 459.00, 1728.50	137.00, 372.00, 1535.75	< 0.001[1]
Gender	934				0.48[2]
F		40% (41)	43% (361)	43% (402)	
M		60% (62)	57% (470)	57% (532)	
Weight, kg	934	2.70, 3.00, 3.50	5.10, 8.30, 14.00	4.30, 7.35, 13.00	< 0.001[1]
Height	885	46.5, 49.0, 52.0	61.0, 74.0, 100.0	58.0, 70.0, 97.0	< 0.001[1]
Body surface area, m^2	887	0.19, 0.20, 0.21	0.29, 0.41, 0.62	0.26, 0.38, 0.60	< 0.001[1]
Type	934				< 0.001[2]
Primary		100% (103)	87% (720)	88% (823)	
Reoperation		0% (0)	13% (111)	12% (111)	
RACHS	934				< 0.001[2]
1		0% (0)	5% (40)	4% (40)	
2		21% (22)	52% (433)	49% (455)	
3		26% (27)	27% (224)	27% (251)	
4		17% (17)	7% (59)	8% (76)	
5/6		11% (11)	3% (22)	4% (33)	
Uncategorized		25% (26)	6% (53)	8% (79)	
CPB time, min	934	51, 77, 94	46 63 86	46 64 87	0.021[1]
Clamp time, min	934	24.5, 49.0, 64.0	23.0, 43.0, 63.0	23.0, 44.0, 63.0	0.42[1]
DHCA time, min	934	0.0, 0.0, 11.5	0.0, 0.0, 0.0	0.0, 0.0, 0.0	< 0.001[1]
Length of stay, days	934	15.5, 22.0, 37.0	9.0, 15.0, 25.0	9.0, 15.0, 26.0	< 0.001[1]
Preop LOS, days	918	2 5 9	1 2 5	1 2 6	< 0.001[1]
Postop LOS, days	918	10.0, 16.5, 29.0	7.0, 11.0, 19.0	7.0, 11.0, 20.0	< 0.001[1]
Result	934				0.14[2]
Death		9% (9)	5% (40)	5% (49)	
Discharged		88% (91)	94% (778)	93% (869)	
Still in hospital		3% (3)	2% (13)	2% (16)	

a b c represent the lower quartile a, the median b, and the upper quartile c for continuous variables. N is the number of non-missing values. Numbers after proportions are frequencies

Tests used: [1]Wilcoxon test, [2]Pearson test

Results

There were 934 index operations included in the analysis. Neonates accounted for 11% (103) of the patients. Some patients contributed more than one operation to the data. The youngest patient in the analysis was zero days old. The smallest patient requiring surgery with the use of CPB was 1.25 kg. Table 1 shows the detailed descriptive statistics of the study patients. The operative RACHS category distribution was different for neonates compared to post-neonates, while in neonates 11% underwent category 5/6 operation and 17% category 4 operations, compared to 3% and 7% in post-neonates, respectively. Neonates also had a higher percentage of uncategorized operations, 25% versus 6% in post-neonates. The primary outcome of in-hospital death occurred in 9% (9) neonates and 5% (40) post-neonatal children; this difference did not reach statistical significance in unadjusted univariable testing, p value = 0.14. The median postoperative length of stay was 16.5 days for neonates, and 11 days for post-neonatal children, in unadjusted univariable testing the p value was < 0.001.

Adjusting for gender, preoperative length of stay CPB time, aortic clamp time, DHCA time, reoperation, and RACHS category, age, weight, and neonatal status were not found to be independent predictors of in-hospital death or prolonged hospital stay (> 14 days). In fact, only RACHS category and CPB time were the statistically significant predictors of in-hospital mortality, p value 0.0085 and 0.0023, respectively (Table 2). On the other hand, preoperative length of stay, CPB time, aortic clamp time, DHCA time, and RACHS category were independent significant predictors of prolonged hospital stay, p values shown in Table 3.

Table 2 Wald statistics of logistic regression, outcome: in-hospital death

Factor	Chi-square	d.f.	*p*
Age	0.06	1	0.8
Neonate	0.06	1	0.8
Gender	0.00	1	0.9
Weight	0.23	1	0.6
Preoperative LOS	0.08	1	0.8
Reoperation	2.39	1	0.122
Bypass time (min)	9.27	1	*0.0023*
Aortic clamp time (min)	0.84	1	0.3580
DHCA time (min)	0.25	1	0.6
RACHS	15.47	5	*0.0085*

d.f. degrees of freedom, *LOS* length of stay, *DHCA* deep hypothermic circulatory arrest, *RACHS* Risk Adjustment in Congenital Heart Surgery

Discussion

The common practice of corrective surgery for major congenital heart disease lesions during neonatal and young infant life has been established since 1990; however, still many patients are denied care or significantly delayed due to the dogma that the risk of surgery is too high due to the young age or small weight. We have shown that in crude terms, it may appear that neonates have higher in-hospital mortality and prolonged length of stay, in fact with analysis adjusted for the complexity of the operation that does not bare truth. In addition to adjusting for complexity by the RACHS category, we believe that CPB time and DHCA time are also a surrogate for complexity. CPB time may also be a surrogate for operative difficulties or complications.

The limitations of this study include a lack of reliable data about extra-cardiac comorbidity, prematurity, and chromosomal or genetic anomalies. Therefore, it is difficult to assertively comment on the effect of these variables. However, it is more than likely that an important contribution does exist for these and other variables [12]. It is also difficult to account for the urgency of the operation. We included a variable for the preoperative length of stay in hopes of at least partially accounting for some of these effects. We found that the patients with the shortest postoperative length of stay were those who did not have very short or very long preoperative stay. We hypothesize that patient with preoperative length of stay less than 1 day may be a surrogate for urgency and that prolonged preoperative length of stay may be a surrogate for comorbidity requiring medical treatment in preparation for surgery.

We were unable to comment on patients with significant prematurity and extreme small weight as well as patients who underwent patent ductus ligation, as they

Table 3 Wald statistics of logistic regression, outcome: postoperative LOS > 14 days in survivors

Factor	Chi-square	d.f.	*p*
Age	6.42	4	0.17
Nonlinear	1.36	3	0.7
Neonate	0.13	1	0.7
Gender	0.17	1	0.7
Weight	0.31	1	0.6
Preoperative LOS	23.55	1	< 0.0001
Reoperation	0.2	1	0.7
Bypass time (min)	13.87	1	0.0002
Aortic clamp time (min)	14.85	4	0.005
Nonlinear	12.57	3	0.006
DHCA time (min)	10.23	1	0.0014
RACHS	16.17	5	0.006

d.f. degrees of freedom, *LOS* length of stay, *DHCA* deep hypothermic circulatory arrest, *RACHS* Risk Adjustment in Congenital Heart Surgery were not included in this analysis, as stated in the methods.

Conclusions

We did not find age or weight to be independent predictors of in-hospital death or prolonged hospital stay. Except for severe prematurity and prohibitive genetic or metabolic disease, patients with CHD should get appropriate and expeditious surgical care regardless of age and weight.

Abbreviations

CHD: Congenital Heart Disease; CPB: Cardiopulmonary bypass; DHCA: Deep hypothermic circulatory arrest; RACHS-1: Risk Adjustment in Congenital Heart Surgery, edition 1

Acknowledgements

Not applicable.

Authors' contributions

OOA conducted the literature search; designed the study; was responsible for the data collection and analysis and interpretation of data; conducted the statistical analysis; and drafted the manuscript. The author read and approved the final manuscript.

References

1. Martin GR, Jonas RA (2018) Surgery for congenital heart disease: improvements in outcomes. Am J Perinatol 35(6):557–560
2. Pawade A, Waterson K, Laussen P, Karl TR, Mee RB (1993) Cardiopulmonary bypass in neonates weighing less than 2.5 kg: analysis of the risk factors for early and late mortality. J Card Surg. 8:1–8
3. Al-Radi OO (2016) "Low body weight and failure to gain weight are risk factors for heart surgery in children"- doctors should stop saying that to parents. Semin Thorac Cardiovasc Surg. 28(1):e1–e2
4. Kalfa D, Krishnamurthy G, Duchon J, Najjar M, Levasseur S, Chai P, Chen J, Quaegebeur J, Bacha E (2014) Outcomes of cardiac surgery in patients weighing <2.5 kg: effect of patient-dependent and -independent variables. J Thorac Cardiovasc Surg 148(6):2499–506.e1
5. Curzon CL, Milford-Beland S, Li JS, O'Brien SM, Jacobs JP, Jacobs ML et al (2008) Cardiac surgery in infants with low birth weight is associated with increased mortality: analysis of the Society of Thoracic Surgeons Congenital Heart Database. J Thorac Cardiovasc Surg. 135:546–551
6. Jenkins KJ, Gavreau K, Newburger JW, Spray TL, Moller JH, Iezzoni L (2002) Consensus-based method for risk adjustment for surgery for congenital heart disease. J Thorac Cardiovasc Surg 123:110–118
7. Matte GS, del Nido PJ (2012) History and use of del Nido cardioplegia solution at Boston Children's Hospital. J Extra Corpor Technol 44(3):98–103 Erratum in: J Extra Corpor Technol. 2013 Dec;45(4):262
8. R Core Team (2019) R: A language and environment for statistical computing. In: R Foundation for Statistical Computing, Vienna URL https://www.R-project.org/
9. FE Harrell Jr (2019). rms: Regression modeling strategies. R Package Version 5.1-3.1. https://CRAN.R-project.org/package=rms
10. FE Harrell Jr. With contributions from Charles Dupont and many others. (2019). Hmisc: Harrell Miscellaneous. R package version 4.2-0. https://CRAN.R-project.org/package=Hmisc
11. ElMahrouk AF, Ismail MF, Hamouda T, Shaikh R, Mahmoud A, Shihata MS, Alradi O, Jamjoom A (2019) Extracorporeal membrane oxygenation in postcardiotomy pediatric patients-15 years of experience outside Europe and North America. Thorac Cardiovasc Surg. 67(1):28–36. https://doi.org/10.1055/s-0037-1608962 Epub 2017 Dec 12
12. Ma MH, He W, Benavidez OJ (2019) Congenital heart surgical admissions in patients with trisomy 13 and 18: frequency, morbidity, and mortality. Pediatr Cardiol. 40(3):595–601

4

Endoscopic versus open harvesting of radial artery for CABG

Mohamed Abdel Hafez Fouly

Abstract

Background: Endoscopic harvest of the radial artery avoids long forearm incisions and has better cosmesis compared to the open technique. The objective of this study was to compare the short-term results and wound-related complications of endoscopic radial artery harvest versus open technique.

Results: From 2013 to 2017, 800 patients had coronary artery bypass grafting; 88 patients of them had radial artery harvesting (11%). Two groups were included in the study according to the surgeon preference, endoscopic radial harvest (group 1, $n = 30$; 3.75% of total CABG patients) and open harvest (group 2, $n = 58$; 7.25% of total CABG patients). Group 1 had more males (25 (83.33%) vs. 35 (60.34%); $p = 0.028$). There was no difference in the preoperative comorbidities between both groups. The duration of the harvest was significantly longer in group 1 (median 40 min ranges from 38 to 42 min vs. 49 min ranges from 47 to 52 min in groups 1 and 2, respectively; $p < 0.001$). The operative time was longer in group 1 (median 302.5 min ranges from 295 to 310 min vs. 277 min ranges from 273 to 280 min in groups 1 and 2, respectively; $p < 0.001$). The hospital stay in the endoscopic radial artery harvest group was significantly shorter than that of open technique (median 7 days ranges from 6 to 7 days vs. 7.5 days ranges from 7 to 9 days; $p < 0.001$). There was no significant difference in the postoperative complications between both groups. One case (3.3%) was transformed from the endoscopic to open technique due to uncontrolled bleeding. Endoscopic technique was associated with more patients presenting with hand numbness (6 cases; 20% versus 3 cases 5.2%) and radial nerve injury (2 cases; 6.6% versus none), while open technique showed more cases of local hematoma (8 cases; 13.8% versus 1 case; 3.3%) and wound infection (6 cases; 10.34% versus none); $p > 0.05$.

Conclusion: Endoscopic radial artery harvest is associated with shorter harvest time and shorter hospital stay. Endoscopic radial artery harvest is a safe technique with good short-term outcomes. Longer follow-up is recommended.

Keywords: Endoscopic radial artery harvest, Coronary artery bypass grafting, Radial artery graft

Background

Radial artery graft is associated with good long-term outcomes when used to bypass critical coronary artery stenosis in a young patient [1, 2]. The radial artery has several advantages as a conduit in coronary artery bypass grafting (CABG). The radial artery can be used as an alternative to the right internal mammary artery (RIMA) in certain circumstances as in diabetic, obese patients and patients with chronic obstructive pulmonary disease (COPD) where bilateral harvesting of the internal mammary arteries increases the risk of sternal infection [3]. The radial artery is more prone to spasm from the competitive flow because of the thick muscular wall; therefore, it is advised to put the radial artery on critical lesions with the very faint native antegrade flow [4]. The proximal end of the radial artery can be anastomosed directly to the aorta or as a composite T or Y graft to the internal mammary artery [5].

Two techniques were described for the harvesting of the radial artery: open and endoscopic. Open harvest of the radial artery involves large longitudinal forearm incision with the potential of longer harvest time and more wound-related complications [6]. Endoscopic vessel harvesting was introduced in 1990, where it was used for harvesting of the saphenous vein. Then in 2001, it was used in the harvesting of the radial artery. By the year 2005, it was used over a large scale for the harvesting of

Correspondence: mhafez1982.gf@gmail.com
Cardiothoracic, Cairo University, Cairo, Egypt

both saphenous vein and radial artery, and now, about 80% of CABG patients at USA hospitals have both saphenous vein and radial artery harvested endoscopically [7].

Methods

Study design and patients

This research paper is a retrospective cohort study that was conducted in King Faisal Specialized Hospital over 5 years, starting from January 2013 till January 2017. During this period, 800 patients had CABG; 11% of them (n = 88) had radial artery conduits. The data of 88 patients who underwent elective CABG with radial artery as an arterial conduit were collected. The patients were divided into two groups; group 1 included patients who had endoscopic radial artery harvest (n = 30; 3.75% of total CABG patients), and group 2 included the patients who had open radial artery harvest (n = 58; 7.25% of total CABG patients). Patients were assigned to either group according to the surgeon's preference and the availability of the endoscope.

The data collected included age, sex, and comorbidities, such as hypertension and diabetes. Operative data included the duration of the radial artery harvest and the operative time. Postoperative data included the complications in the form of wound hematoma, reexploration, wound infection, local neurological complications from nearby dorsal radial nerve injury with numbness on the dorsum of the hand, and its reflection on hospital stay.

Data collection was approved by the Institutional Review Board at King Faisal Specialized and Research Center, and the patient's consent to participate in research was obtained during procedure consent.

Inclusion criteria

We included patients who had elective three or four vessels CABG and less than 60 years old. The preoperative Allan test was performed and showed equivocal dependence of the arterial supply of the hand on both radial and ulnar artery. We used the radial artery of the nondominant hand. The radial artery was used to graft the obtuse marginal (OM) with a critical lesion of the circumflex artery, and the proximal end of the radial artery was anastomosed directly to the aorta.

Exclusion criteria

We excluded patients who had an emergency CABG or a concomitant procedure CABG. Patients who had radial dependent hand circulation and those who had sequential radial grafting or T or Y radial anastomosis to LIMA were excluded.

Surgical procedures

Endoscopic harvesting

Endoscopic harvesting was performed using the VASOVIEW® Endoscopic Vessel Harvesting System (MAQUET Cardiovascular, Santa Clara, CA.). A 3-cm longitudinal incision is made just proximal to the wrist crease over the radial artery that is identified by its pulsation (Fig. 1). Then, direct dissection locally through the lateral fascia to identify the radial artery and its venae comitantes, which are dissected as one pedicle to avoid direct trauma of the radial artery. The endoscope with the conical tip is advanced directly over the radial artery to allow the insertion of the port (Fig. 2). The port was inflated with air to create a seal. CO_2 was insufflated at a pressure of average 10–12 mmHg and a flow rate of about 4 L/min to create a tunnel [6]. Dissection using the conical tip started from the

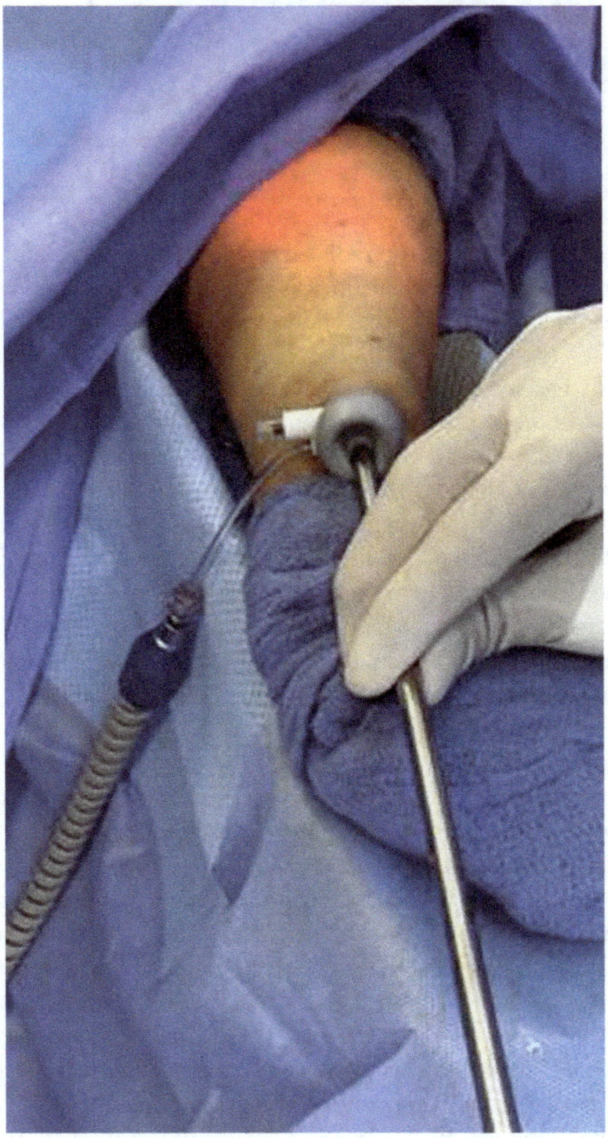

Fig. 1 The endoscopic port with the conical tip inserted in the forearm

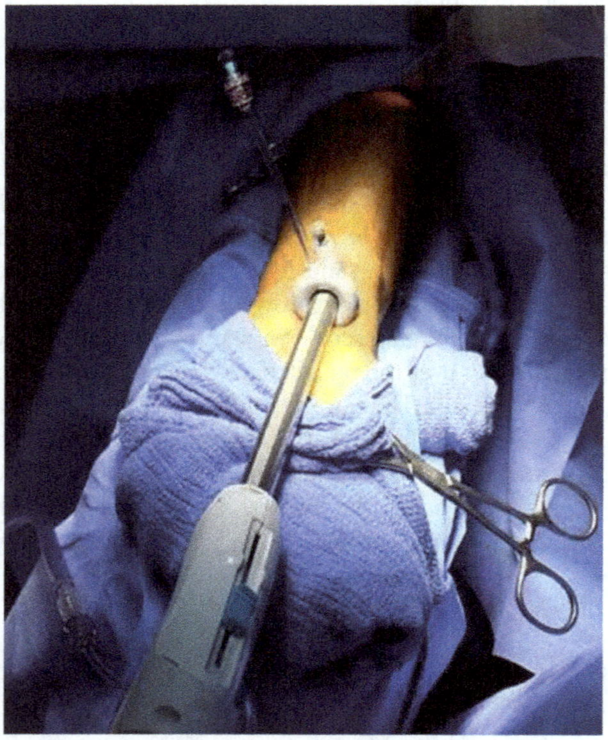

Fig. 2 The VasoView cannula inserted through the forearm

posterior aspect of the radial artery at first then the anterior aspect. The conical tip was removed from the end of the endoscope, and the endoscope was placed into the VasoView® HemoPro™ Endoscopic Vessel Harvesting Cannula. Fasciotomy was performed using direct energy force. Dissection of the tissues was performed by grasping it between both jaws of the cannula together with pulling and rotation of the tool to apply direct tension. The branches were captured between both Jaws by pulling the Toggle into the middle position. The radial artery pedicle can be divided and ligated in the antecubital fossa with an 11-blade using a vessel loop endoscopic technique [8]. The radial artery is prepared by direct flushing with papaverine and clipping of the branches by direct clip applier [8].

Open harvesting

Conventional open radial artery harvesting technique was performed using the method described by Reyes and colleagues through a forearm incision along the course of the radial artery of the nondominant hand starting from the felt pulsation of the artery till its origin from the brachial artery. It was harvested as one pedicle with its venae comitantes with less manipulation of the graft to avoid direct blunt trauma. Dissection of the pedicle was performed by using low-intensity monopolar electrocautery, and the control of the side branches was done using vascular clips [9]. Closure of the forearm was done over a direct drain with one layer of subcutaneous tissue using Vicryl without closure of the fascia to prevent compartmental syndrome if hematoma formed. After closing, a direct elastic bandage was applied and wrapped around the forearm [9].

In both techniques, dissection was done without heparin, and division of the radial artery was done after heparinization. After finishing harvesting, a direct drain was inserted beside the wrapping of the forearm which was done with direct elastic stocking after the closure of the forearm incision.

Statistical analysis

All analyses were performed using STATA 16 software (Stata-Corp, College Town, TX, USA). Continuous variables were described as median (50th percentile) and 25th–75th percentile and were compared between group 1 (endoscopic radial artery harvest) and group 2 (open radial artery harvest) using the Wilcoxon rank-sum test. Categorical variables were presented as number and percent and were compared using the chi-square or Fisher exact test if the expected frequency is less than 5. The analysis was bilateral. A p value of less than 0.05 was considered significant.

Results

Group 1 (n = 30) had 25 males (83.33%) which were significantly higher than group 2 (n = 58; 35 (60.34%); p = 0.028). There was no significant difference in preoperative comorbidities between both groups (Table 1). The duration of the harvest was significantly shorter in group 1 (median 40 min vs. 49 min in groups 1 and 2, respectively; $p < 0.001$) (Fig. 3). The operative time was longer in group 1 (median 302.5 min vs. 277 min in groups 1 and 2, respectively; $p < 0.001$) (Fig. 4 and Table 2). One patient was transformed into an open approach as one branch of radial artery avulsed during dissection with arterial bleeding that obscured the field of vision through the endoscopic camera. The hospital stays in endoscopic harvesting were significantly shorter than those of open harvesting ($p <$ 0.001). Although they did not reach a significant level, the complication rate was higher in group 2 except hand numbness, which occurred more frequently in group 1 (20% vs. 5.2%; $p = 0.057$) (Table 3).

Table 1 Preoperative patient's characteristics

	Group 1 (n = 30)	Group 2 (n = 58)	p
Age (years)	52 (48–57)	55 (48–58)	0.275
Male	25 (83.33%)	35 (60.34%)	0.028
Diabetes mellitus	21 (70%)	46 (76.31%)	0.331
hypertension	19 (63.33%)	42 (72.41%)	0.381
Renal failure	1 (3.33%)	6 (10.34%)	0.415
Previous stroke	2 (6.67%)	3 (5.17%)	> 0.99

Continuous variables are presented as median and 25th–75th percentiles and categorical variables as number and percent

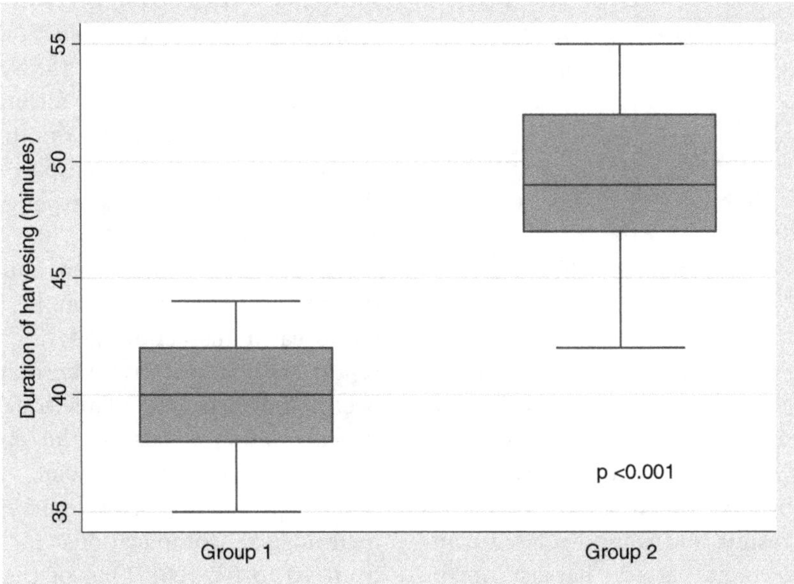

Fig. 3 Comparison of the harvest time between both groups

Discussion

The radial artery is being used as a second or third arterial conduit after internal thoracic arteries in CABG patients [10, 11]. The radial artery has an advantage over the saphenous vein with a better long-term patency rate [11, 12]. Radial artery harvest is relatively easy compared to other arterial conduits since its distal end is subcutaneous, and its pulsation can be felt easily; additionally, it has a large diameter, which facilitates both proximal and distal anastomosis [13]. Moreover, the radial artery has a satisfactory length [14], the forearm wound is less prone to infection compared to the leg wound, and the neurological complications are less frequent [15, 16]. The availability of calcium channel blockers that protect the graft from arterial spasm increased the importance of radial artery harvesting and potentiated its role as one of the vital arterial grafts [17]. Open radial artery harvesting creates a long forearm scar with local wound complications. Recently, a new technique of endoscopic harvesting was widely adopted with better cosmetic results and a decrease in the rate of forearm complications [18, 19]. However, endoscopic harvesting requires a more extended practice compared to the open technique; this is why it must be done by a well-trained practitioner who may be a non-physician [20]. This is well presented during our study in the rate of complications at the endoscopic technique that was high in the beginning as it was a new technique for us with less experience; meanwhile, after we reached a good position in the learning curve, the rate of complications started to decrease.

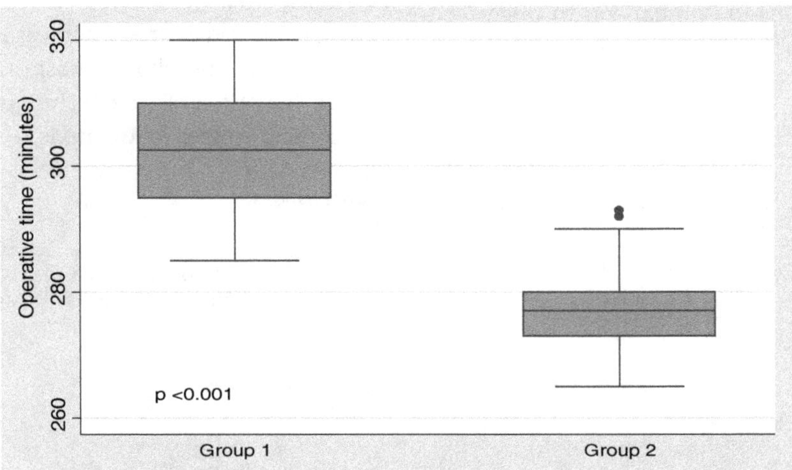

Fig. 4 Comparison of the operative time between both groups

Table 2 Operative data comparison between the two groups

	Group 1 (*n* = 30)	Group 2 (*n* = 58)	*p*
Duration of harvest (min)	40 (38–42)	49 (47–52)	< 0.001
Operative time (min)	302.5 (295–310)	277 (273–280)	< 0.001
Number of grafted vessels			0.353
Three	24 (80%)	51 (87.93%)	
Four	6 (20%)	7 (12.07)	

Continuous variables are presented as median and 25th–75th percentiles and categorical variables as number and percent

Endoscopic radial artery harvesting was introduced in King Faisal Specialized Hospital in 2011, and in January 2012, this technique became regularly used. It was performed using the VASOVIEW® Endoscopic Vessel Harvesting System. The objective of this study was to compare the short-term results and wound-related complications of endoscopic radial artery harvest versus open technique.

Although endoscopic radial artery harvest is less time consuming than the open technique, the whole timing of the CABG operation was longer in the endoscopic group. This time discrepancy is attributed to the sequential endoscopic radial artery and saphenous vein harvest with one VasoView; however in open technique, there are two teams harvesting both conduits at the same time.

In our study, we compared the short-term results of both endoscopic radial artery harvest and open technique in the form of local complications as forearm hematoma and infection and its effect on hospital stay. The rate of local complications was higher in the open group (hematoma and infection), the rate of hematoma was 13.85% in open group versus 3.35% in the endoscopic group, and for infection, it was 10.35% in the open group with zero cases in endoscopic technique. This is similar to other studies, and the largest case-control study of endoscopic radial artery harvesting reported fewer complications in comparison to open technique [21]. Other studies have shown the same, including a significant decrease in other complications such as hematomas and infections [22, 23].

Superficial radial nerve (SRN) injury and local hand numbness occurred more during endoscopic harvesting (20% versus 5.2%), mostly due to excessive cauterization that occurs in the terminal part of the radial artery near the wrist reflecting less experience of harvesting. SRN runs laterally of the RA in the distal forearm and provides sensation to the volar and dorsal part of the first two fingers. This nerve may be encountered during distal forearm dissection [24, 25]. One randomized trial reporting postoperative neurological complications had been published [19]. This trial reported fewer neurological complications in the endoscopic harvest technique versus open radial artery harvest group. Endoscopic radial artery harvest reduced the risk of neurological complications in one prospective study from 10 to 0% [26]. One of the complications that occurred more frequently was chest reexploration from clipped branches of radial artery that were harvested endoscopically (6.75 vs. 1.7%) because of our less experience of the endoscopic technique with excessive nearby cauterization without leaving adequate stump for clipping of the branches.

Finally, there was a statistical significance between both groups in the length of hospital stay in favor of endoscopic technique ($p < 0.001$) because of less postoperative wound complications in endoscopic group with less need to stay in hospital to manage these complications.

Table 3 Comparison of the operative outcomes between both groups

	Group 1 (*n* = 30)	Group 2 (*n* = 58)	*p*
Hematoma	1 (3.33%)	8 (13.79%)	0.158
Wound infection	0	6 (10.34%)	0.075
Radial nerve injury	2 (6.67%)	0	0.114
Hand numbness	6 (20%)	3 (5.171%)	0.057
Chest re-exploration	2 (6.67%)	1 (1.72%)	0.267
Hospital stay (days)	7 (6–7)	7.5 (7–9)	< 0.001

Continuous variables are presented as median and 25th–75th percentiles and categorical variables as number and percent

Limitation of the study

The major limitations are the retrospective design and the small size of endoscopic harvesting sample as it is a new technique that requires trained persons, besides no long-term follow up for the patients as regards of graft patency for both groups.

Conclusions

Endoscopic radial artery harvest is associated with shorter harvest time and shorter hospital stay. Endoscopic radial artery harvest is a safe technique with good short-term outcomes. Longer follow-up is recommended.

Abbreviations

BTT: Blunt tip trocar port; CABG: Coronary artery bypass graft; COPD: Chronic obstructive pulmonary disease; DIAG: Diagonal artery; ITA: Internal thoracic artery; LAD: Left anterior descending artery; OM: Obtuse marginal artery; PDA: Posterior descending artery; RCA: Right coronary artery; RIMA: Right internal mammary artery; SRN: Superficial radial nerve

Acknowledgements

None to declare.

Author's contribution

Single author DR MAHF was responsible for the data collection, analysis of results, and final conclusion. The author read and approved the final manuscript.

References

1. Parolari A, Rubini P, Alamanni F et al (2000) The radial artery: which place in coronary operation? Ann Thorac Surg 69:1288–1294
2. Acar C, Ramsheyi A, Pagny JY et al (1998) The radial artery for coronary artery bypass grafting: clinical and angiographic results at five years. J Thorac Cardiovasc Surg 116:981–989
3. J Tatoulis, BF Buxton, JA Fuller, AG Royse. The radial artery as a graft for coronary revascularization: techniques and follow-up, Advances in cardiac surgery, Vol 11, : Mosby, St Louis (1999), pp. 99-128.
4. Acar C, Jebara VA, Portoghese M, Beyssen B, Pagny JY, Grare P et al (1992) Revival of the radial artery for coronary artery bypass grafting. Ann Thorac Surg 54:652–660
5. Calafiore AM, Di Giammarco G, Luciani N, Maddestra N, Di Nardo E, Angelini R (1994) Composite arterial conduits for a wider arterial myocardial revascularization. Ann Thorac Surg 58:185–190
6. Navia JL, Brozzi N, Chiu J et al (2012) Endoscopic versus open radial artery harvesting for coronary artery bypass grafting. J Cardiovasc Surg (Torino) 53: 257–263
7. Allen KB, Cheng B, Cohn W, Connolly MW, Edgerton J, Falk V, Martin J, Ohtsuka T, Vitali RM: Endoscopic vascular harvest in coronary artery bypass grafting surgery: a consensus statement of the International Society of Minimally Invasive Cardiothoracic Surgery (ISMICS). Innovations. ,2005: 51-60.
8. Kim G, Jeong Y, Cho Y et al (2007) Endoscopic radial artery harvesting may be the procedure of choice for coronary artery bypass grafting. Circ J 71: 1511–1515
9. Reyes A, Frame R, Brodman RF (1995) Technique for harvesting the radial artery as a coronary artery bypass graft. Ann Thorac Surg. 59:118–126
10. Acar C, Buxton B, Norsworthy C, Eizenberg N, Taggart D et al (1999) Radial artery. In: Buxton B, Frazier OH, Westaby S (eds) Ischemic heart disease surgical management. Mosby, London, pp 151–157
11. Desai ND, Cohen EA, Naylor CD, Fremes SE (2004) A randomized comparison of radial-artery and saphenousvein coronary bypass grafts. N Engl J Med 351:2302–2309
12. Collins P, Webb CM, Chong CF, Moat NE (2008) Radial artery versus saphenous vein patency randomized trial. Five-year angiographic follow-up. Circulation 117:2859–2864
13. Cable DG, Caccitolo JA, Pearson PJ et al (1998) New approaches to prevention and treatment of radial artery graft vasospasm. Circulation 98: II15–II21 discussion II21-2
14. Rodriguez E, Ormont ML, Lambert EH et al (2001) The role of preoperative radial artery ultrasound and digital plethysmography prior to coronary artery bypass grafting. Eur J Cardiothorac Surg 19:135–139
15. Allen RH, Szabo RM, Chen JL (2004) Outcome assessment of hand function after radial artery harvesting for coronary artery bypass. J Hand Surg Am 29: 628–637
16. Meharwal ZS, Trehan N (2001) Functional status of the hand after radial artery harvesting: results in 3,977 cases. Ann Thorac Surg 72:1557–1561
17. Brodman RF, Hirsh LE, Frame R (2002) Effect of radial artery harvest on collateral forearm blood flow and digital perfusion. J Thorac Cardiovasc Surg 123:512–516
18. Casselman FP, Meir ML, Cammu G, Wellens F, Geest RD et al (2004) Initial experience with an endoscopic radial artery harvesting technique. J Thorac Cardiovasc Surg 128:463–466
19. Patel AN, Henry AC, Hunnicutt C, Cockerham CA, Willey B et al (2004) Endoscopic radial artery harvesting is better than the open technique. Ann Thorac Surg 78:149–153
20. Connolly MW, Torrillo LD, Stauder MJ, Patel NU, McCabe JC et al (2002) Endoscopic radial artery harvesting: result of first 300 patients. Ann Thorac Surg 74:502–506
21. Shapira OM, Eskenazi BR, Hunter CT, Anter E, Bao Y, Murphy R, Lazar HL, Shemin RJ (2006) Endoscopic versus conventional radial artery harvest – is smaller better? J Card Surg. 21:329–335. https://doi.org/10.1111/j.1540-8191.2006.00266.x
22. Kim G, Jeong Y, Cho Y, Lee J, Cho J (2007) Endoscopic radial artery harvesting may be the procedure of choice for coronary artery bypass grafting. Circ J. 71:1511–1515. https://doi.org/10.1253/circj.71.1511
23. Patel AN, Henry AC, Hunnicutt C, Cockerham CA, Willey B, Urschel HC Jr (2004) Endoscopic radial artery harvesting is better than the open technique. Ann Thorac Surg 78:149–153. https://doi.org/10.1016/j.athoracsur.2004.03.001 Discussion 149–153
24. Royse AG, Royse CF, Shah P, Williams A, Kaushik S, Tatoulis J (1999) Radial artery harvest technique, use and functional outcome. EurJ Cardiothorac Surg. 15:186–193
25. Meharwal ZS, Trehan N (2001) Functional status of the hand after radialartery harvesting: results in 3977 cases. Ann Thorac Surg. 72:1557–1561
26. Patel AN, Henry AC, Hunnicutt C, Cockerham CA, Willey B, Urschel HC Jr (2004) Endoscopic radial artery harvesting is better than the open technique. Ann Thorac Surg. 78:149153. https://doi.org/10.1016/j.athoracsur.2004.03.001

5

The outcome of surgical repair of anomalous origin of the left coronary artery from the pulmonary artery (ALCAPA) in infants

Leena Moshref[1*], Rana Moshref[1], Mazen Faden[2] and Osman Al-Radi[1,3]

Abstract

Background: Anomalous origin of the left coronary artery from the pulmonary artery (ALCAPA) is a rare congenital malformation in infants presenting with angina, dyspnea, and excessive perspiration invoked by crying and feeding. The aim of this study was to evaluate the factors affecting morbidity and the use of extracorporeal membrane oxygenation (ECMO) and to assess the quality of life post-repair.

Methods: In this retrospective study, information about five infants who underwent ALCAPA repair was collected from the databases of two tertiary referral cardiac centers (King Abdulaziz University Hospital and King Faisal Specialist Hospital & Research Center, Jeddah, Saudi Arabia) from 2011 to 2018. The patients were diagnosed using echocardiography, and data including mitral insufficiency and ejection fraction were assessed preoperatively and postoperatively. Quality of life was assessed using a questionnaire-based interview.

Results: The median (range) age at the time of repair was 95 (34–144) days, and the median weight was 4.9 (3–5.7) kg. Two patients underwent the Takeuchi procedure, and three patients underwent left coronary artery reimplantation and translocation to the aorta. The median preoperative ejection fraction was 25 (12.5–45)%, and at the last follow-up, the median EF of the three survivors was 59 (50–70)%. There was no significant change in mitral insufficiency grade postoperatively. Two patients had ECMO support and died postoperatively. The infants who died were younger (< 75 days) and had lower weight (< 4.5 kg) at the time of intervention. Patients who survived showed good quality of life were asymptomatic and had heart function within the normal range.

Conclusion: Echocardiography and CT angiogram are effective tools for ALCAPA diagnosis in pediatric patients. Low weight at time or repair was associated with increased morbidity and ECMO did not increase survival.

Keywords: Anomalous left coronary artery from the pulmonary artery, Mitral regurgitation, Ejection fraction, Extracorporeal membrane oxygenation

Background

Bland and colleagues defined a symptom complex in infants presenting with angina, dyspnea, excessive perspiration, dizziness, and paleness invoked by crying and feeding, which they named Bland-White-Garland syndrome [1]. It mimics heart failure and often accompanies significant mitral valve regurgitation (MR) and might be mistaken as colic, reflux, or bronchiolitis [2, 3]. Bland-White-Garland syndrome or anomalous origin of the left coronary artery from the pulmonary artery (ALCAPA) is a rare congenital malformation that accounts for 0.25–0.5% of all congenital cardiac anomalies [3, 4]. It is classified into two types: infantile or adult. The infantile variety is associated with a poor prognosis if not treated surgically because of the lack of coronary collaterals. In the adult variety, collaterals are present or have developed; thus, adequate blood supply to the myocardium is present [4].

* Correspondence: leenahatem0987@gmail.com
[1]Department of Surgery, King Abdulaziz University, Jeddah, Kingdom of Saudi Arabia
Full list of author information is available at the end of the article

This syndrome is usually diagnosed by echocardiography (ECHO) and CT scan [5]. Few patients survive past childhood without surgical repair, and up to 90% of the survivors die suddenly at a mean age of 35 years [6]. In patients who survive until adulthood, the coronary steal phenomenon and retrograde left-sided coronary flow are the bases of developing chronic subendocardial ischemia, which may lead to left ventricular dysfunction, ischemic mitral regurgitation, malignant ventricular arrhythmias, and sudden cardiac death. The average age for sudden cardiac death is 31 years, and that for a life-threatening presentation is 33 years [7]. The common origin of the carotid arteries (COCA) is a frequent pattern of aortic arch vessels and is the single most common cause of tracheobronchial compression by a congenital cardiovascular anomaly [8].

To our knowledge, there have been no recent studies conducted in the western region of Saudi Arabia regarding the prevalence of ALCAPA, its associated anomalies, and surgical interventions. In this study, we attempted to determine the factors affecting the use of extracorporeal membrane oxygenation (ECMO) and the mortality and to assess the quality of life after ALCAPA repair. Quality of life was assessed in terms of mental and physical development.

Methods

In this retrospective study, patients were recruited from the databases of two tertiary referral cardiac centers (King Abdulaziz University Hospital and King Faisal Specialist Hospital & Research Center, Jeddah, Saudi Arabia) from 2011 to 2018. Patients aged less than 1 year and who underwent repair of the anomalous left coronary artery from the pulmonary artery were included. The study was approved by the ethics review committee of King Abdulaziz University Hospital, reference number (179-18). The study was conducted according to the ethical guidelines conforming to the declaration of Helsinki, and patients' parents/guardians consented to participate; therefore, a written consent was obtained.

The patients' parameters including age at surgery, associated anomalies, type of surgery, and duration were recorded. The postoperative parameters included complications, duration of ventilation, the need for extracorporeal membrane oxygenation (ECMO), length of intensive care unit (ICU) stay, and inotropic use and duration. Additionally, hospital stay and follow-up (durations, complications, and interventions) were assessed. ECHOs of patients were documented pre- and postoperatively and included the degree of mitral regurgitation, ejection fraction, and fractional shortening.

Surgical technique

The surgical approach was through a median sternotomy. The pericardium was opened and suspended, followed by excision of the thymus. Cardiopulmonary bypass was started and immediately the branched pulmonary arteries were snuck down.

Takeuchi procedure (cases 1 and 5)

The main pulmonary artery was transversely cut, and the left anomalous coronary artery was identified arising from the non-facing sinus very close to the commissure of the pulmonary valve. A large button was harvested from the left anomalous coronary artery, and adequate mobilization of the vessel was achieved. There was insufficient distance or tissue for that vessel to reach the ascending aorta; therefore, pericardial tissue was taken and was formulated into a tube-like structure that was anastomosed to the ostium of this anomalous left coronary artery and the ascending aorta after creating a window in the left inferior border of the ascending aorta. The anastomosis was performed using the 7-0 Proline continuous suture. Then, the posterior wall of the main pulmonary artery was augmented, and re-anastomosis of the pulmonary arteries was completed. The patients were weaned off bypass successfully. Chest tube and pacer wire were inserted. In case 1, peritoneal dialysis lines were inserted, and the chest was closed using a patch. In case 5, the chest was closed by sternal wires.

Left coronary artery reimplantation (cases 2, 3, and 4)

Single left coronary was re-implanted onto the aorta, and patch pulmonary artery repair was performed. Chest tube and pacer wire were inserted. The chest was closed using a patch. In case 3, a direct ventricular septal defect (VSD) closure was performed, and case 4 underwent mitral valve (MV) repair.

Postoperative follow-up

Patients were followed up by echocardiography at 1 day, 1 and 4 months, and 1, 2, and 3 years postoperatively. The follow-up was conducted by pediatric cardiologists and included echocardiography (EF, MR, and FS), and the parameters were measured on the M-mode.

The quality of life was assessed using a questionnaire-based interview. The questionnaire was validated by two consultants. The questionnaire was telephone based and consisted of open-ended and multiple-choice questions. It aimed to assess the quality of life postoperatively, and it recorded the following data: the achievement of milestones, medications, symptoms, and complications.

Statistical analysis

Data were analyzed in SPSS version 20 (IBM Corporation, Chicago, IL, USA). Continuous data were presented as median, and range and categorical data as number and percentage. Categorical data were compared using Fisher's exact test and numerical data by Mann-Whitney test. Paired t test was used to compare preoperative and postoperative parameters. Kaplan-Meier method was used to assess the survival rate at the latest follow-up.

Table 1 Preoperative patients' characteristic

Case	Gender	Age (days)	Weight (kg)	Height (cm)	Associated anomalies	Mitral valve	EF (%)	FS (%)	Admitting Diagnosis
1	Female	95	4.9	60	–	Mild MR	25	12.5	Referred with depressed LV systolic function
2	Male	109	4.9	60	–	Mild to moderate MR with 2 jets	12.5	12.1	Cardiogenic shock and severe LV dysfunction
3	Male	34	3	52	Perimembranous VSD Biventricular dilatation Thickened pulmonary valve	Mild MR	28	14	Referred with heart failure and severe LV dysfunction
4	Female	75	4.5	44	Mild TR Dilated LV	Severe MR with 2 jets	45	25	Sepsis
5	Female	144	5.7	62	Severely dilated LV	Moderate MR	22	10	Respiratory distress Suspected myocarditis

EF ejection fraction, *FS* fraction shortening, *LV* left ventricle, *MR* mitral regurgitation, *TR* tricuspid regurgitation, *VSD* ventricular septal defect

Results

Preoperative assessment

Five infants (less than 1 year), with a male to female ratio 2:3, who underwent ALCAPA repair, were included in this study. The median age was 95 days (range, 34 to 144 days) . The median weight was 4.9 kg (range, 3 to 5.7 kg). The patients were diagnosed based on echocardiography (ECHO) findings and CT angiogram. The median of the preoperative ejection fraction was 25% (range, 12.5–45%). Mitral regurgitation degree was mild in 2 patients, mild-to-moderate in 1 patient, moderate in 1 patient, and severe in 1 patient. Echocardiography measurements along with patients' height and weight are illustrated in Table 1.

Surgical intervention

Cardiopulmonary bypass median time was 118 min (range, 52 to 157 min), and ischemic time was 50 min (range, 24 to 111 min) (Table 2).

Postoperative assessment

Postoperatively, inotropes (milrinone and epinephrine) were administered to all the patients. Furosemide and spironolactone were administered to 60% (3/5) of patients, who survived eventually. Two patients (cases 1 and 2) had delayed closure due to severe left ventricular dysfunction. ECMO was used in two patients who died eventually. The median duration of ventilation was 3 days (range, 2 to 5 days), and the median duration of ICU stay was 8 days (range, 2 to 12 days). The median postoperative hospital stay was 11 days (range, 2 to 15 days). The mortality rate was 40% (2/5) in patients who had ECMO support. Postoperative details are shown in Table 3.

Follow-up assessment

Median follow-up was 10 months. The infants who died were younger and had lower weight at the time of intervention ($p = 0.08$ and 0.07, respectively), and they had multiple congenital anomalies (ventricular septal defect, tricuspid regurgitation, and pulmonary valve thickening).

Survival rate was 60% (3/5) at 3 years' follow-up. Ejection fraction improved during follow-up compared to the preoperative value (p value = 0.02) (Fig. 1). Mitral regurgitation degree preoperatively was mild in 1 patient, mild to moderate in 1 patient, and moderate in 1

Table 2 Operative details of patients who underwent ALCAPA repair

Case	Operation procedure	Surgery time (min)	CPB time (min)	Ischemic time (min)	Operative events
1	Takeuchi procedure (LCA augmentation by bovine pericardium graft then anastomosed to the aorta)	260	157	111	–
2	LCA reimplantation to aorta, patch PA repair	100	52	27	–
3	LCA reimplantation to the aorta, patch PA repair, and direct VSD closure	176	129	70	Arrested for 8 min. Hemodynamic instability with high lactate High doses of inotropes (dobutamine and epinephrine)
4	LCA reimplantation to the aorta, patch PA repair, and MV repair	180	118	50	Hypotension, bradycardia, and bleeding Blood transfusion Arrested and CPR was done for 2 min
5	Takeuchi procedure	101	73	24	–

ALCAPA anomalous left coronary artery from the pulmonary artery, *CPB* cardiopulmonary bypass, *CPR* cardiopulmonary resuscitation, *LCA* left coronary artery, *MV* mitral valve, *PA* pulmonary artery, *VSD* ventricular septal defect

Table 3 Postoperative outcomes after ALCAPA repair

Case	MV duration (days)	ECMO	Inotropes and (duration; days)	ICU stay (days)	Time to sternal closure (days)	Postoperative complications	Mortality	Hospital stay (days)	Follow-up duration
1	3	No	Milrinone (15), epinephrine (4)	9	1	Severe left ventricular dysfunction Sternal reopening	Alive	15	10 months
2	5	No	Epinephrine (2), milrinone (12)	12	1	Severe ventricular dysfunction Sternal reopening Upper chest wall abscess (1 month)	Alive	12	53 months
3	2	Yes	Milrinone (2)	2	2	Bleeding Surgical reexploration Pacemaker inserted Multiorgan failure	Dead	2	2 days
4	4	Yes	Epinephrine (4), norepinephrine (4), milrinone (3)	5	5	Bleeding Cardiac catheterization showed dissection of coronary arteries. Surgical re-exploration, anastomosis revision, and LIMA to LAD Multiorgan failure	Dead	5	5 days
5	3	No	Milrinone (6), epinephrine (6)	8	None	Left lower lung collapse.	Alive	11	28 months

ECMO extracorporeal membrane oxygenation, *ICU* intensive care unit, *LAD* left anterior descending artery, *LIMA* left internal mammary artery, *MV* mechanical ventilation

patient, compared to postoperatively 2 patients were mild and 1 patient was moderate degree ($p > 0.99$).

One patient (case 2) had postoperative cardiac MRI to assess the coronary arteries and function and revealed subendocardial infarction of the mid- and distal antero-lateral wall with poor function. Ten months postoperatively, the patient had a cardiac CT which showed normal coronaries with no stenosis. No other complications or admissions were noted after that.

Quality of life assessment

Quality of life questionnaire was assessed in three patients. As shown in Table 4, all patients were asymptomatic, with 1–2 medications and normal milestones.

Discussion

ALCAPA is a rare congenital disease associated with poor prognosis in infants [4]. There are different surgical techniques for repair. The coronary transfer is the current technique of choice for the repair of ALCAPA [9], and it has an acceptable survival rate [10]. In this study, two patients underwent the Takeuchi procedure, and three patients had LCA reimplantation to the aorta and patch PA repair. The patients who underwent Takeuchi procedure survived while two patients who underwent LCA reimplantation had ECMO support and could not survive.

Surgeries were usually undertaken in acute settings as the most common presentation was acute heart failure and depressed LV function [11]. In addition, three

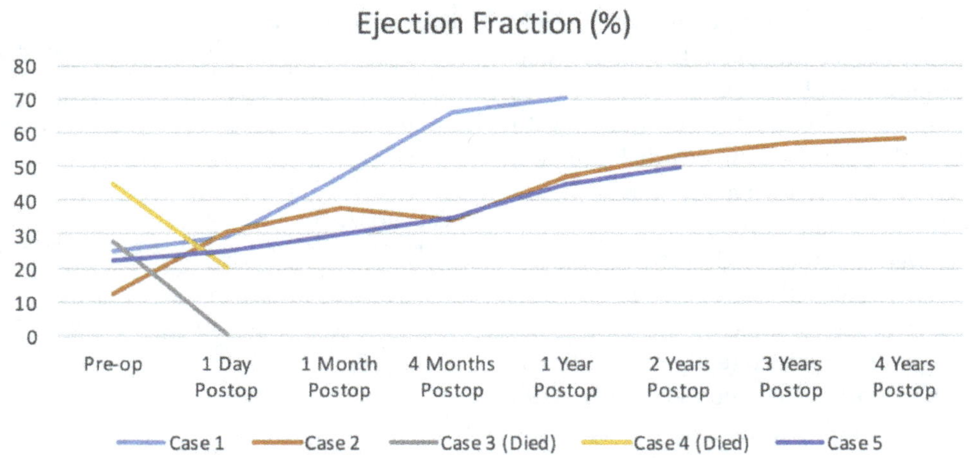

Fig. 1 Ejection fraction pre and post repair

Table 4 Quality of life assessment

Case	Age (years)	Alive Yes/no	Symptomatic Yes/no	Yes, what are symptoms	Medication Yes/no	What medications	Milestones			
							Social and emotional	Language/ communication	Cognitive	Movement/physical development
1	5.3	Yes	No	–	Yes	Aspirin	Up to age.	Normal and up to age.	Up to age in school	Fully active and no restriction of movement.
2	6.3	Yes	No	–	Yes	Digoxin	Up to age.	Normal and up to age.	Up to age in school	Fully active and no restriction of movement.
5	3.2	Yes	No	–	Yes	Captopril and aspirin	Up to age.	Normal and up to age.	Up to age.	Fully active and no restriction of movement.

patients had associated anomalies preoperatively; one patient had VSD with a mildly thickened pulmonary valve and the other two patients had dilated LV, and one of them had tricuspid regurgitation. In a study conducted by Laux and colleagues, the most encountered cardiac anomaly associated with this condition was coarctation of the aorta, followed by tetralogy of Fallot with or without pulmonary atresia [12]. One patient had simultaneous mitral valve repair, and several researchers recommend performing simultaneous mitral annuloplasty in patients who have moderate and severe mitral regurgitation at the time of ALCAPA repair [13].

Younger and low weight patients did not survive the repair even though they were on ECMO during the postoperative period. Joshi and colleagues reported their experience in the off-pump repair of ALCAPA [14] as an alternative to the conventional repair that avoids the use of the circulatory support and its associated morbidity. On the other hand, the use of mechanical circulatory support in patients with difficult weaning from cardiopulmonary bypass achieved a high survival rate with good long-term recovery in another study [15]. The poor ECMO outcome in our study could be attributed to the small patient's number and the associated patients' related factors. Younger age at presentation indicates a severe form of the disease.

Among the survived patients, the EF improved markedly in the last follow-up compared to the preoperative value. This finding was consistent with a study conducted over 40 years in patients aged less than 1 year and showed a preoperative EF < 35% in 71% patients, and the last follow-up EF > 50% in 84% [16]. Infants with ALCAPA presents with depressed myocardial function due to poor collaterals and restoring myocardial blood flow improved the function markedly.

All living patients were asymptomatic with no late sequelae, which was consistent with other studies [17, 18]. In our study, the survival rate of patients was 60% at the 3-year follow-up. A better survival rate of 98% at the 20-year follow-up was reported in another study [19]. Survival varies widely in the literature, and this could be attributed to different baseline characteristics and the volume of the centers.

Limitations of the study

The number of participants included in the study is small, and multiple surgical techniques were utilized. The follow-up period was not fixed. Moreover, the authors found difficulty in finding an assessment of the quality of life questionnaire in infants and toddlers because the available questionnaires were validated and are applicable to pediatric and adult patients and, thus, were not relevant for this study.

Conclusion

Echocardiography and CT angiography are effective diagnostic tools for ALCAPA in pediatric patients. Morbidity occurred more frequently in low weight infants, and ECMO use did not increase survival. Patients who survived had a good quality of life and were asymptomatic with a normal range of heart function. Quality of life is rarely assessed in ALCAPA cases which are usually discovered in infants, so we recommend further studies in this area.

Abbreviations

ALCAPA: Anomalous left coronary artery from the pulmonary artery; ECMO: Extracorporeal membrane oxygenation; EF: Ejection fraction; MR: Mitral regurgitation

Acknowledgements

The authors would like to thank the patients' families who agreed to participate in the study.

Authors' contributions

LM carried out the drafting of the manuscript and carried out the statistical analysis. RM participated in writing the manuscript and collecting the data. MF helped to draft the manuscript. OR came out with the idea and helped in editing the manuscript. All authors read and approved the final manuscript.

Author details

[1]Department of Surgery, King Abdulaziz University, Jeddah, Kingdom of Saudi Arabia. [2]Department of Anesthesia and Critical Care, King Abdulaziz University, Jeddah, Kingdom of Saudi Arabia. [3]Cardiovascular Department, King Faisal Specialist Hospital & Research Center-General Organization, Jeddah, Kingdom of Saudi Arabia.

References

1. Bland EF, White PD, Garland J (1933) Congenital anomalies of the coronary arteries (report of an unusual case associated with cardiac hypertrophy). *Am Heart J.* 8:787–789. https://doi.org/10.1016/S0002-8703(33)90140-4

2. Huddleston CB, Balzer DT, Mendeloff EN (2001) Repair of anomalous left main coronary artery arising from the pulmonary artery in infants: long-term impact on the mitral valve. Ann Thorac Surg 71(6):1985–1988; discussion 1988-9. https://doi.org/10.1016/s0003-4975(01)02518-8
3. Brotherton H, Philip RK (2008) Anomalous left coronary artery from pulmonary artery (ALCAPA) in infants: a 5-year review in a defined birth cohort. Eur J Pediatr 167(1):43–46. https://doi.org/10.1007/s00431-007-0423-1
4. Pfannschmidt J, Ruskowski H, de Vivie ER (1992) Bland-White-Garland syndrome. Clinical aspects, diagnosis, therapy. Klin Padiatr 204(5):328–334. https://doi.org/10.1055/s-2007-1025367
5. Zhang H-L, Li S-J, Wang X et al (2017) Preoperative evaluation and midterm outcomes after the surgical correction of anomalous origin of the left coronary artery from the pulmonary artery in 50 infants and children. Chin Med J (Engl) 130(23):2816–2822. https://doi.org/10.4103/0366-6999.219156
6. Pisacane C, Pinto SC, De Gregorio P et al (2006) "Steal" collaterals: an echocardiographic diagnostic marker for anomalous origin of the left main coronary artery from the pulmonary artery in the adult. J Am Soc Echocardiogr 19(1):107.e3–107.e6. https://doi.org/10.1016/j.echo.2005.09.024
7. Tavakoli R, Jamshidi P, Yamani N, et al. Direct re-implantation of left coronary artery into the aorta in adults with anomalous origin of left coronary artery from the pulmonary artery (ALCAPA). J Vis Exp. 2017;(122). doi: https://doi.org/10.3791/55590.
8. Ehren H, Wells TR, Landing BH (1985) Association of common origin of the carotid arteries with anomalous origin of the left coronary artery from the pulmonary artery. Pediatr Pathol 4(1-2):59–66. https://doi.org/10.3109/15513818509025903
9. Lange R, Vogt M, Hörer J et al (2007) Long-term results of repair of anomalous origin of the left coronary artery from the pulmonary artery. Ann Thorac Surg 83(4):1463–1471. https://doi.org/10.1016/j.athoracsur.2006.11.005
10. Hoashi T, Kagisaki K, Okuda N et al (2013) Indication of Takeuchi technique for patients with anomalous origin of the left coronary artery from the pulmonary artery. Circ J 77(5):1202–1207. https://doi.org/10.1253/circj.cj-12-1321
11. Florent C, Vouhe PR, Khoury W et al (1988) Anomalous left coronary artery arising from the pulmonary artery: a series of 27 infants undergoing operation in the first years of life. J Cardiothorac Anesth 2(4):445–449. https://doi.org/10.1016/0888-6296(88)90224-4
12. Laux D, Bertail C, Bajolle F et al (2014) Anomalous left coronary artery connected to the pulmonary artery associated with other cardiac defects: a difficult joint diagnosis. Pediatr Cardiol 35(7):1198–1205. https://doi.org/10.1007/s00246-014-0916-4
13. Xu JP, Guo HW, Hu SS et al (2006) Results of surgical correction in patients with anomalous origin of the coronary artery from the pulmonary artery. Zhonghua Wai Ke Za Zhi 44(22):1525–1528
14. Joshi SV, Naik AV, Bhalgat PS et al (2016) An experience with off pump technique for repair of anomalous left coronary artery from pulmonary artery (ALCAPA). Indian Heart J 68(5):704–708. https://doi.org/10.1016/j.ihj.2016.02.002
15. del Nido PJ, Duncan BW, Mayer JE Jr et al (1999) Left ventricular assist device improves survival in children with left ventricular dysfunction after repair of anomalous origin of the left coronary artery from the pulmonary artery. Ann Thorac Surg. 67(1):169–172. https://doi.org/10.1016/s0003-4975(98)01309-5
16. Lange R, Cleuziou J, Krane M et al (2018) Long-term outcome after anomalous left coronary artery from the pulmonary artery repair: a 40-year single-centre experience. European Journal of Cardio-Thoracic Surgery 53(4):732–739. https://doi.org/10.1093/ejcts/ezx407
17. Kudumula V, Mehta C, Stumper O et al (2014) Twenty-year outcome of anomalous origin of left coronary artery from pulmonary artery: management of mitral regurgitation. Ann Thorac Surg 97(3):938–944. https://doi.org/10.1016/j.athoracsur.2013.11.042
18. Rodriguez-Gonzalez M, Tirado AM, Hosseinpour R et al (2015) Anomalous origin of the left coronary artery from the pulmonary artery: diagnoses and surgical results in 12 Pediatric Patients. Tex Heart Inst J 42(4):350–356. https://doi.org/10.14503/THIJ-13-3849
19. Naimo PS, Fricke TA, d'Udekem Y et al (2016) Surgical intervention for anomalous origin of left coronary artery from the pulmonary artery in children: a long-term follow-up. Ann Thorac Surg 101(5):1842–1848. https://doi.org/10.1016/j.athoracsur.2015.11.020

6

Role of dexmedetomidine infusion after coronary artery bypass grafting

Tamer Hamouda[1,2], Mohamed Ismail[1,3], Tamer Hamed Ibrahim[4], Hesham Ewila[5] and Ahmed Elmahrouk[1,6*]

Abstract

Background: Postoperative pain has negative consequences on patients' outcomes after cardiac surgery. Routine management with opioid and or non-steroidal anti-inflammatory medications has several disadvantages. Dexmedetomidine is a selective α2 agonist used for sedation and analgesia. The use of dexmedetomidine for postoperative pain management and decreasing delirium and agitation in cardiac surgery patients is a matter of debate. Our objective was to determine the role of an early administration of dexmedetomidine in decreasing opioid use post-cardiac surgery and its effects on the quality of postoperative recovery.

Results: Medical records of 120 patients admitted to the cardiac surgery intensive care unit (CSICU) after coronary artery bypass grafting (CABG) in two cardiac centers between December 2015 and December 2016 were reviewed. Patients were divided into two groups. Group A included 55 patients who received dexmedetomidine in a dose of 0.2–0.4 mcg/kg/h on admission to CSICU, and group B included 65 patients who did not receive dexmedetomidine. The primary outcome was the pain score immediately after extubation, and the secondary outcomes included post-extubation sedation and pain scores for 12 h.

There were significant decrease of the pain scores in dexmedetomidine group that continues through the 3rd, 6th, 8th, and 12th hour readings after surgery with mean modified Ramsay scores 0.1 ± 0.0, 0.89 ± 2.05, 0.35 ± 0.1, and 0.12 ± 1.1 respectively compared to 0.46 ± 1.15, 3.46 ± 2.93, 0.98 ± 1.90, and 0.12 ± 1.1 in group B ($p < 0.001$), significant decrease in cumulative morphine received ($p < 0.001$, OR = 909, 95% CI 0.05–0.19), favorable reduction in heart rate in dexmedetomidine group (80 ± 1.9 b/min) compared to 96 ± 8.8 b/min in the other group ($p = 0.017$), and smoother recovery from general anesthesia.

Conclusion: Administration of dexmedetomidine in the early postoperative period can be safe. It may reduce the use of opioids, has sedative, analgesic, and sympatholytic effects that could play a useful role during the management of coronary artery bypass patients, and may improve postoperative recovery.

Keywords: Dexmedetomidine, Coronary artery bypass grafting, Postoperative pain, Alpha 2 agonists

Background

Postoperative pain after cardiac surgery has a negative impact on the outcome, in addition to the patients' experience. Tachycardia, hypertension, arrhythmias, and myocardial ischemia are frequent postoperative findings. Most postoperative pain management protocols are opioid-based, which have a dose-dependent analgesic effect [1].

* Correspondence: ahmed.elmahrouki1@med.tanta.edu.eg; Ael-mahrouk@kfshrc.edu.sa; a_marouky@hotmail.com
[1]Cardiovascular Department, King Faisal Specialist Hospital and Research Center, Jeddah, Saudi Arabia
[6]Cardiothoracic Surgery Department, Faculty of Medicine, Tanta University, Tanta, Egypt
Full list of author information is available at the end of the article

On the other hand, opioids have a number of undesired side effects, including nausea, vomiting, decreased gastrointestinal motility, respiratory depression, drowsiness, and hemodynamic effect with large doses [2]. Moreover, non-opioids analgesics, such as non-steroidal anti-inflammatory drugs and acetaminophen, may be a useful complement to opioids for postoperative pain relief. Additionally, non-opioid analgesics can reduce the need for opioids and minimize its side effects. However, the efficiency of these medications can be limited, as it can seriously affect the patients postoperatively because of their effect on bleeding and renal function [3].

Dexmedetomidine (DEX) is a highly selective α2 receptor agonist that provides better sedation, analgesic, and anxiolytic effect. This property is considered unique among sedatives used for intensive care units generally [4, 5]. Many studies on DEX in postoperative high-risk non-cardiac patients showed that those patients required significantly lower sedative agents. Furthermore, dexmedetomidine has a less hemodynamic effect and non-significant respiratory depression [6, 7]. Additionally, patients who received DEX experienced mutual sedation and smooth extubation, and they had lower mortality [7].

Moreover, recent findings show that such patients have a lower incidence of delirium over comparators [8, 9]. On the other hand, other studies argued the effect of DEX in decreasing the incidence of postoperative delirium, especially in older patients [10, 11]. In this retrospective study, we tried to examine the efficacy of post-coronary artery bypass grafting (CABG) DEX infusion in reducing postoperative morphine consumption and in improving the quality of postoperative recovery.

Methods

Design and patients

Data of all patients admitted to the cardiac surgery intensive care unit (CSICU) following CABG, between December 2015 and 2016, were retrieved from the medical records after approval from the local medical ethics committee. Patients' confidentiality was maintained by removing any identifying information from the data set before further usage and analysis. The variables and their values were coded into an alphanumeric format for concealment with few designated persons having the coding key.

A hundred and twenty patients were included in the study. Patients with renal failure, prolonged postoperative intubation for more than 8 h because of hemodynamic instability or bleeding, and patients who had re-exploration were excluded.

Patients were divided into two groups: group A included 54 patients who received postoperative DEX infusion for sedation, and group B included 66 patients who did not receive DEX.

Study protocol and outcomes

All patients were intubated, ventilated, and sedated by propofol intravenous (IV) infusion 25–50 µg/kg/min. On admission to CSICU, vital signs were recorded, and group A patients were started on DEX IV infusion 0.2–0.4 µg/kg/h. while patients in group B were maintained only on propofol infusion.

Vital signs, including heart rate (HR), oxygen saturation, and end-tidal carbon dioxide, were continuously monitored, and blood pressure was monitored both invasively and non-invasively. Patients were started on acetaminophen 1 g IV every 6 h, and 2–3 mg of morphine were administered intravenously if the pain was suspected in case of unexplained tachycardia and hypertension when the patients were still intubated.

We reviewed the difference in total morphine consumption and vital data between the two groups while patients were intubated. Our protocol was to start weaning the patients from sedation and prepare for extubation 2 h after admission to CSICU and after ensuring the stable hemodynamic and full return of muscle power, so once these criteria were met, propofol and DEX infusion were turned off, and patients were extubated after full recovery.

Our primary outcome was the pain score assessed by the primary nurse and physician immediately after extubation. The pain was evaluated according to the numeric pain intensity scale (NPIS), ranging from no pain (0) to severe non-tolerable pain (10).

We reviewed the pain scores and vital signs every hour in all patients for the first 12 h post-extubation in addition to sedation score which was assessed by modified Ramsay score (MRS) and ranged from 1 to 6 as follows: 1 = anxious/agitated, 2 = cooperative oriented, 3 = responds to commands only, 4 = asleep with brisk response to light glabellar tap (LGT), 5 = sluggish response to (LGT), 6 = asleep no response to (LGT).

Our protocol was to administer 2–3 mg of morphine to the patient once the pain score is ≥2, and the total morphine consumption in the first 12 h post-extubation in both groups was reviewed, and that was our secondary outcome in addition to the vital data and sedation scores in the first 12 h after extubation.

Statistical analysis

Statistical analysis was performed using SPSS 15 for Windows (IBM Corp, Chicago, IL, USA). Continuous data were presented as mean ± standard deviation and categorical data as count and percent. *T* test was used to compare the continuous variables, and chi-squared test or fisher exact test was used for categorical variables when appropriate. The trend of pain severity was investigated by a repeated measure analysis of variance (ANOVA) model. Freedom from the first dose of morphine was plotted using the Kaplan-Meier survival curve and compared between both groups using a log-rank test.

Results

One hundred and twenty patients with a mean age of 56 ± 10.1 years were included in the study. The mean left ventricular ejection fraction (LVEF) was 40 ± 9.4% in the DEX group compared to 44 ± 7.3% in group B ($p = 0.75$). The average time of anesthesia was 312 ± 66 min in group (A) and 309 ± 42 min in group (B) ($p = 0.54$). Patients stayed in the intensive care unit (ICU) after surgery with a mean time of 2.9 ± 1.1 days and a range of 2 to 4 days.

Fifty-four patients had intravenous DEX started on admission to the intensive care unit, and 66 patients were started on propofol. Analysis of baseline variables of the patients was presented in Table 1, which showed no significant differences between the two groups.

The severity of pain was measured by 10 points in NPIS in different time intervals: 1st, 3rd, 6th, 12th, 18th, and 24th hours (Table 2).

Patients experienced a period of analgesia after surgery. The most severe pain had a point that was less than 3. By the 6th hour after surgery, the pain started to appear gradually and became more severe. The severity of pain diminished until the disappearance at the 18th hour after surgery ($p < 0.001$).

In the first hour after the operation, the trend of pain severity was equal in both groups. The effect of analgesia continues in those who received dexmedetomidine until the 3rd hour after surgery, while in the control group, the pain severity was increasing. The patients in the DEX group had statistically significant lower pain severity compared to the control group throughout the first postoperative day (p value < 0.001) (Fig. 1).

The assessment was done every hour during intubation and 2-hourly after extubation; the mean sedation score was analyzed all through intubation (Table 3). We observed that intubation time was 6 ± 2.3 h in the DEX group compared to group B with 8 ± 7.9 h ($p = 0.231$). The mean arterial pressure had increased in both groups within the first 1 h and dropped within the first 2 h then became stable in the DEX group with a lower heart rate than the other group.

In the DEX group, 10% of patients needed to receive morphine for pain compared to 95% of the patients in the other group ($p < 0.001$, OR = 909, 95% CI 0.05–0.19). Moreover, the dose of received morphine sulfate was lower in the DEX group (1.0 ± 1.2 mg) compared to 2.9 ± 1.8 mg in the other group ($p < 0.001$).

The time of prescription of the 1st dose of morphine sulfate could be considered as a proxy for the beginning of intolerable pain (pain score between 4 and 5) (Fig. 2). The pain became relatively unbearable 6 h after finishing the surgery. No significant difference between the two groups was noticed using the log-rank test ($p = 0.09$). The pattern of receiving the first dose of morphine sulfate was similar in both groups.

Discussions

This study demonstrated that early infusion of DEX following CABG operations was associated with a reduction of morphine usage, a decrease in pain severity, and improvement of sedation, which encouraged early extubation. Pain control is crucial after cardiac surgery. The release of catecholamine causes the increase of the peripheral vascular resistance, heart rate, and risk of myocardial infarction, arrhythmias, and mortality. From our observations, we noticed a transient rise in main arterial pressure (MAP) during the 1st postoperative hour in both groups, followed by a decrease in MAP.

Arain and associates [12] found a brief increase in blood pressure in the DEX group, which was related to activation of α2 agonist on the smooth muscle of the vessel wall, which leads to transient vasoconstriction and increased in mean arterial pressure. We have noticed this in both groups. However, we thought these initial hemodynamic changes in MAP and HR were most probably related to post-surgical stress, the surgical procedures itself, or pre-existing hypertension as it happened in both groups [13]. The decrease in MAP and HR was

Table 1 Comparison of the preoperative, operative, and postoperative data between groups (continuous data are presented as mean and standard deviation or median and categorical data as number and percent)

	Group A ($n = 54$)	Group B ($n = 66$)	p value
Age (years)	54 ± 9.5	57 ± 8.3	0.181
Weight (kg)	85 ± 10	80 ± 9.3	0.530
Height (cm)	1.61 ± 9	165 ± 3	1.511
Ejection fraction	40 ± 9.4	44 ± 7.3	0.752
Duration of anesthesia (min)	312 ± 66	309 ± 42	0.541
Operative time (min)	248 ± 18	251 ± 92	0.572
Bypass time (min)	110 ± 38.5	105 ± 40.3	0.641
ICU stay/days	2 ± 0.5	3 ± 0.1	0.512
Intubation time (hours)	6 ± 2.3	8 ± 7.9	0.231
MAP (mmHg)	77.93 ± 5.9	74.53 ± 8.3	0.561
Heart rate	80 ± 1.9	96 ± 8.8	0.017
Modified RS (median)	2	3	0.802
Pain intensity score median	1	2	0.113

cm centimeters, *min* minutes, *ICU* intensive care unit, *MAP* mean arterial pressure, *HR* heart rate, *Modified RS* modified Ramsay score

Table 2 Pain score in different time interval after cardiac surgery (data are presented as mean and standard deviation)

Group	1st hour	3rd hour	6th hour	8th hour	12th hour	24th hour
Group A ($n = 54$)	0.39 ± 1.25	0.1 ± 0.0	0.89 ± 2.05	0.35 ± 0.1	0.12 ± 1.1	0.0 ± 0.90
Group B ($n = 66$)	1.08 ± 0.67	0.46 ± 1.15	3.46 ± 2.93	0.98 ± 1.90	0.30 ± 0.2	0.0 ± 0.96

related to more gradual central effect of DEX in patients who received it, while the reduction of MAP for patients who did not receive DEX and depended on morphine as main analgesic most probably was related to decreasing catecholamine and direct vasodilatation effect of morphine considering that there was no significant difference in the number of patients receiving inotropes and vasodilators between the two groups.

Our findings were in line with Liu and coworkers' [14] meta-analysis, which stated that DEX lead to a shorter length of intubation, but it can be associated with bradycardia in patients after cardiac surgery compared with propofol. This tendency to lower the heart rate and systolic blood pressure with decreased incidence of tachycardia and arrhythmias have a cardioprotective effect, as stated by another meta-analysis by Gong and coauthors [15].

On the other hand, Mukhtar and colleagues [16] concluded in their study that intraoperative DEX infusion attenuated the hemodynamic and neuroendocrine response to surgical trauma and cardiopulmonary bypass. The same findings were declared by Priye and associates [17], who concluded that DEX infusion, even those without the loading dose, have a safe, effective adjuvant analgesic effect. It can reduce narcotic consumption without undesirable hemodynamic effects in cardiac surgery patients.

Shehabi and coworkers [11] found that DEX reduced vasopressors' requirement after cardiac surgery with effective analgesia sedation, less hypertension, and more bradycardia versus morphine regimen. In our study, we did not find any difference between the two groups with regard to MAP and HR ($p = 0.561$ and 0.017, respectively). Barletta and associates [18] stated that DEX decreased cardiac index and HR for patients undergoing lengthy procedures which remained reduced at the time of discharge; our results did not support this conclusion as there was no significant difference between the two groups in HR. On the other hand, Maldonado and coworkers [19] concluded that DEX was associated with a lower rate of respiratory depression. It caused a higher rate of adverse hemodynamic events, which might be a concern in a hemodynamically unstable patient, but we did not observe any adverse effect on hemodynamic stability; this can be attributed to the low number of patients who needed inotropic support or vasodilator during the post-operative period in our cohort. Moreover, we have estimated opioid administration as analgesics postoperatively, which could reflect passively on the patients' hemodynamics post-CABG. We observed that 10% of the patients were in need of opioids in the DEX group. These patients could be considered to have a low pain threshold or the post-operative managing doctors had a low threshold to give his patients more analgesia.

It worth mentioning that, while 95% of the control group were depended on opioids, 5% only of them only received non-steroidal anti-inflammatory (NSAID), according to the

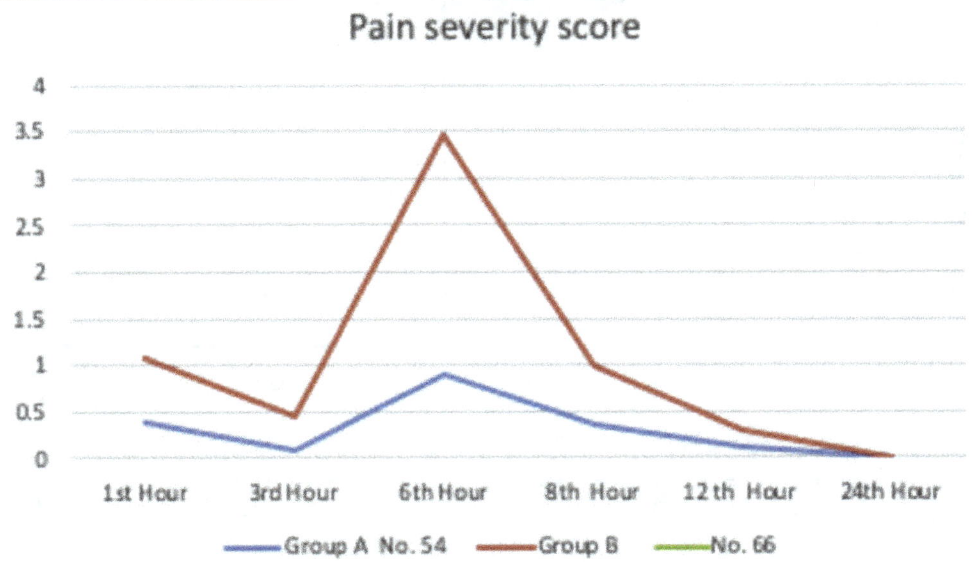

Fig. 1 Changes of pain severity score in study groups

Table 3 Sedation score during intubation and after extubation (data are presented as the mean)

	During intubation	Immediately after extubation	2 h after extubation	4 h after extubation	6 h after extubation	8 h after extubation
Group A (*n* = 54)	5.2	3.2	2.9	2.7	2.2	2.3
Group B (*n* = 66)	4.5	2.1	2.1	2	2.1	2.1

assessment of the post-operative ICU doctors who considered most of these patients with high pain threshold, and so, NSAID was enough to control their pain. Moreover, the dose of opioids given in the DEX group was significantly less than those of the other group [20, 21].

The pattern of pain in both groups was almost the same, which means that DEX does not alter the trend of the pain but decreased the intensity, and both groups needed to receive analgesics at the same point according to pain score between 4 and 5. These results agreed with Cheng and associates' study [22].

Some authors mentioned that the use of DEX decreased the length of ICU stay in comparison with the use of other sedative and analgesics like midazolam and morphine, and we did not observe in our study significant differences in ICU stay as it was 2 ± 0.5 and 3 ± 0.1 days ($p = 0.512$). There are many factors other than pain and analgesics which could influence the ICU stay, including the patient's hemodynamics, which can be affected by other etiologies other than pain.

From the clinical point of view, Lin and coworkers [9] suggested that DEX gave a suitable condition through which it facilitated weaning process from mechanical ventilator as it did not depress spontaneous ventilation, as well as it decreased the risk of delirium, ventricular tachycardia, and hyperglycemia following cardiac surgery; however, it could cause significant bradycardia. In our study, there was no significant difference between the two groups in intubation time.

Study limitations

The primary limitation of the study is the retrospective nature, and several factors may have affected the outcomes other than the treatment. A randomized clinical trial is required to adjust for the measured and unmeasured variables that could confound the results. However, because the administration of DEX in our cohort was not related to patients' specific risk factors, the two groups had comparable baseline data.

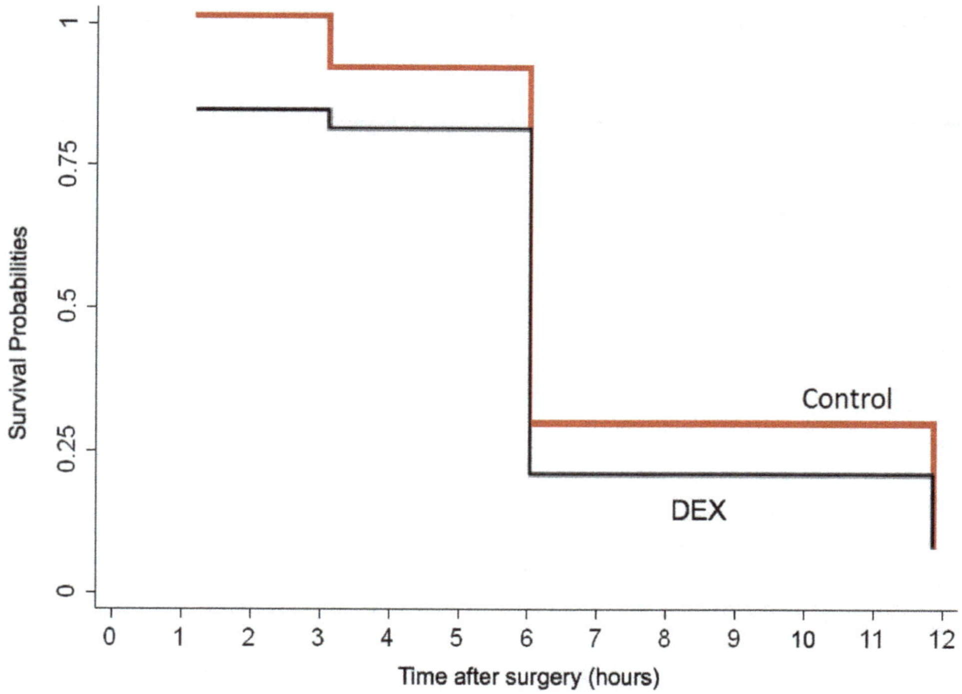

Fig. 2 Kaplan-Meier curve for estimation of the time to receive the morphine

Conclusion

Administration of dexmedetomidine in the early postoperative period can be safe. It may reduce the use of opioids, has sedative, analgesics, and sympatholytic effects that could play a useful role during the management of coronary artery bypass patients, and may improve postoperative recovery.

Abbreviations

CABG: Coronary artery bypass grafting; CSICU: Cardiac surgery intensive care unit; DEX: Dexmedetomidine; HR: Heart rate; ICU: Intensive care unit; LGT: Light glabellar tap; LVEF: Left ventricular ejection fraction; MAP: Main arterial pressure; MRS: Modified Ramsay score; NPIS: The numeric pain intensity scale; NSAID: Non-steroidal anti-inflammatory

Acknowledgements

Not applicable.

Authors' contributions

TH conducted the literature search and data collection and drafted the manuscript. MI designed the study, analysis, and interpretation of data and drafted the manuscript. TI conducted the statistical analysis and interpretation of data and drafted the manuscript. HE conducted the statistical analysis and data collection and conducted the literature search and interpretation of data. AE supervised the study and conducted the review of data, was involved in the study design, analysis, and interpretation of data, and drafted the manuscript (corresponding author). All authors have read and approved the manuscript.

Author details

[1]Cardiovascular Department, King Faisal Specialist Hospital and Research Center, Jeddah, Saudi Arabia. [2]Cardiothoracic Surgery Department, Faculty of Medicine, Benha University, Benha, Egypt. [3]Cardiothoracic Surgery Department, Faculty of Medicine, Mansoura University, Mansoura, Egypt. [4]Department of Anaesthesia, Faculty of Medicine, Ain Shams University, Cairo, Egypt. [5]Department of Anaesthesia, Faculty of Medicine, Suez Canal University, Ismailia, Egypt. [6]Cardiothoracic Surgery Department, Faculty of Medicine, Tanta University, Tanta, Egypt.

References

1. Wijeysundera DN, Naik JS, Beattie WS (2003) Alpha-2 adrenergic agonists to prevent perioperative cardiovascular complications: a meta- analysis. Am J Med 114(9):742–752
2. Biccard BM, Goga S, de Beurs J (2008) Dexmedetomidine and cardiac protection for non-cardiac surgery: a meta-analysis of randomised control trials. Anaesthesia 63(1):4–14
3. Hoy SM, Keating GM (2011) Dexmedetomidine: a review of its use for sedation in mechanically ventilated patients in an intensive care setting and for procedural sedation. Drugs. 71:1481–1501
4. Christensen A (2009) Update on dexmedetomidine for adult ICU sedation. Conn Med 73:469–472
5. Szumita PM, Baroletti SA, Anger KE, Wechsler ME (2007) Sedation and analgesia in the intensive care unit: evaluating the role of dexmedetomidine. Am J Health Syst Pharm 64:37–44
6. Afonso J, Reis F (2012) Dexmedetomidine: current role on anaesthesia and intensive care. Rev Bras Anestesiol 62:118–133
7. Muntazar M, Kumar FC (2004) Cardiac arrest, a preventable yet a possible risk of dexmedetomidine: fact or fiction? Anesthesiology 101(6):1478–1479
8. Abd Aziz N, Chue MC, Yong CY, Hassan Y, Awaisu A, Hassan J, Kamarulzaman MH (2011) Efficacy and safety of dexmedetomidine versus morphine in post-operative cardiac surgery patients. Int J Clin Pharm 33: 150–154
9. Lin YY, He B, Chen J, Wang Z (2012) Can dexmedetomidine be a safe and efficacious sedative agent in post cardiac surgery patients? Critical car 16 R:169
10. Li X, Yang J, Nie XL, Zhang Y, Li XY, Li LH, Ma D (2017) Impact of dexmedetomidine on the incidence of delirium in elderly patients after cardiac surgery: a randomized controlled trial. PLoS One 12(2):e0170757
11. Shehabi Y, Grant P, Wolfenden H, Hammond N, Bass F, Campbell M, Chen J (2009) Prevalence of delirium with dexmedetomidine compared with morphine-based therapy after cardiac surgery: a randomized controlled trial (DEXmedetomidine COmpared to Morphine-DEXCOM Study). Anesthesiology 111(5):1075–1084
12. Arain SR, Ruehlow RM, Uhrich TD, Ebert TJ (2004) The efficacy of dexmedetomidine versus morphine for postoperative analgesia after major inpatient surgery. Anesth Analg 98(1):153–158
13. Ismail M, El-Mahrouk A, Hamouda T, Radwan H, Haneef A, Jamjoom A (2017) Factors influencing postoperative atrial fibrillation in patients undergoing on-pump coronary artery bypass grafting, single center experience. J Cardiothorac Surg 12:40
14. Liu X, Xie G, Zhang K, Song S, Song F, Jin Y, Fang X (2017) Dexmedetomidine vs propofol sedation reduces delirium in patients after cardiac surgery: a meta-analysis with trial sequential analysis of randomized controlled trials. J Crit Care 38:190–196
15. Gong Z, Ma L, Zhong YL, Li J, Lv J, Xie YB (2017) Myocardial protective effects of dexmedetomidine in patients undergoing cardiac surgery: a meta-analysis and systematic review. Exp Ther Med 13(5):2355–2361
16. Mukhtar AM, Obayah EM, Hassona AM (2006) The use of dexmedetomidine in paediatric cardiac surgery. Anaesthesia and Analgesia 103:52–56
17. Priye S, Jagannath S, Singh D, Shivaprakash S, Reddy DP (2015) Dexmedetomidine as an adjunct in postoperative analgesia following cardiac surgery: a randomized, double-blind study. Saudi J Anaesth 9(4): 353–358
18. Barletta JF, Miedema SL, Wiseman D, Heiser JC, KJ MA (2009) Impact of dexmedetomidine on analgesic requirements in patients after cardiac surgery in a fast-track recovery room setting. Pharmacotherapy 29:1427–1432
19. Maldonado J, van der Starre PJ and Wysong A: Postoperative sedation and the incidence of ICU delirium in cardiac surgery patients. Presented at the American Society of Anaesthesiologists, Annual Meeting. San Francisco, CA, Anesthesiology.2003; 99:A465
20. Elmahrouk A, Hamouda T, Kasab I, Ismail M, Jamjoom A (2017) Short term outcome of conventional versus off-pump coronary artery bypass grafting for high-risk patients. J Egypt Soc Cardiothorac Surg 26(1):24–29
21. Zientara A, Matter-Ensner S, Mariotti S, Seifert B, Graves K, Dzemali O, Genoni M (2016) Dexmedetomidine provides effective pain modulation and rapid extubation during perioperative fast-track management in patients after off-pump coronary artery bypass grafting. Thorac Cardiovasc Surg 64:OP101
22. Cheng H, Li Z, Young N, Boyd D, Atkins Z, Ji F, Liu H (2016) The effect of dexmedetomidine on outcomes of cardiac surgery in elderly patients. J Cardiothorac Vasc Anesth 30(6):1502–1508

7

Total anomalous pulmonary venous drainage repair: the effect of anatomical type and pulmonary vein stenosis on outcomes

Osman O. Al-Radi[1,2*], Ahmed Elmahrouk[2,3], Mohamed Ismail[2,4], Abdelmonem Helal[5,6] and Tamer Hamouda[2,7]

Abstract

Background: Surgical repair of total anomalous venous drainage (TAPVD) is lifesaving. The operative mortality is reported between 4 and 35%. Anatomical type, obstructed presentation, associated single ventricle, and heterotaxy syndromes are thought to influence short- and long-term outcomes. The effect of simple versus sutureless repair for primary surgery is unclear. This study reports the outcomes of the surgical repair and the effect of these variables in a contemporary setting.

Results: Between 2011 and 2019, all patients undergoing surgical repair for TAPVD were included. Operative mortality, length of hospital stay, and long-term survival were reported. The effect of anatomical type, surgical technique, obstruction, and associated lesions was assessed. Pearson's test, Wilcoxson's test, and generalized linear regression with Poisson distribution were used.

Forty-nine patients from two centers underwent TAPVD repair. The operative mortality was 4%. Postoperative pulmonary vein stenosis occurred in three patients, and reoperation was done in one patient. Survival free from reoperation was 98%, 98%, and 90% at 1, 24, and 60 months in the absence of pulmonary vein stenosis. However, all three patients who developed pulmonary vein stenosis died, at 0.5, 2.7, and 6.3 months of follow-up, respectively. We were unable to detect a significant effect of anatomical type, preoperative obstruction, associated single ventricle, or heterodoxy syndrome on operative mortality or long-term freedom from death or reoperation. Patients who presented with obstruction and infracardiac or supracardiac TAPVD had longer hospital stay.

Conclusion: TAPVD repair outcomes are excellent except for patients who develop postoperative pulmonary venous stenosis. Anatomical type, obstructed presentation, associated single ventricle, or heterotaxy are not significant predictors of survival.

Keywords: Total anomalous pulmonary venous drainage, Pulmonary vein stenosis

Background

Surgical correction is a lifesaving treatment for total anomalous pulmonary venous drainage (TAPVD). The operative mortality of surgery varies widely in the literature between 4 and 35% [1–4]. Anatomical type [5], stenosis of the drainage pathway [6], surgical technique [6–12], and time era all are reported to have an important effect of short- and long-term outcomes. Associated single ventricle anomalies carry a particularly poor prognosis [13]. The advent of the so-called sutureless techniques is thought to prevent stenosis and have an impact on long term outcomes [14, 15]. Pulmonary vein stenosis is a dreaded and relentless complication reported with all types of surgical techniques [9]. The use of modern postoperative measures including high-frequency jet ventilation (HFJV) and extracorporeal membrane oxygenation (ECMO) is thought to be helpful in some cases with obstructed TAPVD [16–18]. However, air embolism has

* Correspondence: oradi@kau.edu.sa
[1]Department of Surgery, Faculty of Medicine, King Abdulaziz University, PO Box 80215, Jeddah 21589, Saudi Arabia
[2]Cardiovascular Department, King Faisal Specialist Hospital and Research Center, Jeddah, Saudi Arabia
Full list of author information is available at the end of the article

been reported as a complication of aggressive ventilation that may be specific to sutureless repair [19].

This study describes the outcomes of surgical repair of TAPVD and the effect of anatomical and surgical factors.

Methods

Patients who underwent surgical repair of TAPVD from September 1, 2011, to December 13, 2019, were included. The data were collected retrospectively using an encrypted online database [20]. Five surgeons in two centers contributed to this cohort of patients. Follow-up was obtained by review of electronic records and direct contact of the treating physicians and the parents if recent data were not available in the records. The diagnosis was established by detailed echocardiographic studies and augmented with computed tomography and magnetic resonance imaging when the diagnosis and anatomical type was not clear by echocardiography.

The surgical methods included the use of cardiopulmonary bypass (CPB) with antegrade blood or Del Nido cardioplegia [21], and occasional periods deep hypothermic circulatory arrest. Direct suture technique between the posterior wall of the left atrium and the pulmonary venous confluence was the preferred technique. In the presence of small pulmonary veins or multiple venous confluences, sutureless techniques by suturing the incised left atrial wall to in situ pericardium around the incised pulmonary veins were used [14]. The draining vertical vein was ligated or divided when possible. In cases of infracardiac TAPVD or where the drainage vein was stenotic, it was left untouched. In cases of cardiac TAPVD, the dilated coronary sinus was completely unroofed and the atrial septation was recreated with a patch of autologous pericardium. If the pulmonary veins were small or stenotic, sutureless technique was applied. ECMO and HFJV were used only when necessary. Delayed sternal closure was also utilized if needed [22].

Statistical methods

The data were described as frequency and percent for categorical variables, and median and quartiles for continuous variables. The normality and linearity or continuous variables were assessed, and transformation or statistical methods suitable for such variables was used when necessary. The outcome measures of interest were operative mortality (OM) defined as death due to any cause during the index admission, postoperative length of stay (LOS) in the hospital, and long-term survival. The need for reoperation for pulmonary vein stenosis was recorded. The effect of anatomical type, simple versus sutureless repair technique, associated single ventricle lesions, and heterotaxy syndromes as well as demographic variables was assessed. For OM, due to its rarity, Pearson chi-square with continuity correction or Wilcoxon test was used for categorical and continuous variables, respectively. For LOS, the analysis was limited to survivors and a multivariable generalized linear regression model with Poisson distribution was used. For long-term survival, Kaplan-Meier survival analysis was used for the graphical description of freedom from death or reoperation. Log-rank test was used to test for significant associations. All statistical analyses were done using the R statistical system with Hmisc and rms packages [23–25].

Results

In the study period, 49 patients underwent primary TAPVD repair. The anatomical type distribution was supracardiac in 51% (25), cardiac in 18% (9), infracardiac in 16% (8), and mixed in 14% (7) of the patients. Single ventricle lesions and heterotaxy syndromes were each present in 12% (6) of the patients. According to risk adjustment in congenital heart surgery (RACHS-1) risk categorization, patients who underwent surgery before 30 days of age were classified as category 4, 22% (11), and those who were 30 days of age or older were classified as category 2, 78% (39) regardless of anatomical type or associated lesions [24]. Approximately one third of the patients, 29% (14), presented with obstructive symptoms and required emergency surgery. The frequency of presentation with obstruction was significantly higher in infracardiac TAPVD (87.5%) compared to the other types (11–12%), P value < 0.001. Moreover, the median age at operation was significantly younger in patients with infracardiac TAPVD, P value = 0.01. There were two main surgeons contributing 67% (33) and 16% (8) of the patients, respectively. The remaining three surgeons contributed less patients. Table 1 shows the details of the patient demographics grouped by anatomical type of TAPVD.

The CPB and aortic cross-clamp times were higher for mixed type TAPVD, P value < 0.001. However, delayed sternal closure was highest in infracardiac TAPVD, P value < 0.001. There were two deaths during the hospital stay, one for infracardiac and one for cardiac TAPVD, and overall OM was 4% (2/49) and was not significantly different between neonates and older children, P value = 0.9; the anatomical TAPVD types, P value 0.55; or presentation with obstruction, P value 0.8. Completeness of follow-up was 96%, and there were two late deaths at 6 and 49 months. One of the late deaths was related to pulmonary vein stenosis in a patient who presented 6 months after surgery to the emergency department at a peripheral hospital and was not fit for transport to a cardiac surgical facility. The cause of death in the other patient who died at 49-month follow-up is unknown. Three patients were diagnosed with postoperative

Table 1 Descriptive statistics by TAPVD type (N = 49)

	Cardiac, N = 9	Infracardiac, N = 8	Mixed, N = 7	Supracardiac, N = 25	Combined, N = 49	P value
Age in days	$_{79.0}\,128.0\,_{153.0}$	$_{23.5}\,32.5\,_{47.5}$	$_{25.5}\,65.0\,_{135.5}$	$_{59.0}\,124.0\,_{267.0}$	$_{38.0}\,87.0\,_{157.0}$	**0.01**[1]
Gender						
F	77.78% (7)	12.50% (1)	42.86% (3)	36.00% (9)	40.82% (20)	**0.046**[2]
M	22.22% (2)	87.50% (7)	57.14% (4)	64.00% (16)	59.18% (29)	
Weight in kg	$_{3.55}\,3.90\,_{4.20}$	$_{2.53}\,3.00\,_{3.55}$	$_{3.43}\,3.80\,_{4.55}$	$_{3.60}\,4.60\,_{6.50}$	$_{3.26}\,4.00\,_{5.00}$	0.162[1]
BSA in m^2	$_{0.23}\,0.24\,_{0.27}$	$_{0.18}\,0.18\,_{0.20}$	$_{0.21}\,0.24\,_{0.27}$	$_{0.22}\,0.25\,_{0.31}$	$_{0.20}\,0.24\,_{0.27}$	**0.009**[1]
Single ventricle						
No	100.00% (9)	87.50% (7)	100.00% (7)	80.00% (20)	87.76% (43)	0.304[2]
Yes	0.00% (0)	12.50% (1)	0.00% (0)	20.00% (5)	12.24% (6)	
Heterotaxy						
No	88.89% (8)	87.50% (7)	100.00% (7)	84.00% (21)	87.76% (43)	0.725[2]
Yes	11.11% (1)	12.50% (1)	0.00% (0)	16.00% (4)	12.24% (6)	
Obstructed						
No	55.56% (5)	12.50% (1)	85.71% (6)	92.00% (23)	71.43% (35)	**< 0.001**[2]
Yes	44.44% (4)	87.50% (7)	14.29% (1)	8.00% (2)	28.57% (14)	
RACHS						
2	88.89% (8)	50.00% (4)	57.14% (4)	88.00% (22)	77.55% (38)	0.06[2]
4	11.11% (1)	50.00% (4)	42.86% (3)	12.00% (3)	22.45% (11)	
Hospital						
A	55.56% (5)	87.50% (7)	57.14% (4)	52.00% (13)	59.18% (29)	0.355[2]
B	44.44% (4)	12.50% (1)	42.86% (3)	48.00% (12)	40.82% (20)	
Surgeon						
A	22.22% (2)	50.00% (4)	14.29% (1)	4.00% (1)	16.33% (8)	0.293[2]
B	66.67% (6)	25.00% (2)	71.43% (5)	80.00% (20)	67.35% (33)	
C	11.11% (1)	12.50% (1)	14.29% (1)	8.00% (2)	10.20% (5)	
D	0.00% (0)	12.50% (1)	0.00% (0)	4.00% (1)	4.08% (2)	
E	0.00% (0)	0.00% (0)	0.00% (0)	4.00% (1)	2.04% (1)	

$_a\,b\,_c$ represent the lower quartile a, the median b, and the upper quartile c for continuous variables. Numbers after proportions are frequencies
[1]Kruskal-Wallis test
[2]Pearson test

Table 2 Operative and outcome statistics (N = 49)

	Cardiac, N = 9	Infracardiac, N = 8	Mixed, N = 7	Supracardiac, N = 25	Combined, N = 49	P value
CPB time (min)	$_{43.0}\,64.0\,_{64.0}$	$_{65.0}\,84.0\,_{103.5}$	$_{78.5}\,100.0\,_{114.0}$	$_{42.0}\,53.0\,_{69.0}$	$_{45.0}\,64.0\,_{83.0}$	**< 0.001**[1]
Aortic clamp time (min)	$_{23.00}\,35.00\,_{43.00}$	$_{28.50}\,44.50\,_{63.25}$	$_{54.50}\,62.00\,_{84.00}$	$_{25.00}\,32.00\,_{37.00}$	$_{26.00}\,35.00\,_{48.00}$	**< 0.001**[1]
DHCA used	0.00% (0)	25.00% (2)	0.00% (0)	16.00% (4)	12.24% (6)	0.287[2]
Sutureless repair	11.11% (1)	12.50% (1)	14.29% (1)	4.00% (1)	8.16% (4)	0.745[2]
Delayed Sternal Closure	22.22% (2)	87.50% (7)	0.00% (0)	16.00% (4)	26.53% (13)	**< 0.001**[2]
ECMO	11.11% (1)	12.50% (1)	0.00% (0)	0.00% (0)	4.08% (2)	0.267[2]
Operative death	0.00% (0)	12.50% (1)	0.00% (0)	4.00% (1)	4.08% (2)	0.546[2]
Stenosis	11.11% (1)	12.50% (1)	0.00% (0)	4.00% (1)	6.12% (3)	0.658[2]
Reoperation	0.00% (0)	0.00% (0)	0.00% (0)	4.00% (1)	2.04% (1)	0.806[2]

$_a\,b\,_c$ represent the lower quartile a, the median b, and the upper quartile c for continuous variables. Numbers after proportions are frequencies
[1]Kruskal-Wallis test
[2]Pearson test

pulmonary vein stenosis at 2 weeks, 6 months, and 49 months after the primary surgery. The patient diagnosed at 2 weeks postoperatively was a patient with supracardiac TAPVD who was discovered to have retroesophageal course of the venous confluence draining vein [26]. She underwent reoperation during the same hospital admission and remains asymptomatic at 5 months' follow-up after the reoperation. The patient who was diagnosed at 6 months is the same patient who was reported above as a late death and did not undergo reoperation. The third patient with presumed pulmonary vein stenosis had infracardiac TAPVD. Her initial presentation was with obstructed TAPVD and had a complicated postoperative course and was not fit to undergo reoperation (Table 2).

Over long-term follow-up, pulmonary vein stenosis was significantly associated with death or reoperation, Fig. 1, *P* value < 0.001. However, the anatomical type of TAPVD and repair technique were not significantly associated with freedom from death or reoperation, Figs. 2 and 3, respectively. The presence of preoperative obstructed TAPVD also did not affect the long-term freedom from death or reoperation, *P* value 0.5.

Obstructed presentation was significantly associated with prolonged hospital stay in survivors, *P* value = 0.002, Fig. 4. The prolonged hospital stay was also significantly associated with infracardiac and supracardiac TAPVD types and with body surface area in a non-linear fashion, Fig. 4. Single ventricle anomalies, heterotaxy syndrome, and age at operation were not significant predictors of postoperative hospital stay, Fig. 4.

Discussion

In a recent meta-analysis of 26 studies involving over 2700 patients, Wu et al. concluded that primary sutureless repair was associated with less post-operative pulmonary vein stenosis and need for reoperation; however, there was no difference in early late or overall survival [10]. In line with that, we did not find any significant association between the repair technique and freedom from death or reoperation; the determination of whether the type of surgical technique is associated with postoperative stenosis and long-term outcomes is in need for prospective randomized trials and cannot be made from retrospective studies.

There were only two deaths before hospital discharge and two late deaths; therefore, we were not able to perform a multivariable analysis for survival. However, in univariable analysis, we did not find that neonatal age, weight, TAPVD anatomical type, or presentation with obstruction were significantly associated with operative or long-term death. This contrasts with the findings of the larger and more long-term studies like Yong et al. [13] and Sakamoto et al. [4] which showed that neonatal age, weight less than 2 kg, and mixed TAPVD were factors associated with reduced survival.

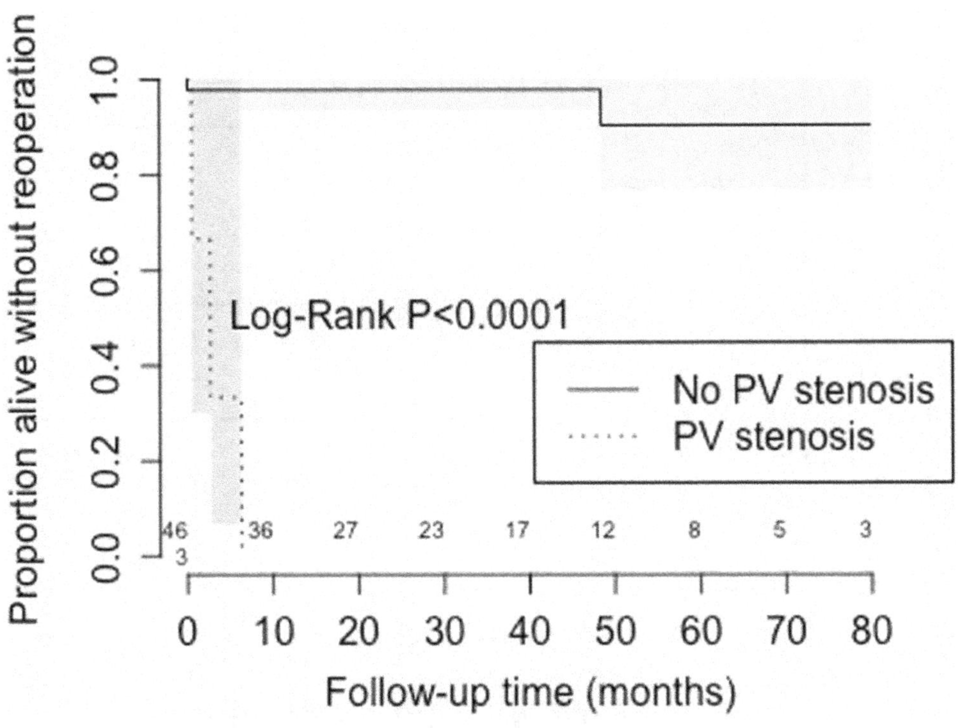

Fig. 1 Kaplan-Meier freedom from death or reoperation in patients who developed postoperative pulmonary vein stenosis and those who did not

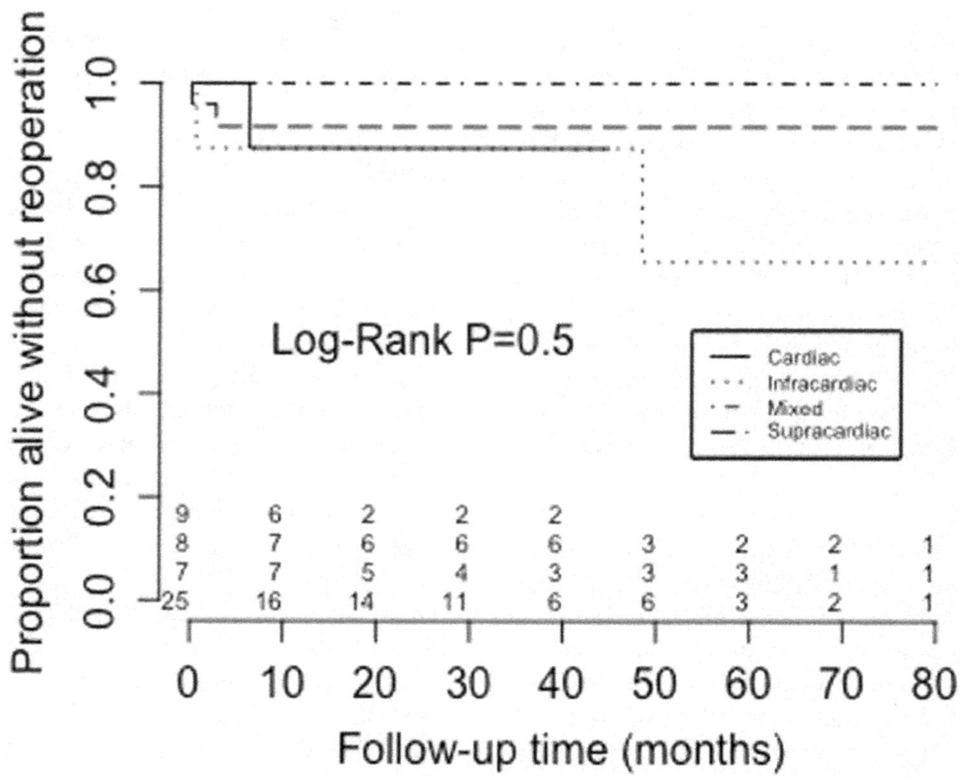

Fig. 2 Kaplan-Meier freedom from death or reoperation shown by TAPVD anatomical types

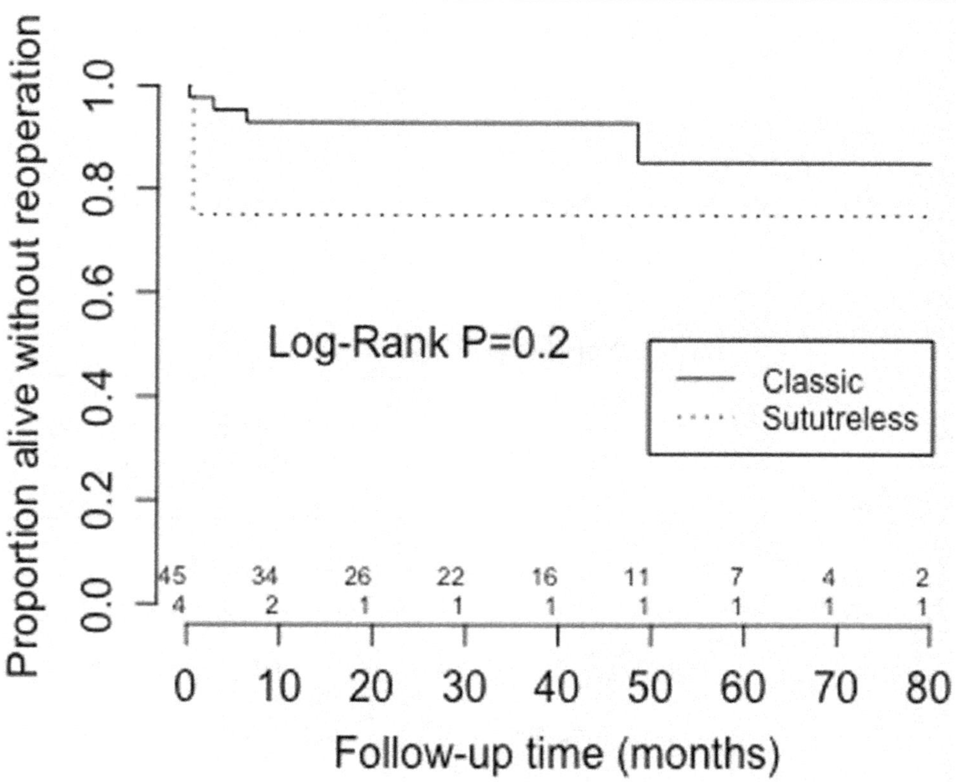

Fig. 3 Kaplan-Meier freedom from death or reoperation in classic and sutureless repair patients

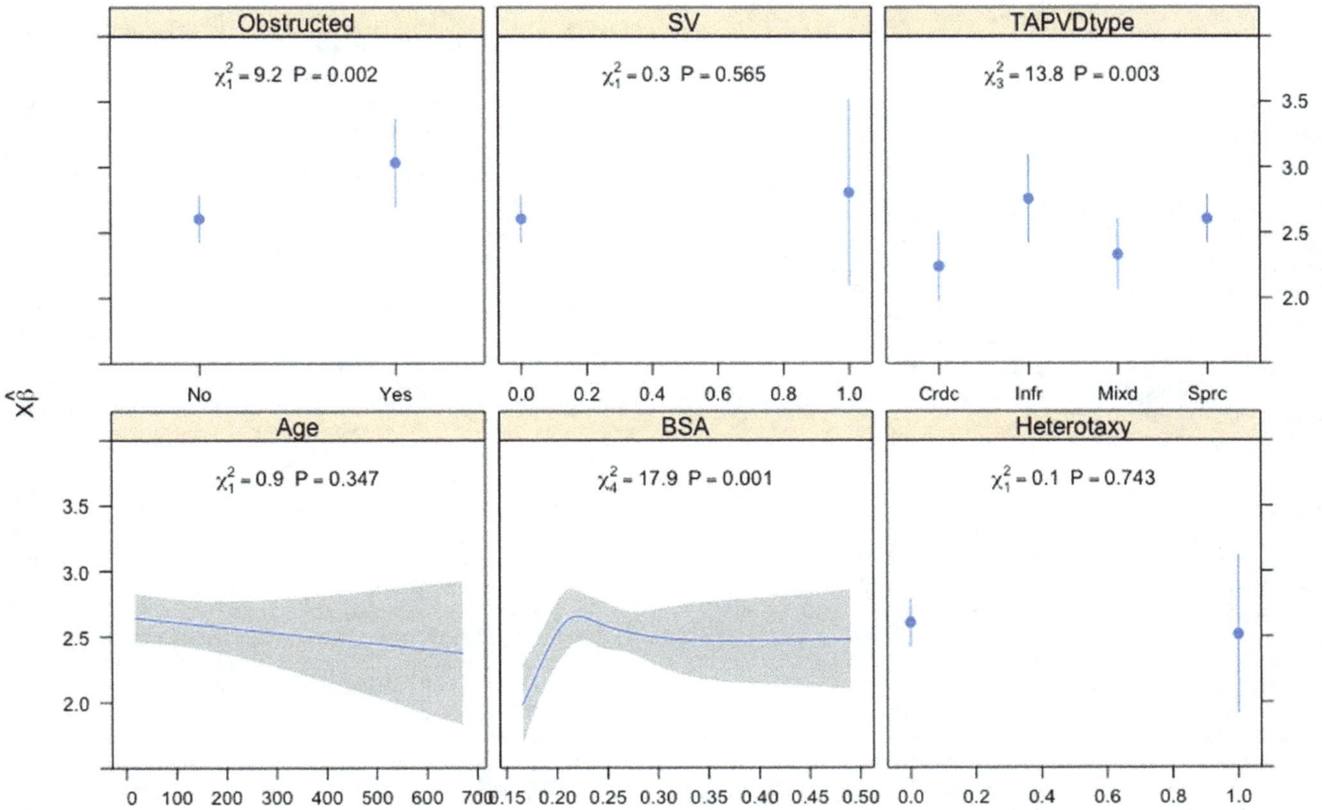

Fig. 4 Predictors of postoperative length of stay using a generalized linear model with Poisson distribution. Test shown is Wald statistic of model analysis of variance. SV: single ventricle anomalies, TAPVDtype: anatomical TAPVD type, Crdc: cardiac TAPVD, Infr: infracardiac TAPVD, Mixd: mixed TAPVD, Sprc: supracardiac TAPVD, BSA: body surface area

The current study has shown that pulmonary vein stenosis is an important predictor of long-term freedom from death or reoperation. It is our current belief that if surgery can be done avoiding postoperative pulmonary vein stenosis, then the outcomes should be very good regardless of other factors [27, 28].

The presence of TAPVD in association with heterotaxy syndromes and single ventricle anomalies is believed to be a poor prognostic indicator, and some would deny such patients' surgical care. In the current study, we did not find that to be justifiable. This is consistent with the reporting of outcomes of patients who underwent TAPVD repair with single ventricle anomalies and then went on to receive a Fontan operation, Yong et al. [13]. The outcomes of patients who had TAPVD repair then Fontan operation were comparable to Fontan patients without TAPVD repair.

The present study is limited by its retrospective nature and small number of patients and outcomes. However, it represents the complete experience of two surgical centers over an 8-year period with near-complete follow-up.

Conclusion

Surgical correction of TAPVD is a lifesaving operation and is applicable to patients who present with this anomaly regardless of age, weight, anatomical type, heterotaxy, or single ventricle anomalies. Preoperative obstruction of the pulmonary venous pathway is likely a significant factor in the patient reaching or failing to reach the operative setting; however, once the repair is performed, preoperative obstruction does not affect long-term outcome but may prolong the hospital stay. It is the development of postoperative pulmonary vein stenosis that significantly reduces freedom from death and reoperation.

Abbreviations

CPB: Cardiopulmonary bypass; ECMO: Extracorporeal membrane oxygenation; HFJV: High-frequency jet ventilation; LOS: Length of stay; OM: Operative mortality; RACHS-1: Risk adjustment in congenital heart surgery; TAPVD: Total anomalous venous drainage

Acknowledgements

Not applicable.

Authors' contributions

OOA conducted the literature search; designed the study; performed the data collection, analysis, and interpretation of data; conducted the statistical analysis; and drafted the manuscript. AE supervised the study and conducted the review of data, involved in the study design, analyzed and interpreted the data, and drafted the manuscript. MI designed the study, analyzed and interpreted the data, and drafted the manuscript. AH conducted the statistical analysis, performed the data collection, conducted the literature search, and interpreted the data. TH conducted the literature search, analyzed and interpreted the data, performed the data collection, and drafted the manuscript. All authors have read and approved the final manuscript.

Author details
[1]Department of Surgery, Faculty of Medicine, King Abdulaziz University, PO Box 80215, Jeddah 21589, Saudi Arabia. [2]Cardiovascular Department, King Faisal Specialist Hospital and Research Center, Jeddah, Saudi Arabia. [3]Cardiothoracic Surgery Department, Faculty of Medicine, Tanta University, Tanta, Egypt. [4]Cardiothoracic Surgery Department, Faculty of Medicine, Mansoura University, Mansoura, Egypt. [5]Department of Paediatrics, Paediatric Cardiology Division, Faculty of Medicine, Cairo University, Giza, Egypt. [6]Department of Paediatrics, Paediatric Cardiology Division, King Faisal Specialist Hospital and Research Center, Jeddah, Saudi Arabia. [7]Cardiothoracic Surgery Department, Faculty of Medicine, Benha University, Benha, Egypt.

References

1. Harada T, Nakano T, Oda S, Kado H (2019) Surgical results of total anomalous pulmonary venous connection repair in 256 patients. *Interact Cardiovasc Thorac Surg*. 28(3):421–426. https://doi.org/10.1093/icvts/ivy267
2. Kogon B, Fernandez J, Shashidharan S, Kanter K, Alsoufi B (2017) A 30-year experience with mixed-type total anomalous pulmonary venous connection: a word of caution. *Cardiol Young*. 27(5):870–876. https://doi.org/10.1017/S1047951116001414
3. Lemaire A, DiFilippo S, Parienti J-J et al (2016) Total anomalous pulmonary venous connection: a 40 years' experience analysis. Thorac Cardiovasc Surg. 65(01):009–017. https://doi.org/10.1055/s-0036-1588007
4. Sakamoto T, Nagashima M, Umezu K et al (2018) Long-term outcomes of total correction for isolated total anomalous pulmonary venous connection: lessons from 50-years' experience†. *Interact Cardiovasc Thorac Surg*. 27(1): 20–26. https://doi.org/10.1093/icvts/ivy034
5. Edwards JE, Helmholz HF (1956) A classification of total anomalous pulmonary venous connection based on developmental considerations. *Proc Staff Meet Mayo Clin*. 31(6):151–160
6. Nabar A, Dalvi B (1998) Obstructive total anomalous pulmonary venous drainage. *Indian J Pediatr*. 65(1):35–45. https://doi.org/10.1007/bf02849692
7. Alsoufi B (2014) Modified primary sutureless repair technique of total anomalous pulmonary venous connection. *World J Pediatr Congenit Heart Surg*. 5(2):302–305. https://doi.org/10.1177/2150135113519452
8. Kim H, Sung SC, Choi KH, Lee HD, Kim G, Ko H (2018) Primary sutureless repair of total anomalous pulmonary venous connection: suture-and-open technique. *Ann Thorac Surg*. 106(5):e273–e276. https://doi.org/10.1016/j.athoracsur.2018.05.026
9. Tremblay C, Yoo S-J, Mertens L et al (2018) Sutureless versus conventional pulmonary vein repair: a magnetic resonance pilot study. *Ann Thorac Surg*. 105(4):1248–1254. https://doi.org/10.1016/j.athoracsur.2017.11.015
10. Wu Y, Wu Z, Zheng J et al (2018) Sutureless technique versus conventional surgery in the primary treatment of total anomalous pulmonary venous connection: a systematic review and meta-analysis. *J Cardiothorac Surg*. 13(1):69. https://doi.org/10.1186/s13019-018-0756-z
11. Yun T-J, Coles JG, Konstantinov IE et al (2005) Conventional and sutureless techniques for management of the pulmonary veins: evolution of indications from postrepair pulmonary vein stenosis to primary pulmonary vein anomalies. *J Thorac Cardiovasc Surg*. 129(1):167–174. https://doi.org/10.1016/j.jtcvs.2004.08.043
12. Yanagawa B, Alghamdi AA, Dragulescu A et al (2011) Primary sutureless repair for "simple" total anomalous pulmonary venous connection: midterm results in a single institution. *J Thorac Cardiovasc Surg*. 141(6):1346–1354. https://doi.org/10.1016/j.jtcvs.2010.10.056
13. Yong MS, Zhu MZL, du Plessis K et al (2019) Long-term outcomes of the Fontan operation in patients with total anomalous pulmonary venous drainage. *Ann Thorac Surg*. 108(4):1234–1241. https://doi.org/10.1016/j.athoracsur.2019.04.073
14. Najm HK, Caldarone CA, Smallhorn J, Coles JG (1998) A sutureless technique for the relief of pulmonary vein stenosis with the use of in situ pericardium. *J Thorac Cardiovasc Surg*. 115(2):468–470. https://doi.org/10.1016/S0022-5223(98)70294-6
15. Lacour-Gayet F, Rey C, Planché C (1996) Pulmonary vein stenosis. Description of a sutureless surgical procedure using the pericardium in situ. *Arch Mal Coeur Vaiss*. 89(5):633–636
16. Ross FJ, Joffe D, Latham GJ (2017) Perioperative and anesthetic considerations in total anomalous pulmonary venous connection. *Semin Cardiothorac Vasc Anesth*. 21(2):138–144. https://doi.org/10.1177/1089253216672012
17. ElMahrouk AF, Ismail MF, Hamouda T, Shaikh R, Mahmoud A, Shihata MS, Alradi O, Jamjoom A (2019) Extracorporeal membrane oxygenation in postcardiotomy pediatric patients-15 years of experience outside Europe and North America. Thorac Cardiovasc Surg. 67(1):28–36. https://doi.org/10.1055/s-0037-1608962 Epub 2017 Dec 12
18. Dohain AM, Abdelmohsen G, Elassal AA, ElMahrouk AF, Al-Radi OO (2019) Factors affecting the outcome of extracorporeal membrane oxygenation following paediatric cardiac surgery. Cardiol Young. 20:1–9. https://doi.org/10.1017/S1047951119002634 [Epub ahead of print]
19. Alghamdi AA, Coles JG, Holtby H, Al-Radi OO (2010) Massive air embolism after the repair of obstructed total anomalous pulmonary venous drainage: an unusual complication. *J Card Surg*. 25(5):582–584. https://doi.org/10.1111/j.1540-8191.2010.01065.x
20. Williams WG. CCSDB: Congenital Cardiac Surgery Database. ccsdb.org.
21. del Nido PJ (1997) Myocardial protection and cardiopulmonary bypass in neonates and infants. *Ann Thorac Surg*. 64(3):878–879. https://doi.org/10.1016/s0003-4975(97)00696-6
22. Elassal AA, Eldib OS, Dohain AM, Abdelmohsen GA, Abdalla AH, Al-Radi OO (2019) Delayed sternal closure in congenital heart surgery: a risk-benefit analysis. *Heart Surg Forum*. 22(5):E325–E330. https://doi.org/10.1532/hsf.2471
23. Core R (2019) Team. R: a language and environment for statistical computing. Vienna, Austria: R Foundation for Statistical. Computing https://www.R-project.org/
24. Jr FEH (2019) Dupont with contributions from C, others many. Hmisc, Harrell Miscellaneous. https://CRAN.R-project.org/package=Hmisc
25. Jr FEH. Rms: regression modeling strategies.; 2019. https://CRAN.R-project.org/package=rms.
26. Rodriguez ML, Caldarone CA, Toeg H, Maharajh G (2019) Retroesophageal infracardiac total anomalous pulmonary venous drainage. World J Pediatr Congenit Heart Surg. 10(3):367–369. https://doi.org/10.1177/2150135117731893
27. Mohamed Fouad Ismail, Amr A. Arafat, Tamer E. Hamouda, Amira Esmat El Tantawy, Azzahra Edrees, Abdulbadee Bogis, Nashwa Badawy, Alaa B. Mahmoud, Ahmed Farid Elmahrouk & Ahmed A. Jamjoom : Junctional ectopic tachycardia following tetralogy of fallot repair in children under 2 years Journal of Cardiothoracic Surgery volume 13, Article number: 60 (2018)
28. Ismail MF, Elmahrouk AF, Arafat AA, Hamouda TE, Alshaikh BA, Shihata MS, Jamjoom AA, Al-Radi OO Evolution of the Norwood operation outcomes in patients with late presentation. The Journal of Thoracic and Cardiovascular Surgery https://doi.org/10.1016/j.jtcvs.2019.07.154

8

Minimally invasive aortic valve replacement with central cannulation: A cost-benefit analysis in a developing country

Mohammed Sanad[1,2] and Hatem Beshir[1,3*]

Abstract

Background: Minimally-invasive approaches to aortic valve replacement (MIAVR) are technically and logistically demanding. However, few centers have started using these approaches with standard equipment because of the limited resources. We sought to report intra- and postoperative clinical outcomes and address health resource utilization after MIAVR.

Results: A total of 102 eligible patients who had aortic valve replacement were enrolled in a prospective, multicenter cohort study conducted from June 2015 to December 2017. Fifty patients underwent aortic valve surgery via upper inverted T-shaped hemi-sternotomy (MS), and 52 patients were operated using full sternotomy (FS) in two centers in a developing country. Central cannulation was performed in all cases. Major adverse cardiac events, pain, and wound complications were compared. A cost analysis was performed, and exposure and feasibility for cannulation were assessed. The mean length of MS skin incision was 5.82 ± 0.67 cm. Cumulative cross-clamp time was insignificant between both groups (91.87 ± 34.41 versus 94.91 ± 33.96 min; $p = 0.66$). MS exhibited shorter ventilation time (6.18 ± 1.86 versus 10.68 ± 12.78 h; $p = 0.029$) and intensive care stays (33.27 ± 19.75 versus 49.42 ± 47.1 h; $p = 0.037$). Major adverse cardiac events (MACEs) were compared, and MS group exhibited fewer transfusions (1.18 ± 0.89 versus 1.7 ± 0.97 units; $p = 0.002$), fewer pulmonary complications (1 (2%) versus 2 (3.8%); $p < 0.001$), and less sternotomy wound infection (1 (2%) versus 5 (9.6%); $p = 0.048$). Total operative mortality of 4.46% was recorded ($n = 5$). Significant cost reduction was recorded favoring MS; central cannulation saved $907.16 and carried a total cost reduction of $580 (9.3%) when compared with the FS approach ($p < 0.0001$).

Conclusions: With a lack of logistics in developing countries, MIAVR not only has a cosmetic advantage but carries a significant reduction in blood use, respiratory complications, pain, and cost. MIAVR can be feasible, with a rapid learning curve in developing centers.

Keywords: Aortic valve replacement, Minimally invasive cardiac surgery, Mini-sternotomy, Central cannulation

* Correspondence: hatem.beshir@alexmed.edu.eg; hatem_beshir@msn.com
Previous presentations Presented as a poster presentation D38 during the proceedings of the 18th annual meeting of the international society of the minimally invasive cardiothoracic surgery (ISMICS 18), June 2018 in Vancouver, Canada. Presented as a poster presentation #470 during the proceedings of the 26th annual meeting of the Asian Society for Thoracic and Cardiovascular Surgery (ASCVTS 18), May 2018 in Moscow, Russia. Results Presented orally at the 15th annual congress of update in cardiology and cardiovascular surgery (UCCVS 2019), March 2019 in Antalya, Turkey.
[1]Department of Cardiothoracic Surgery, Faculty of Medicine, Mansoura University Hospitals, D17, F5. 60, El Gomhoria Street, Qism 2, Mansoura, Dakahlia 35516, Egypt
[3]Department of Cardiothoracic Surgery, Egypt Ministry of Health and Population, Alexandria Directorate, Alexandria, Egypt
Full list of author information is available at the end of the article

Background

In developing countries, rheumatic heart disease remains the leading cause of aortic valve disease, and surgical aortic valve replacement (SAVR) through full sternotomy is the standard approach [1].

Several minimally invasive techniques for cardiac surgery had been presented to our country since 2011 to lessen the intrusiveness of the surgical procedures, reduce pain, and shorten hospital stays while sustaining equivalent quality and safety of SAVR with a better quality of life and few complications as compared with conventional SAVR while maintaining cost-effectiveness.

Multiple impediments face cardiac surgery in developing nations. The lack of subsidy, high expenses linked to surgical equipment, and lengthier training curve make minimally invasive SAVR difficult as a standard of care and place a burden on the healthcare systems.

Multiple techniques for minimal invasive SAVR were proposed to decrease the length of skin incision and sternal involvement. Upper J-shaped sternotomy, inverted T-shaped mini-sternotomy, C-shaped sternotomy, and right anterior thoracotomy (RAT) approaches were described [2].

Two strategies of arterial cannulation were proposed: the retrograde route with femoral arterial cannulation and the antegrade route via direct ascending aorta cannulation. Cannulation of the groin was designated for refining exposure during surgery, but irrespective of the higher cost, in some instances, this tactic may lead to infection, lymphoid fistula, arterial wall dissection, distal limb ischemia, and increased risk of neurological complications [3].

The aim of this study was to compare the surgical outcomes and cost-effectiveness of SAVR with central cannulation using mini-sternotomy (MS) to full sternotomy in a developing country without additional equipment.

Methods

This prospective multicenter cohort study was conducted between June 2015 and December 2017 and included 112 adult patients who underwent surgical aortic valve replacement in 2 institutions. We followed the declaration of Helsinki regarding studies on human subjects [4].

The patients were operated by two surgical teams who performed surgery in both centers. Both surgical teams were oriented with conventional and minimally invasive surgical approaches.

There were 102 eligible cases who underwent isolated aortic valve replacement. Cases with valve calcifications and chronic endocarditis were included. Re-operative cases, emergency operation, patients with thoracic deformities, low ejection fraction (EF) (less than 40%), active infective endocarditis, porcelain aorta, and EuroSCORE II predicted mortality more than 10%, and those who had concomitant cardiac surgery were excluded to create two equal groups. Two years of follow-up were conducted, and the vital status was reported.

Twelve patients were excluded from our sample; two cases were excluded from the MS group for concomitant ascending aorta replacement, and ten cases were excluded from the FS group; three had re-operative SAVR, and 7 cases had a concomitant ascending aorta replacement.

The MS group included 50 patients, and the FS group had 52 patients. We analyzed the operative, short-term hospital outcomes, mid-term outcomes, and cost-effectiveness analysis of each technique.

Preoperative stratification

Computerized tomography (CT) was performed preoperatively to all cases to assess the aortic root position, the alpha angle, and the sternal to root distance. Candidate patients for the mini-sternotomy approach required more than 50% of the aortic root behind the sternum [2]. CT is of crucial importance for the exclusion of porcelain aorta and has a better role in stratification of cases eligible for the right anterior mini-thoracotomy approach.

The patients were stratified into two groups according to their definitive surgical route based on surgeons' preference:

1. *Mini-sternotomy (MS)* included 50 patients in whom SAVR was done via upper inverted T-shaped hemi-sternotomy.
2. *Full sternotomy (FS)* included 52 patients with conventional SAVR using full median sternotomy.

Anesthetic protocol

Under full invasive monitoring, the anesthetic protocol encompassed induction with fentanyl (1–10 μg/kg), atracurium besylate (0.4–0.5 mg/kg) for muscle relaxation, and propofol infusion (100–300 μg/kg/h) for the maintenance of anesthesia to endorse early extubation. Pain medication included pethidine hydrochloride in the intensive care unit (ICU) and oral acetaminophen (500 mg) while in the ward.

Surgical technique

Following general anesthesia, the FS group had a full sternotomy, while the MS group underwent a 5–7 cm upper sternotomy skin incision followed by a 10 cm upper inverted T hemi-sternotomy using a primary sternal blade for longitudinal osteotomy and a redo blade for the transverse sternotomy [2] at the level of the third intercostal space. The conventional group had a classical full median sternotomy.

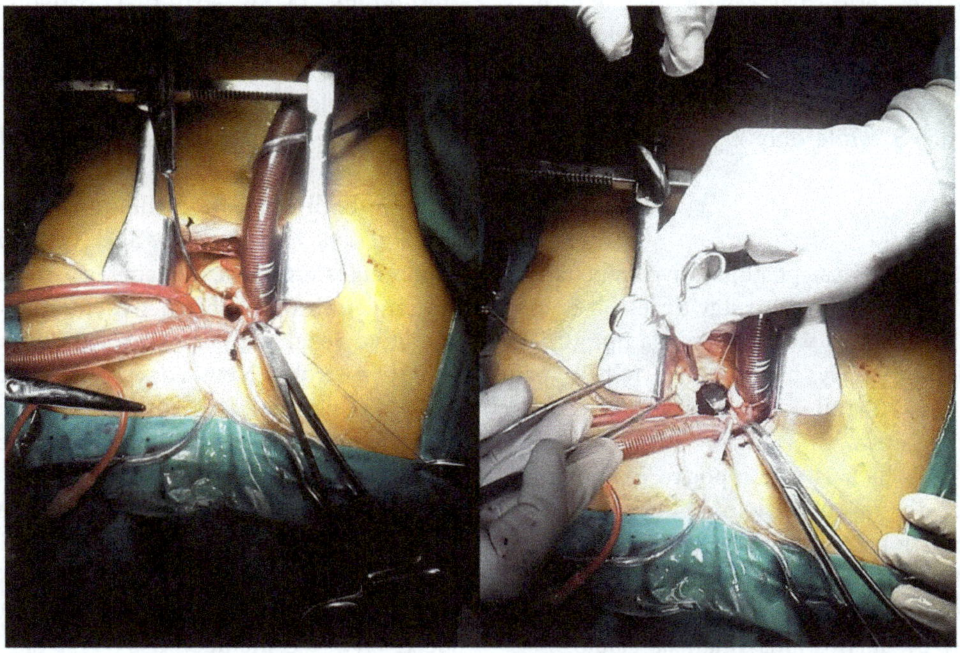

Fig. 1 Intraoperative view of the surgical field with aortic cross-clamp, central cannulation, pulmonary artery vent, and full exposure to the aortic valve with the view of the valve prosthesis in place (right)

The pericardium was retracted to expose the aorta until the origin of the innominate artery. This approach allows the ascending aorta to come forward to obtain better exposure. Two concentric 2-0 polypropylene purse-string sutures were taken at the anterolateral aspect of the ascending aorta as high as possible (Fig. 1).

The cardioplegia cannula was inserted to maintain the least distance of 1 cm between the cross-clamp and the aortic cannulation site.

Cardiopulmonary bypass was instituted after systemic heparinization using central aortic and dual-stage venous cannulation in all cases. Induced systemic arterial hypotension < 90 mmHg was required during cannulation.

Myocardial protection was established using a standard central aortic cross-clamp followed by antegrade aortic root or direct coronary cold cardioplegia with moderate systemic hypothermia 28–32 °C. Venting was performed via catheterizing the right superior pulmonary vein or the pulmonary artery. The rest of SAVR was completed as the standard of care after evaluation of the valve pathology using an appropriately sized bioprosthesis or mechanical aortic valve prosthesis.

Before weaning off bypass, a single subxiphoid chest drain was used from a 1 cm transverse skin incision and

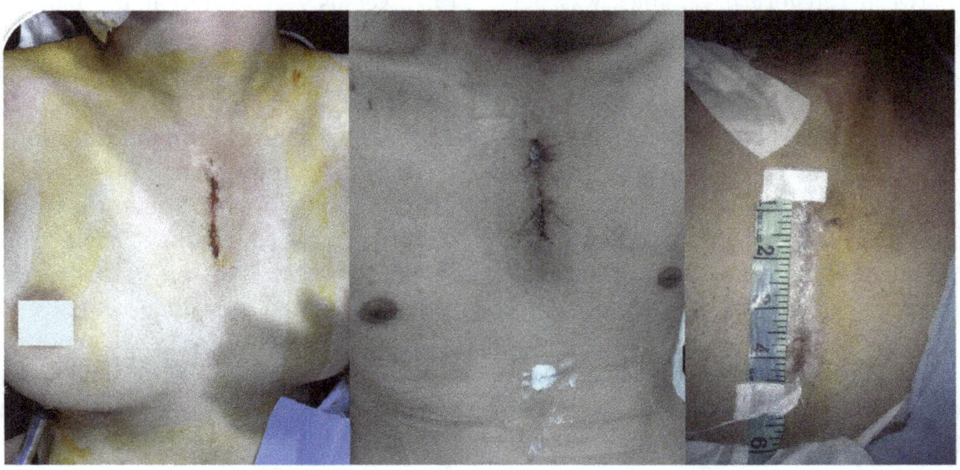

Fig. 2 The incision for minimally invasive aortic valve replacement

inserted through the pericardial cavity. In the case of pleural collection, a separate intercostal drain was inserted if needed (Fig. 2).

Following hemostasis, 4 to 6 stainless steel wires were used for closure of FS, while only 2 wires were used in the MS group.

Study endpoints

The primary endpoint was postoperative mechanical ventilation (MV) and intensive care stay times (in hours). The secondary endpoints were cross-clamp (CCT), cumulative cardiopulmonary bypass time (CBP), pain score after 12 h (1–10), all-cause mortality, need for transfusion, cost analysis, and major adverse cardiac events (MACE) [5], which is a composite endpoint including cardiac death, myocardial infarction, secondary intervention/reoperation, ventricular arrhythmia, renal failure or multi-organ failure, and outcome after 2 years of follow-up. Total cost breakdown was logged for all patients conferring the institutions' financial catalogs.

Statistical analysis

Based on a pilot study of 10 patients of each technique, the mean hours of ICU stays were found to be 35.7 ± 16.5 h in MS versus 45.87 ± 36.78 h in FS. The least significant total sample size of 94 patients was calculated to have a study power of 85% with an alpha error of 5%, a beta error of 15%, and an effect size of (Hedges' g = (45.87 − 35.7)/29.520274 = 0.344509).

A total of 112 patients were enrolled, of which 102 patients met eligibility criteria. The data were tabulated and analyzed using the IBM SPSS software version 22.0 (IBM Inc., Chicago, IL, USA). Qualitative data were described using numbers and percents. Continuous variables were assessed for normality; normal variables were reported as mean ± standard deviation (SD), while non-normal variables were reported as the median and interquartile range (IQR).

A comparison between categorical variables was performed using the chi-square test (χ^2-test). When more than 20% of the cells have expected count less than 5, correction for chi-square was conducted using Fisher's exact test or Monte Carlo correction. Confidence intervals (95% CI) were calculated. For normally distributed data, a comparison between two independent populations was made using the independent *t* test. For abnormally distributed data, we used the Mann-Whitney *Z* test and Wilcoxon signed-ranks tests.

Results

Our study was conducted on 112 patients, who were operated for aortic valve replacement during the study period, and divided into 2 groups. Fifty-two patients were operated through inverted T-shaped ministernotomy (MS); sixty-two patients were operated through a full median sternotomy (FS).

Demographic data

The baseline characteristics of our sample are mentioned in Tables 1 and 2. There was no significant difference between both groups regarding the preoperative patients' characteristics including age, gender, hypertension, hypercholesterolemia, diabetes mellitus, creatinine clearance, chronic obstructive pulmonary disease, preoperative renal dialysis, extra-cardiac arteriopathy, preoperative stroke, New York Heart Association (NYHA) class, preoperative EF%, preoperative angina, recent infarction, old infarction, urgency of the operation, preoperative EuroSCORE, valve lesion, valve pathology, preoperative atrial fibrillation, preoperative complete heart block, and preoperative hemoglobin level.

Patients who underwent MIAVR had less body mass index (BMI) than the FS group (p = 0.002 and 0.001, respectively). We included a 54-year-old female morbidly obese diabetic and a hypertensive patient who had a BMI of 60.2 kg/m^2 (obesity class III) who underwent isolate AVR using MS (Fig. 3).

Operative and postoperative outcomes

All patients were operated for aortic valve replacement. Operative outcomes are mentioned in Table 3.

MS exhibited a significantly less skin incision length of 5.82 ± 0.67 cm versus 27.52 ± 2.71 cm (p = 0.001). No significant differences were observed as regards CCT and CPB times among both groups (p = 0.58 and 0.66).

Patients were monitored postoperatively as the standard of care. Postoperative complications are compared in Table 4. In the FS group, 68.3% had severe postoperative pain, compared with MS group, where 92% experienced mild pain at the visual analog scale at 12 postoperative hours. MS significantly reduced MV time (6.18 ± 1.86 versus 10.68 ± 12.78 h, p = 0.035), ICU stay (33.27 ± 19.75 versus 49.42 ± 47.1 h, p = 0.037), and blood transfusions (1.18 ± 0.89 versus 1.7 ± 0.97 units, p = 0.002). MS patients exhibited fewer pulmonary complications (pneumonia, reintubation, and pleural effusions) (p < 0.001), less superficial wound infections (p = 0.048), and no deep sternotomy wound infection (DSWI).

Resternotomy was indicated for bleeding in 7 patients. MS group showed less incidence of postoperative hemopericardium but without statistical significance. Four patients required sternal rewiring. A total all-cause operative mortality of 5 cases was reported (4.46%).

MS group had 2 mortalities; the first was a 58-year-old female diagnosed with severe aortic stenosis complicated with congestive heart failure (LVEF 42%). She was admitted to ICU on moderate inotropic support with low cardiac output, and mortality occurred on the

Table 1 Baseline clinical characteristics for the studied sample

		Mini-sternotomy (MS) (n = 50)		Full sternotomy (FS) (n = 52)		p
Age (years)	(Mean ± SD)[a]	41.1 ± 10.3		46.4 ± 10.3		0.72
	Min, max	28, 62		25, 71		
Gender	Male	37	(74)	33	(63.5)	0.29
Weight (kg)	(Mean ± SD)	78.1 ± 20.4		89.9 ± 13.5		0.02
Height (cm)	(Mean ± SD)	171.2 ± 10.3		171.4 ± 8.2		0.49
BMI (kg/m^2)	(Mean ± SD)	26.98 ± 6.7		31.1 ± 5.7		0.001
BSA	(Mean ± SD)	1.88 ± 0.24		2.02 ± 1.7		0.001
Angina status	CCS 1	18	(36.0)	7	(13.5)	< 0.001
	CCS 2	24	(48.0)	11	(21.2)	
	CCS 3	8	(16.0)	33	(63.5)	
	CCS 4	0	(0.0)	1	(1.9)	
Dyspnea status	NYHA 1	5	(10)	0	(0)	
	NYHA 2	28	(56)	8	(15.4)	< 0.001
	NYHA 3	17	(34)	42	(80.8)	
	NYHA 4	0	(0)	2	(3.8)	
EuroSCORE %	(Mean ± SD)	1.99 ± 1.43		2.05 ± 1.77		0.64
Congestive cardiac failure	Never	50	(100)	50	(96.2)	0.49
	Past	0	(0)	2	(3.8)	
Diabetes mellitus[b]	Diet control	0	(0)	1	(1.9)	0.76
	Oral therapy	3	(6)	3	(5.8)	
	Insulin	2	(4)	3	(5.8)	
Hypertension		11	(22)	18	(34.6)	0.21
Hypothyroidism		0	(0)	1	(1.9)	0.24
Dyslipidemia		2	(4)	7	(13.5)	0.14
Smoking	Ex-smoker	9	(18)	14	(26.9)	0.53
	Active smoker	4	(8)	3	(5.7)	
GI tract	Liver dysfunction	1	(2)	1	(1.9)	1
Renal	Cr > 200 umol/l	0	(0)	3	(5.8)	0.24
Respiratory	Asthma	1	(2)	0	(0)	0.49
	COPD	1	(2)	1	(1.9)	
CVD	Stroke	1	(2)	1	(1.9)	1
PVD	Arteriopathy	1	(2)	2	(3.8)	1
Preoperative arrhythmia	Atrial fibrillation (AF)	1	(2)	1	(1.9)	1
Hemoglobin	(Mean ± SD)	13.5 ± 1.37		13.24 ± 1.79		0.35
	Min, max	10.2, 16.2		9.8, 17		
S. creatinine (mg/dl)	(Mean ± SD)	0.98 ± 0.39		0.84 ± 0.39		0.09
	Min, max	0.5, 3		0.2, 14		
Creatinine clearance (ml/min)	(Mean ± SD)	69.2 ± 22.63		77.72 ± 35.69		0.37
S. bilirubin	(Mean ± SD)	0.74 ± 0.37		0.48 ± 0.18		0.13
Coronary angiography		12	(24)	42	(80.8)	< 0.001

BMI body mass index; *COPD* chronic obstructive pulmonary disease; *MI* myocardial infarction; *PVD* peripheral vascular disease (or extracardiac arteriopathy) as indicated by claudication, amputation for arterial insufficiency, aortoiliac occlusive disease reconstruction, peripheral vascular bypass surgery, angioplasty or stent, or documented abdominal aortic aneurysm; *EuroSCORE* European System for Cardiac Operative Risk Evaluation; *CVD* cerebrovascular disease; *PVD* peripheral vascular disease or extracardiac arteriopathy

[a]The values are the number of patients with the percentage in brackets or the mean ± standard deviation or the median and interquartile range in brackets

[b]Basal serum glucose > 200 mg/dl at three consecutive measurements before surgery

Table 2 Echocardiographic data

		Mini-sternotomy (MS) (n = 50)		Full sternotomy (FS) (n = 52)		p
LVEF (%)	Fair (30–49%)[#]	5	(10)	7	(13.5)	0.58
	Good (> 50%)	45	(90)	45	(86.5)	
Aortic stenosis	n (%)	36	(72)	45	(86.5)	0.32
Aortic valve area (cm^2)	(Mean ± SD)	1.24 ± 0.37		1.15 ± 0.53		0.72
Preoperative peak Gr. on the valve (mmHg)	(Mean ± SD)	71 ± 19.7		74.7 ± 23.7		0.38
Preoperative mean Gr. on the valve (mmHg)	(Mean ± SD)	43 ± 12.5		47 ± 17.9		0.68
Reason for operation	Severe valve pathology	22	(44)	0	(0)	< 0.001
	Anatomical	25	(50)	46	(88.5)	
	Angina	2	(4)	5	(9.6)	
	Unknown	1	(2)	1	(1.9)	

LVEF left ventricular ejection fraction, *Gr* gradient, *mmHg* millimeters of mercury
[#]Cases with LVEF < 40% were excluded as per exclusion criteria

second postoperative day. The second case was a 48-year-old male with aortic stenosis who was discharged to the ward following the third postoperative day with a stable condition, and mortality was encountered on the eighth postoperative day.

FS group had 3 mortality cases; the first was a 71-year-old male with severe aortic stenosis and LVEF of 40%. Low cardiac output and LVEF of 32% were encountered, and mortality occurred on the eighth postoperative day. The second case was a 65-year-old obese male smoker who was diagnosed with severe aortic regurgitation and impaired LVEF of 42%. Mortality was recorded following prolonged mechanical ventilation because of chest infection and sepsis. The third case was a 48-year-old non-smoker diabetic female who had delayed recovery requiring reintubation and mechanical ventilation. She developed right-sided pneumonia. Sputum culture yielded Klebsiella species. She developed ventricular fibrillation for which she received cardioversion. Mortality was declared on the eighth postoperative day.

One late mortality was recorded upon follow-up of a 58-year-old female with a good left ventricular function who underwent SAVR using the MS approach 1 year following surgery due to cardiac arrest at home without

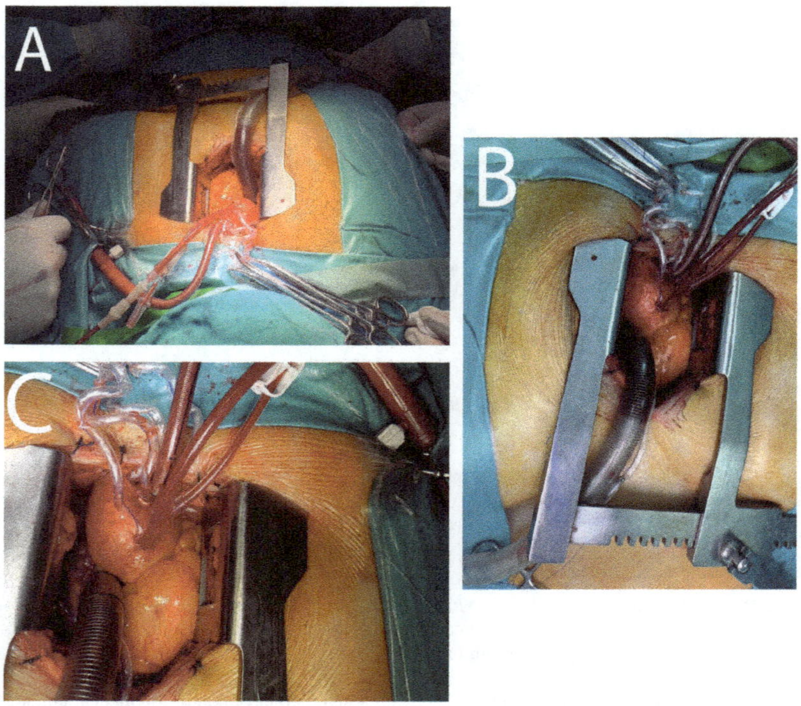

Fig. 3 Exposure for minimally invasive aortic valve replacement in a morbidly obese female patient of BMI=60.2 kg/m^2

Table 3 Operative data for the studied sample

		Mini-sternotomy (MS) (n = 50)		Full sternotomy (FS) (n = 52)		p
Length of skin incision (cm)	(Mean ± SD)	5.82 ± 0.67		27.64 ± 2.71		0.001
Implant type	Mechanical	38	(76)	28	(53.8)	0.16
	Biological	12	(24)	24	(46.2)	
Implant size (mm)	19	4	(8)	9	(17.3)	0.31
	21	20	(40)	23	(44.2)	
	23	16	(32)	16	(30.8)	
	25	8	(16)	3	(5.8)	
	27	2	(4)	1	(0.2)	
Cumulative bypass time (min)	(Mean ± SD)	91.87 ± 34.41		94.91 ± 33.96		0.66
	Min, max	43, 180		50, 215		
Cumulative cross-clamp time (min)	Mean ± SD	68.88 ± 29.63		65.78 ± 24.36		0.58
	Min, max	70.2, 35		30, 165		
Minimum core temperature (°C)	Mean ± SD	31.02 ± 2.39		30.47 ± 1.17		0.14
	Min, max	31, 27		27, 32		
Inotropic support	High	0	(0)	3	(5.7)	0.445
	Moderate	1	(2)	2	(3.8)	
	Minimal	24	(48)	26	(50)	
	None	25	(50)	21	(38.7)	

Cm centimeters, *mm* millimeters, *SD* standard deviation, *°C* degree celcius

prior symptoms. None of the mortality cases required reexploration or encountered bleeding.

Cost analysis

All costs were converted to the corresponding US dollar rate using the inpatient hospital service Consumer Price Index (CPI). The total cost for admission and operation was calculated to discharge (direct cost). Indirect costs for sick leaves were not calculated.

Looking at the breakdown of costs (Table 5), significant cost reduction was recorded favoring MS approach as regards blood product cost (17.75%, $p < 0.0001$), ICU stay (34.48%, $p < 0.0001$), ward admission (15.46%, $p < 0.0001$), and total cost reduction of $580 (9.35%, $p < 0.0001$).

Discussion

The lack of stable supplies is the foremost issue limiting us from performing minimally invasive cardiac surgery. Supplies may not be existing at all, or out of stock. As we are a government-funded institution, our supply chain is affected by the assets of the country, which are currently in a poor state.

In order to conquer some of these problems, we have had to espouse groundbreaking stratagems in other resource-poor settings to make our patients' profit splendor of minimally invasive cardiac surgery. Minimal invasive surgery offers benefits more than being only cosmetically appealing. It has comparable results to the conventional FS [1].

Our study was novel in that it utilized itemized facility costs for the procedure for each technique. Our facility divided costs based on direct patient care (including blood, laboratory, theater, room, supplies, therapy, imaging, and miscellaneous costs).

It is clear from multiple studies [3] that antegrade perfusion through the ascending aorta has several advantages as being more physiological and reduces the risk of embolization, iatrogenic aortic dissection, and groin incisions with associated complications. We used the advantage of antegrade perfusion along the minimally invasive SAVR.

A recent Cochrane review [6] encompassed seven trials with 511 participants from 7 countries. The effects of minimally invasive limited upper MS on SAVR as compared with FS were investigated [7–13].

In our study, we found that CBP and CCT times were not significantly different between both techniques. Notably, total operative time was significantly longer in the MS group in our first cases. In accordance with our results, there was no evidence of an increase CBP with AVR performed via an upper MS (mean difference (MD) 3.02 min, 95% CI − 4.10, 10.14; participants = 311; studies = 5; low quality). There was no evidence of an increase in aortic CCT (MD 0.95 min, 95% CI − 3.45, 5.35; participants = 391; studies = 6; low quality) [7, 9–11, 13].

Table 4 Postoperative data

		Mini-sternotomy (MS) (*n* = 50)		Full sternotomy (FS) (*n* = 52)		*p* (95% CI)
ICU and hospital stay						
Ventilation time (days)	(Mean ± SD)	1 ± 0.1		1.17 ± 0.83		0.188 (− 0.417, 0.831)
	Min, max	1, 1		1, 6		
Ventilation time (h)	(Mean ± SD)	6.18 ± 1.86		10.68 ± 12.78		0.029 (− 6.63, − 1.09)
	Min, max	6, 18		4, 90		
ICU stay (nights)	(Mean ± SD)	1.43 ± 0.89		2.1 ± 1.89		0.035 (− 1.29, − 0.492)
	Min, max	1, 6		4, 10		
ICU stay (h)	(Mean ± SD)	33.27 ± 19.75		49.42 ± 47.1		0.037 (− 2.659, − 0.978)
	Min, max	18, 120		4, 240		
Postoperative hospital stay (days)	(Mean ± SD)	6.95 ± 3.83		8.34 ± 4.61		0.105 (− 3.156, 0.297)
	Min, max	2, 25		4, 132		
Postoperative complications		5	(10)	7	(11.3)	0.096
Transfusion number of blood units	(Mean ± SD)	1.18 ± 0.89		1.7 ± 0.97		0.002 (− 0.078, − 0.244)
	Min, max	0, 4		0, 5		
Need for transfusion (cases)	*n* (%)	34	(68)	38	(73.1)	0.052
Resternotomy	Bleeding/tamponade	2	(4)	5	(9.6)	0.437
Sternal resuturing		1	(2)	3	(5.8)	0.627
Arrhythmia	Ventricular fibrillation	0	(0)	3	(5.8)	0.014
	Supraventricular tachycardia	0	(0)	0	(0)	
	Permanent block—pace	2	(4)	1	(0.2)	
Pulmonary complications	Pleural effusion and drainage	1	(2)	2	(3.8)	< 0.001
	Reintubation/ventilation	0	(0)	4	(7.7)	
Neurological complications	Delayed recovery/stroke/other	0	(0)	1	(1.9)	0.138
	TIA	0	(0)	1	(1.9)	
Infective complications	Superficial wound infection	1	(2)	5	(9.6)	0.048 (− 0.194, − 0.179)
	DSWI	0	(0)	1	(1.9)	
Renal complications	Cr > 3	1	(2)	3	(5.7)	0.26
GI complications	Upper GI bleeding	0	(0)	4	(7.7)	0.22
Multi-organ failure	*n* (%)	0	(0)	2	(3.8)	0.34
Discharged to	Died in hospital	2	(4)	3	(5.7)	0.67
	Home	48	(96)	49	(94.2)	
Status at 2 years of follow-up	Alive	47	(94)	49	(94.2)	0.55
	Died in hospital	2	(4)	3	(5.7)	
	Died	1	(2)	0	(0)	

Unlike our study, none of the included studies in this review reported major adverse cardiac and cerebrovascular events as a composite endpoint. There was no evidence of any effect of upper MS on mortality versus FS (risk ratio (RR) 1.01, 95% (CI) 0.36 to 2.82; participants = 511; studies = 7; moderate quality) [9, 12].

We calculated the duration of postoperative MV from the moment of intensive care unit admission to the moment of extubation of the endotracheal tube. We observed a shorter period of postoperative MV in the MS group compared with the FS group. We contemplate that these results were due to the upheld integrity of the thoracic cage, expressly the lower costal margin, which helps in the conservation of the respiratory mechanics. The smaller incision can be convoyed with less pain and easier respiratory movements.

The results of mini-sternotomy are promising regarding decreasing MV and ICU stay, which will have a

Table 5 Mean total cost breakdown

	Mini-sternotomy (MS) (*n* = 50)	Full sternotomy (FS) (*n* = 52)	Difference mean (%) (95% CI)	*p*
Operative costs				
Theater admission	$72.58	$72.58		NS
Oxygenator and tubing	$362.89	$362.89		NS
Cannulae (aortic and two stage venous)	$181.44	$181.44		NS
Drainage system	$38.72	$38.72		NS
Suturing material	$211.67	$211.67		NS
Sternal wire	$60.42	$90.42		NS
Mechanical prosthesis	$604.78	$604.78		NS
Biological prosthesis	$1632.95	$1632.95		NS
Blood	$241.92	$294.32	$52.08 (17.75%) (33.33, 70.83)	< 0.0001
Operating team fees	$2419.2	$2419.2		NS
Postoperative costs				
ICU stay and pharmacy	$529.77	$809.75	$279.23 (34.48%) (223.86, 334.61)	< 0.0001
Ventilator	$78.64	$78.64		NS
Ward	$349.6	$413.32	$63.72 (15.46%) (35.47, 91.98)	< 0.0001
Imaging	$54.25	$62.54	$8.29 (13.25%) (-3.975, 20.56)	0.1832
Laboratory	$415.75	$498.13	$82.38 (16.57%) (54.08, 110.69)	< 0.0001
Total cost (mechanical)	$5621.63	$6201.76	580.13 (9.35%) (351.08, 649.18)	< 0.0001
Total cost (biological)	$6649.81	$7229.93	580.12 (8.02%) (281.61, 719.38)	0.0001

NS non-significant statistically at $p > 0.05$

positive economic impact. Upper inverted T-shaped hemi-sternotomy maintains the integrity of the chest wall, which will improve the chest wall mechanics and facilitate early weaning and ambulation. This is a major advantage of MS over FS other than the cosmetic results and should be the primary target of the approach. In paradox, literature reported no significant effect on MV times (MD – 1.12 h, 95% CI – 3.43 to 1.19; participants = 297; studies = 5; low quality) [7, 8, 10–13].

We observed significantly shorter ICU stay a slightly shorter, but non-significant, duration of the postoperative hospital stay in the MS group. In the literature, there was a small reduction in length of intensive care unit stays as a result of the MS (MD was – 0.57 days, 95% CI – 0.93 to – 0.20; participants = 297; studies = 5; low quality) [9]. However, there was no evidence of an effect on length of hospital stay (MD – 1.31 days, 95% CI – 2.63, 0.01; participants = 297; studies = 5; I2 = 89%; very low quality) [7, 8, 10, 11 13].

In agreement to our results, postoperative blood loss was lower in MS (MD – 158.00 ml, 95% CI – 303.24 to – 12.76; participants = 297;studies = 5; moderate quality). The literature did not attest a drop in DSWI (RR 0.71, 95% CI 0.22 to 2.30; participants = 511; studies = 7; moderate quality) or re-exploration (risk ratio (RR) 1.01, 95% CI 0.48 to 2.13; participants = 511; studies = 7; moderate quality) [5, 6].

Dissimilar to our results, a review reported no change in pain scores by upper MS (standardized mean difference (SMD) – 0.33, 95% CI –0.85 to 0.20; participants = 197; studies = 3; I2 = 70%; very low quality) [8, 10, 11].

Our study did not address pulmonary function test as an endpoint. The literature reported a small increase in postoperative pulmonary function tests with MS (MD 1.98% predicted FEV1, 95% CI 0.62 to 3.33; participants = 257; studies = 4; I2 = 28%; low quality) [6].

MS approach did not reduce perioperative atrial fibrillation (AF) compared with FS (RR 0.60, 95% CI 0.07 to 4.89; participants = 240; studies = 3; moderate quality). All of our patients, except one, were having sinus rhythm [6].

None of the included studies in the Cochrane review reported cost analyses. This was a major advantage of the present study.

More recently, the MAVRIC (manubrium-limited mini-sternotomy versus conventional sternotomy for aortic valve replacement trial) [14] a single-center, single-blind randomized study that compared AVR via manubrium-limited mini-sternotomy using a 5- to 7-cm midline incision (intervention) and conventional FS and had postoperative red cell transfusion as the primary outcome. MIS was allied to higher CBP time and reduced drain losses, but this difference did not translate in a significant reduction in blood transfusion. Additionally, conventional SAVR was found to be more cost-effective (MS had a 5.8% probability of being cost-effective) [14].

Study limitations and strength

There are some imperative shortcomings of this study. The prospective cohort study is non-randomized. The sample size was small, and the calculation was based on a single outcome of the ICU stay. Other vital outcomes were mentioned as secondary outcomes. Despite the orientation of all surgical teams with both approaches, several surgeons still preferred a traditional FS, so there might have been some selection bias as allocation was according to surgeons' preference. The unequal number of groups was another issue. However, the groups were almost matched demographically. Despite the FS group had of higher BMI, we included cases with morbid obesity in the mini-sternotomy group up to 158 kg/BMI 60.2 kg/m^2 without impact on postoperative outcomes. The study might be underpowered to detect significance in the difference in low-frequency events. This may or may not have affected some of the important outcomes such as pulmonary or neurological complications but not the ICU stay. Although we incorporated fast recovery protocols in our ICU, the duration of endotracheal intubation and length of postoperative stay was decided by the individual surgeon. No conversions were recorded.

Aortic surgery via mini-sternotomy has already been done in many centers worldwide, this study introduced MS at our centers with limited resources and achieved excellent outcomes with some benefits.

Evidently, the benefit of MS over FS is still debated, and some outcomes of each are well established as cosmetic superiority, bleeding reduction, postoperative pain, MV, and ICU stays as well as reduced pulmonary complications. In light of low resources, patients in developing countries still should benefit the splendor of MIAVR that has verified reduced budgets.

Conclusions

With the lack of logistics and equipment in developing countries, MIAVR carries a significant reduction of blood product use, respiratory problems, pain, resource utilization, and cosmesis over FS without additional equipment. MIAVR using MS is feasible, with a rapid learning curve, in developing centers.

Abbreviations

BMI: Body mass index; CCT: Cumulative cross-clamp time; CI: Confidence interval; CPB: Cardiopulmonary bypass time; CPI: Consumer price index; DSWI: Deep sternotomy wound infection; EF%: Ejection fraction percentage; FS: Full sternotomy; ICU: Intensive care unit; MACEs: Major adverse cardiac events; MAVRIC: Manubrium-limited mini-sternotomy versus conventional sternotomy for aortic valve replacement trial; MIAVR: Minimally-invasive approaches to aortic valve surgery; MS: Mini-sternotomy/hemi-sternotomy; MV: Mechanical ventilation; NYHA: New York Heart Association class; RAT: Right anterior thoracotomy; RR: Risk ratio; SAVR: Surgical aortic valve replacement; SD: Standard deviation; SMD/MD: Standardized mean difference

Acknowledgements

This trial would not be possible without the enthusiasm and commitment of clinicians, nurses, and our patients.

Authors' contributions

Both authors contributed equally in conceptualization, operating cases. MS presented the data in several international meetings and revised the manuscript; HB performed statistical analysis and writing of the manuscript with MS. All authors have read and approved the final manuscript.

Author details

[1]Department of Cardiothoracic Surgery, Faculty of Medicine, Mansoura University Hospitals, D17, F5. 60, El Gomhoria Street, Qism 2, Mansoura, Dakahlia 35516, Egypt. [2]Department of Cardiothoracic Surgery, Egypt Ministry of Health and Population, Nasser Institute for Research and Treatment, Cairo, Egypt. [3]Department of Cardiothoracic Surgery, Egypt Ministry of Health and Population, Alexandria Directorate, Alexandria, Egypt.

References

1. Glauber M, Ferrarini M, Miceli A (2015) Minimally invasive aortic valve surgery: state of the art and future directions. Ann Cardiothorac Surg 4(1): 26–32
2. Hancock HC, Maier RH, Kasim AS et al (2019) Mini-sternotomy versus conventional sternotomy for aortic valve replacement. J Am Coll Cardiol 73(19):2491–2492
3. Murzi M, Glauber M (2015) Central versus femoral cannulation during minimally invasive aortic valve replacement. Ann Cardiothoracic Surg 4(1): 59–61
4. World Medical Association (2001) World Medical Association Declaration of Helsinki. Ethical principles for medical research involving human subjects. Bull World Health Organ 79(4):373–374
5. Myles PS (2014) Meaningful outcome measures in cardiac surgery. J Extra Corpor Technol 46(1):23–27
6. Kirmani BH, Jones SG, Malaisrie SC, Chung DA, Williams RJNN (2017) Limited versus full sternotomy for aortic valve replacement (Review). Cochrane Database Syst Rev 4:CD011793
7. Aris A, Camara ML, Montiel J, Delgado LJ, Galan J, Litvan H (1999) Ministernotomy versus median sternotomy for aortic valve replacement: a prospective, randomized study. Ann Thorac Surg 67:1583–1587
8. Bonacchi M, Prifti E, Giunti G, Frati G, Sani G (2002) Does ministernotomy improve postoperative outcome in aortic valve operation? A prospective randomized study. Ann Thorac Surg 73:460–465
9. Borger MA, Moustafine V, Conradi L, Knosalla C, Richter M, Merk DR et al (2015) A randomized multicenter trial of minimally invasive rapid deployment versus conventional full sternotomy aortic valve replacement. Ann Thorac Surg 99:17–25
10. Calderon J, Richebe P, Guibaud JP, Coiffic A, Branchard O, Asselineau J et al (2009) Prospective randomized study of early pulmonary evaluation of patients scheduled for aortic valve surgery performed by ministernotomy or total median sternotomy. J Cardiothorac Vasc Anesth 23:795–801
11. Dogan S, Dzemali O, Wimmer-Greinecker G, Derra P, Doss M, Khan MF et al (2003) Minimally invasive versus conventional aortic valve replacement: a prospective randomized trial. J Heart Valve Dis 12:76–80
12. Mächler HE, Bergmann P, Anelli-Monti M, Dacar D, Rehak P, Knez I et al (1999) Minimally invasive versus conventional aortic valve operations: a prospective study in 120 patients. Ann Thorac Surg 67:1001–1005
13. Moustafa MA, Abdelsamad AA, Zakaria G, Omarah MM (2007) Minimal vs median sternotomy for aortic valve replacement. Asian Cardiovascular Thoracic Annals 15:472–475
14. Akowuah E, Goodwin TA, Owens WA, Hancock HC, Rebecca Maier R, Kasim A, Mellor A, Khan K, Murphy G, Mason J (2017) Manubrium-limited ministernotomy versus conventional sternotomy for aortic valve replacement (MAVRIC): study protocol for a randomised controlled trial. Trials. 18:46

Trans-thoracic versus trans-hiatal resection for oesophageal carcinoma: a retrospective comparative study of a single-centre case series

Aram Baram[1,2*] and Hiwa Sherzad[3]

Abstract

Background: Oesophageal carcinoma (EC) is the eighth most common cancer. Surgery is the cornerstone of management for resectable EC. Trans-thoracic oesophagectomy (TTE) and trans-hiatal oesophagectomy (THE) are the two most widely practised procedures. Most of the related controversies are centred on both early and late post-operative complications and mortality (in terms of overall survival and cancer-free survival).
This was a single-centre, retrospective, comparative study analysing the outcomes of two EC resection methods. All 87 patients underwent surgery by the same surgical team over 13 years. Consequently, 87 oesophagectomies with curative intent were performed and divided into the TTE group (group A = 47) and the THE group (group B = 40).

Results: The mean patient age was 65.60 ± 6.30 years in the TTE group and 63.48 ± 9.34 years in the THE group. No significant difference was found in operative time, blood loss or duration of stay in the intensive care unit. The duration of hospital stay was significantly different between the THE and TTE groups (17.25 ± 5.92 vs. 12.93 ± 3.44, respectively; $P \leq 0.001$). In-hospital mortality was higher in the TTE group (9/47, 19.14%) than in the THE group (5/40, 12.5%) ($P = 0.400$). The mean survival rate from our series showed the superiority of group A (TTE) (65.56 months) over group B (THE) (45.01 months), with $P = 0.146$.

Conclusion: No high level of evidence suggests the superiority of one surgical procedure over another. The THE procedure is less time-consuming concerning care and follow-up, and most patients were more satisfied and experienced less pain than with the TTE procedure. Both THE and TTE have comparable post-operative anastomotic complications, and they have no significant long-term survival differences.

Keywords: Oesophageal cancer, Surgical resection, Operative approaches, Cancer-free survival, Long-term outcome

Background

Oesophageal carcinoma (EC) is the eighth most common cancer in the world and is the sixth leading cause of cancer-related mortality worldwide because of its high malignant potential and poor prognosis [1]. The incidence of EC is expected to increase by approximately 140% over the next 10 years, faster than any other solid cancer in the world [2]. EC affects more than 500,000 people worldwide annually [3]. The National Cancer Institute in the USA estimates approximately 18,440 new cases and approximately 16,170 deaths from EC in 2020 [4]. EC is four times more common in men than in women [1]. The incidence rate varies internationally by approximately 21-fold [5]; within the highest risk area, the rate is greater than 100 per 100,000 (Asian EC Belt) [2, 6].

* Correspondence: aram.baramm@gmail.com; aram.baram@univsul.edu.iq
[1]Department of Surgery, School of Medicine, Faculty of Medical Sciences, University of Sulaimani, François Mitterrand Street, Sulaymaniyah 46001, Iraq
[2]Department of Thoracic and Cardiovascular Surgery, Sulaimani Teaching Hospital, Al Sulaymaniyah, Kurdistan Region 46001, Iraq
Full list of author information is available at the end of the article

Two main histopathological types of EC exist; together, they account for approximately 90% of all cases of EC: squamous cell carcinoma and adenocarcinoma [7].

Squamous cell carcinoma, the most common type of EC worldwide [1, 2, 6] and the most common subtype of EC in developing countries [8], evenly affecting the mid and lower oesophagus, has a strong correlation with smoking, alcohol consumption, nutritional deficiencies, chronic inflammation and irritation [2, 9]. Adenocarcinoma is the most common type of EC in Western countries; it has a strong predilection to the lower third of the oesophagus in up to three quarters of cases and is commonly associated with columnar-lined metaplastic epithelium (Barrett's oesophagus), gastroesophageal reflux disease, smoking and obesity [6–9].

Although *Helicobacter pylori* (*H. pylori*) is a well-known risk factor for gastric carcinoma, no significant correlation between *H. pylori* infection and EC has been found in the general population, and it was even found to have a protective effect in oesophageal adenocarcinoma. However, such a correlation was found to be significant in the Middle East [10].

Surgery is the cornerstone of management for early-stage EC [11, 12]. The most common surgical techniques used to date are trans-thoracic oesophagectomy (TTE) (Ivor Lewis procedure) [13], trans-hiatal oesophagectomy (THE) (Orringer procedure) [14], three-field oesophagectomy (McKeown procedure) [15] and minimally invasive oesophagectomy [16].

While surgical resection is the only treatment modality with curative intent, many researchers have proved that nonsurgical management offers better survival benefits, that oesophagectomy has a relatively high index of mortality and that oesophageal cancer is an incurable disease [2].

Surgery still has a powerful impact on overall survival according to multivariable analyses. The death risk of patients treated with curative surgery is significantly lower than that of patients treated with definite chemoradiotherapy. Furthermore, for patients with stage T3N(+) and T4 disease, surgery combined with neoadjuvant treatment is associated with a significantly higher survival rate than surgery alone or definite chemoradiotherapy [11].

Patients who undergo surgery experience significantly longer survival than those who do not; therefore, curative resection should be considered for oesophageal cancer patients who are medically fit for surgery. Neoadjuvant treatment is recommended for surgically resectable stage T3-T4 EC [11].

A propensity-matched analysis showed that 525 patients who were given preoperative therapy followed by surgery had a median survival duration of 32.3 months compared with 21.9 months in patients who refused surgery. In a multivariate analysis, refusal of surgery remained a strong predictor of poor survival (odds ratio, 1.72; $P < 0.001$) [2].

Trans-thoracic oesophagectomy employs excision of the oesophagus through right thoracotomy under direct vision, excision of the tumour and peritumoural lymphatic tissues combined with mobilization of the stomach through midline laparotomy and reconstruction of the anastomosis in the posterior mediastinum [13]. As the patient undergoes both laparotomy and thoracotomy, there might be more post-operative cardiorespiratory complications, such as mediastinitis and sepsis, and post-operative anastomotic leaks, but this procedure provides more satisfactory oncological clearance of peritumoural tissue and lymph nodes [17–20].

Trans-hiatal oesophagectomy employs dilatation of the oesophageal hiatus through midline laparotomy, dissection of the oesophagus by blunt dissection in the posterior mediastinum without thoracotomy, and then, through a longitudinal left cervical incision, the oesophagus is exposed and gastroesophageal anastomosis is performed in the neck [14]. Therefore, it provides less possibility for compromised post-operative cardiorespiratory function and eliminates the risk of mediastinitis, but the oncological outcome is less favourable because of less oncological clearance [17–20].

Three-stage oesophagectomy (McKeown) combines laparotomy and right thoracotomy with cervical dissection and anastomosis [15]. The potential advantage of this procedure over the other two approaches is more comprehensive lymph node dissection and less need to extend the thoracotomy incision since the anastomosis is in the neck, and it avoids the morbidity associated with intrathoracic anastomosis [21, 22].

In minimally invasive oesophagectomy (MIE), laparoscopy and thoracoscopy are used for intraoperative staging, followed by gastric mobilization and intrathoracic oesophagectomy, respectively. Since it was first introduced by Cuschieri et al. in 1992 [16] as a subtotal endoscopic oesophagectomy through the right thoracoscopic approach, many institutions have reported using this technique in association with either laparotomy or thoracotomy or, more recently, with endoscopy, avoiding open techniques completely [23]. Although the initial results were promising, with a comparable outcome to open resection, avoiding thoracotomy will further reduce pulmonary complications associated with an open approach, and better visual control allows favourable oncological quality of resection. However, there is still no convincing evidence that MIE is superior to open oesophagectomy [24].

Considerable controversies exist about the optimal surgical approach. Most are centred on both early and late post-operative complications and mortality (in terms of overall survival and cancer-free survival).

Our study aimed to evaluate the differences in both early and late surgical outcomes of the most commonly performed procedures for oesophageal resection in our facility (trans-thoracic versus trans-hiatal oesophagectomy).

Methods

Study design

This was a single-centre, retrospective, comparative, observational study analysing the outcomes of the two most common methods of EC resection (trans-thoracic versus trans-hiatal oesophagectomy). Patients with retrospective data were included and analysed prospectively. This manuscript has been reported in line with the Strengthening the Reporting of Cohort Studies in Surgery (STROCSS) statement [25].

Setting

This study was conducted in a single academic institution. Between February 2007 and February 2020, 87 oesophageal resections with curative intent were included: TTE (group A = 47) and THE (group B = 40).

All the data were obtained directly from the patients, patients' relatives and medical records. Approval was granted from the Ethical and Scientific Council of our institution. This study was registered at ResearchRegistry.com (researchregistry5755).

Patient characteristics, including demographic data (Table 1), comorbidities, preoperative imaging data (barium swallow, abdominal ultrasound (US) and computed tomography (CT) of the chest and abdomen), cardiorespiratory function (pulmonary function test (PFT), echocardiography and chest radiography) and endoscopic variables from both oesophagogastroduodenoscopy (EGD) and endoscopic ultrasound (EUS), were analysed. As in the beginning of the study positron emission tomography-computed tomography (PET-CT) was not available, we depended on chest CT and EUS findings for the purpose of preoperative clinical staging.

All patients underwent a histopathological examination for EC of the mid and lower oesophagus. Patients with distant metastases were excluded. Patients were staged according to the 8th edition of the TNM (tumour, node and metastasis) staging system.

Operative details, technique, safety margins, type of anastomosis, duration, intraoperative complications and blood loss were analysed.

Post-operative follow-up, intensive care unit stay, total hospital stay and any post-operative complications (wound infection, anastomotic leak and vocal cord paralysis) were recorded. Patients were followed up at regular intervals with an operative consultant every month for up to 3 months, then every 3 months for up to 1 year and then every 6 months for up to 5 years.

Surgical procedures

Patients were thoroughly discussed at multidisciplinary meetings, and decisions regarding the surgical approach were made by the operating surgeon according to his experience and comfortability with the operative approach

Table 1 Patient characteristics

Variables	Category	Group A (TTE) *n* (%) 47, (54.02%)	Group B (THE) *n* (%) 40, (45.97%)	*P* value
Age (Mean ± SD)	Year	65.60 ± 6.30	63.48 ± 9/34	0.212
Age group	40–50	1 (2.1%)	5 (12.5%)	
	51–60	9 (19.1%)	7 (17.5%)	
	61–70	29 (61.7%)	24 (60%)	
	71–80	8 (17%)	4 (10%)	
Gender	Male	30 (63.8%)	27 (67.5%)	0.720
	Female	17 (36.2%)	13 (32.5%)	
Smoking		26 (55.3%)	24 (60%)	0.660
Comorbidities	DM	19 (40.4%)	11 (27.5%)	0.206
	HTN	41 (87.2%)	31 (77.5%)	0.231
	IHD	25 (53.2%)	27 (67.5%)	0.175
	COAD	8 (17%)	14 (35%)	0.055+
Clinical stages	I	3 (6.4%)	1 (2.5%)	0.489
	II	20 (42.5%)	13 (32.5%)	
	III	24 (51.0%)	26 (65.0%)	
Histology	SCC	35 (74.4%)	24 (60%)	0.529
	Adenocarcinoma	12 (25.5%)	16 (40%)	

and patient characteristics (tumour stage, level and comorbidities).

In group A (47 patients), standard trans-thoracic oesophagectomy (Ivor Lewis operation) was performed. In group B (40 patients), standard trans-hiatal oesophagectomy (Orringer procedure) was performed. Standard gastric tubes were used in both groups. All gastroesophageal anastomoses were hand-sewn with a single layer of interrupted absorbable Vicryl (Ethicon Inc., USA). A stapler was not used for the anastomosis of suture lines in this series. No gastric drainage procedure was performed. Finally, a standard feeding jejunostomy tube was inserted into group A patients only. An intercostal drain was inserted into all patients in group A and inserted into select patients in group B. Cervical and abdominal wounds were always drained and closed with standard methods.

Post-operative care

All efforts were made to wean the patient from mechanical ventilation in the immediate post-operative period. All the patients remained in the intensive care unit for a minimum of 24 h and were transferred to the conventional surgical ward accordingly. In cases of failed extubation, a further extubation attempt was made within the subsequent days. Enteral feeding started through the jejunostomy tube on the second or third post-operative day in group A and through the nasoentric tube in group B. Post-operative respiratory physiotherapy was encouraged in the form of incentive spirometry and early mobilization.

Patients were kept nil by mouth for at least 7 days. On the 8th post-operative day, if there were no clinical or radiological signs of a leak, then a liquid diet was allowed within the following days, while a cervical drain was kept in place.

Statistical analysis

The data were collected and entered into an Excel sheet; after coding, they were transferred to Statistical Package for the Social Sciences (SPSS), version 22. IBM Corporation and R environment version 3.2.2 were used for data analysis. Descriptive and quantitative analyses were performed. The relationships between the initial findings and subsequent morbidity and mortality were determined using the chi-square test or Fisher's exact test for nominal variables and Student's t test for quantitative variables. A P value ≤ 0.05 was considered significant. Kaplan-Meier survival curves were used to estimate tumour-free survival.

Results

A total of 87 patients underwent oesophagectomy for oesophageal cancer. Patients were grouped into group A (47 patients (54.02%) TTE) and group B (40 patients (45.97%) THE). Demographic details of both groups are shown in Table 1. Overall, there were no significant differences in demographic characteristics between the groups. The mean patient age was 65.60 ± 6.30 years in the TTE group and 63.48 ± 9.34 years in the THE group.

Male patients predominated in both groups. Chronic obstructive airway disease (COAD) was the most common associated comorbidity in group B (35%) (vs. 17% in group A; P = 0.055+). The most common clinical presentations were dysphagia (solid (96.6%) and liquid (89.7%)) and anorexia (62.1%). The majority of our patients were in stages II (37.9%) and III (57.4%). Three patients from group A had a lymph node (LN) status of N2 and received neoadjuvant chemotherapy (Tables 1, 2 and 3).

The operative details and post-operative courses are shown in Table 4. Differences in operative time, total blood loss during the operation and number of hours of stay in the intensive care unit post-operatively were not significant between the groups. There was a statistically significant difference in the duration of hospital stay post-operatively among patients who received THE vs. TTE (17.25 ± 5.92 vs 12.93 ± 3.44, respectively) ($P \leq 0.001$).

Detailed post-operative complications are shown in Table 5. Hypokalaemia was the most common post-operative complication among TTE patients (57.4%) (versus 22.5% among THE patients; P = 0.001). Although statistically non-significant, we found more anastomotic leaks in the THE group (10/40 (27.5%)) than in the TTE group (11/47 (21.2%)) (P = 0.499). Re-operation was necessary in three patients who received TTE, and the stent was covered in the remainder of patients (7 patients), while 7 patients who received THE were treated conservatively with a T-tube and cervical wound care, and re-operation was performed in four patients. Vocal cord paralysis was noted in 3 patients in the THE group (7.5%) but not in any patient in the TTE group (P = 0.093).

In-hospital mortality was higher in the TTE group (9/47, 19.14%) than in the THE group (5/40, 12.5%) (P = 0.400). Leak was the cause of death (mediastinitis-related sepsis) in 5/9 patients in the TTE group and in 3/5

Table 2 Clinical stage distribution in two groups of patients studied

Tumour stage	Group A	Group B	Total	*P* value
T1N0M0	3 (6.4%)	1 (2.5%)	4 (4.6%)	0.621
T2N0M0	3 (6.4%)	2 (5.0%)	5 (5.7%)	1.000
T2N1M0	9 (19.1%)	12 (30.0%)	21 (24.1%)	0.238
T2N2M0	1 (2.1%)	0 (0%)	1 (1.1%)	1.000
T3N0M0	12 (25.5%)	8 (20.0%)	20 (22.9%)	0.541
T3N1M0	17 (36.2%)	17 (42.5%)	34 (39.1%)	0.546
T3N2M0	2 (4.3%)	0 (0%)	2 (2.3%)	0.497
Total	47 (100%)	40 (100%)	87 (100%)	-

P = 0.557, not significant, Chi-square test

Table 3 Clinical stage distribution in two groups of patients studied

Clinical stage	Group A	Group B	Total	*P* value
Stage I	3 (6.4%)	1 (2.5%)	4 (4.6%)	0.621
Stage II	10 (21.3%)	8 (20.0%)	18 (20.7%)	0.884
Stage IIB	10 (21.3%)	5 (12.5%)	15 (17.3%)	0.280
Stage III	23 (48.9%)	26 (65.0%)	49 (56.3%)	0.132
Stage IIIB	1 (2.1%)	0	1 (1.1%)	1.000
Total	47 (100%)	40 (100%)	87 (100%)	-

P = 0.489, not significant, Fisher exact test

patients in the THE group. Respiratory failure and inability to wean from a ventilator caused death in one patient in the TTE group (2.12%), while in the THE group, pulmonary complications (respiratory failure) were encountered in two patients (5%); one was a consequence of post-operative leaks (P = 0.592). Cardiac complications were noted in 4 (8.5%) patients in the TTE group, three of whom had acute myocardial infarction with sudden cardiac arrest and one who developed acute rapid atrial fibrillation (AF) and was treated medically with anti-arrhythmic medications. In the THE group, cardiac complications were noted in 2 patients (5%) (one with sudden cardiac arrest and another with rapid AF who was treated medically; P = 0.683).

Post-operative dysphagia was noted in both the TTE (7 (14.89%)) and THE (8 (20%)) groups (P = 0.530). The tumour recurrence rate was not different between the groups (TTE 3/47 vs. THE 6/40, P = 0.291).

The estimated survival duration from our series showed that the mean survival duration was longer in group A (TTE) (65.56 months) than in group B (THE) (45.01 months), with P = 0.146 (Fig. 1).

Discussion

The exact incidence of EC in our locality (Iraqi Kurdistan) is unknown due to the lack of a national cancer registry; therefore, there is a strong need to perform research on different types of cancer in our region. The most credible published data from our single-province cancer registry (Hiwa Hospital) over 8 years of observation (2006–2014) showed that the age-specific incidence of EC is approximately 18.77 for males and 13.18 for females/100,000 population/year for those aged older than 65 years [26]. This high rate of incidence is expected, as Iraqi Kurdistan is included within the Asian Esophageal Cancer Belt [26].

EC is a highly aggressive tumour; half of the patients present later with distant metastasis, and only 30–40% of patients are operable at the time of presentation [1, 12]. Surgery is the cornerstone of management for resectable EC [11, 12]. There is no high level of evidence to suggest the superiority of one surgical procedure over another; most of the observations have been from individual studies and small-sample randomized controlled trials. Each surgical approach has its own pros and cons: some advocate TTE for oncological perspective only, while others advocate THE, as it is associated with relatively less early morbidity and mortality. The decision regarding surgical technique is based mostly on the experience of the surgeon and hospital, comorbidities, level and stage of the oesophageal tumour [11, 27]. The choice of approach was surgeon preference guided mainly by nodal staging, MDT, tumour size and extend. The surgical approach for each patient was thoroughly discussed at the multidisciplinary meetings, and decision regarding surgical approach was made by the operating surgeon according to his experience and comfort ability with the operative approach and patients characteristics (tumour stage, level, mediastinal nodal status and comorbidities)

In our series, there was no statistically significant difference between the groups at baseline in terms of demographic or tumour characteristics; however, the rate of COAD was higher in group B (35%) than in group A (17%; P = 0.055+). This higher number of COAD patients in the THE group can be explained by the fact that TTE is associated with higher post-operative cardiorespiratory compromise; therefore, selecting these high-risk patients for THE might eliminate or decrease post-operative respiratory complications [28].

Hulscher et al. [19] conducted a randomized controlled trial that reached level I of evidence regarding the best surgical treatment for EC. THE was associated with a shorter operative duration (3.5 vs. 6 h), less blood loss (1 vs. 1.9 litters), a lower perioperative morbidity

Table 4 Operative details and post-operative course

	Group A (TTE) *n* (%), 47 (54.02%)	Group B (THE) *n* (%), 40 (45.97%)	*P* value
Duration of surgery (min)	172.77 ± 35,67	178.48 ± 36.14	0.462
Blood loss (ml)	619.15 ± 175.25	587.5 ± 234.45	0.474
Intraoperative complications	20 (42.6%)	10 (25%)	0.086
ICU stay (h)	28.51 ± 11.93	30.13 ± 15.86	0.590
Hospital stay (days)	12.93 ± 3.44	17.25 ± 5.92	< 0.001

Table 5 Post-operative complications

Complications	TTE *n* (%), 47 (54.02%)	THE *n* (%), 40 (45.97%)	*P* value
Hypokalaemia	27 (57.4%)	9 (22.5%)	0.001
Wound infection	20 (42.5%)	18 (45%)	0.819
Anastomotic leak	10 (21.2%)	11 (27.5%)	0.499
Pulmonary complications	1 (2.12%)	2 (5%)	0.592
Cardiac complications	4 (8.5%)	2 (5%)	0.683
Vocal cord paralysis	0 (0%)	3 (7.5%)	0.093
In-hospital mortality	9 (19.14%)	5 (12.5%)	0.400
Post-operative dysphagia	7 (14.89%)	8 (20%)	0.530
Tumour recurrence	3 (6.38%)	6 (15%)	0.291

rate (pulmonary complications 27% vs. 57%, chylous leakage 2% vs. 10%) and shorter hospital stay (mean 15 days vs. 19 days, $P \leq 0.001$) than TTE. Within our series, we did not identify a statistically significant difference in operative time (172.77 ± 35.67 vs. 178.48 ± 36.14, respectively; $P = 0.462$), blood loss (619.15 ± 175.25 vs 587.5 ± 234.45, respectively; $P = 0.474$), perioperative morbidity such as pulmonary complications (2.12% vs. 5%, respectively; $P = 0.592$) or cardiac complications (8.5% vs. 5%, respectively; $P = 0.683\%$), between the TTE and THE groups. Chylous leakage was not observed in either group. We observed higher respiratory complications in the THE group, although the difference was not statistically significant, but we found that COAD (in the THE group) was associated with other systemic diseases, especially cardiovascular diseases such as ischaemic heart disease and hypertension.

Early post-operative complications, such as hypokalaemia, were observed more often in the TTE group than in the THE group (57.4 vs. 22.5%, respectively; $P = 0.001$). These later post-operative complications were not reported by many authors; in our case, the possible explanation could be insufficient replacement or loss from the jejunostomy feeding tube we used for group A patients [29]. Concerning in-hospital mortality, although the difference was not statistically significant, the

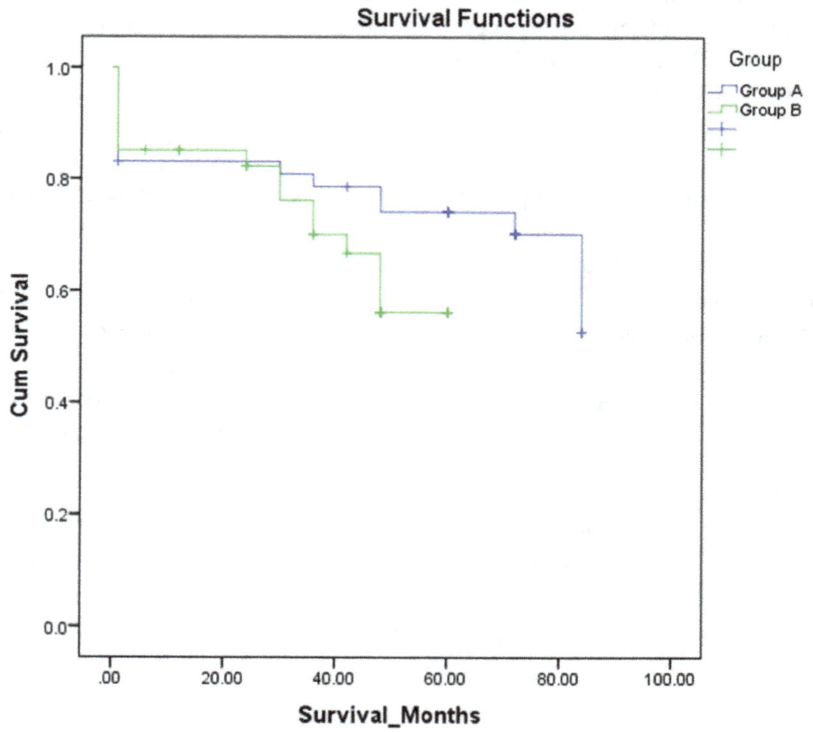

Fig. 1 Kaplan-Meier survival curve shows 5-year survival in both the TTE (group A) and THE (group B) groups

mortality rate was higher in the TTE group (19.14%) than in the THE group (12.5%) (*P* = 0400). Of those patients, 5/9 had anastomotic leak-related sepsis, three died from sudden cardiac arrest (acute myocardial infarction) and one died from respiratory failure. The higher complication rate in the TTE group has been well explained in the literature: a leak in the chest is associated with more severe clinical outcomes, such as mediastinitis and sepsis [28].

Patients who received TTE had a shorter hospital stay than patients who received THE (12.93 ± 3.44 vs. 17.25 ± 5.92, respectively; $P \leq 0.001$). We correlated the longer hospital stay of the THE group in our series with anastomotic leaks, although the leak rate was comparable in our series. In contrast, post-operative leaks after TTE was associated with a more severe clinical course and longer hospital stay. However, in our series, leaks after TTE were managed with a covered stent (7/10), while early post-operative leaks were treated with re-operation. Leaks after THE were treated conservatively (7/11) with the controlled fistula technique, opening of the cervical wound and packing and daily dressing rather than with a stent because of the unavailability of a conventional stent at the cervical location [30].

Gooszen et al. [31] compared the surgical approach and predictors of post-operative anastomotic leaks. The anastomotic leak rate was 19.6%. They found a lower rate of anastomotic leaks with TTE (17.0%) than with THE (21.9) (*P* = 0.025) and that independent predictors of anastomotic leaks were ASA fitness grades III and IV, DM, COAD, history of cardiac arrhythmia and proximal location of the tumour. In our series, the leak rate was 24.1%. Although statistically non-significant, patients who received TTE had a lower rate of leaks than those who received THE (21.3% vs. 27.5%, respectively; *P* = 0.499). We could not find such a relation between these variables and the leak rate in our series.

The higher rate of leaks with THE can been explained, as the reconstruction of a long gastric conduit and narrow thoracic inlet can compromise the vascularity of the conduit, with subsequent ischaemia and venous congestion, necrosis and disruption of the anastomosis [32, 33]. Despite a lower leak rate and shorter hospital stay with TTE, some surgeons (including us) believe that THE with cervical anastomosis will allow a wider resection margin of the oesophagus and less severe post-operative complications [31, 34].

The left recurrent laryngeal nerve (LRLN) paresis rate in our series was 7.5% (TTE 0% vs. THE 7.5%, *P* = 0.095). This higher rate of RLN paresis after THE indicates that RLN is mainly at risk during cervical dissection and reconstruction of the anastomosis. The rate found in our study is comparable to that reported by Gooszen et al. (7.0%) [32] but lower than that reported by Rindani et al. (11.2%) [33], Hulscher et al. (13%) [19] and Liu et al. (10.3%) [35]. All observed that THE was associated with a higher incidence of LRLN paresis.

Post-operative anastomotic stricture with subsequent dysphagia was observed in 14.89% of patients in the TTE group and 20% of patients in the THE group (*P* = 0.530). Three of seven patients (42.8%) in the TTE group and 5/8 (62.5%) in the THE group required one or more sessions of endoscopic dilatation. None of our patients required surgical intervention. This higher rate of anastomotic stricture associated with THE has also been reported by other studies. Boshier et al. [11] conducted a meta-analysis and found a stricture rate of 25.1% among patients in the THE group versus 21.8% among patients in the TTE group. Rindani et al. [35] found a stricture rate of 28% among patients in the THE group vs. 16% among patients in the TTE group and Liu et al. found a stricture rate of 19.8% among patients in the THE group vs. 13.5% among patients in the TTE group [35]. Gastric conduit ischaemia with subsequent post-operative anastomotic leaks, stapled anastomosis, cardiovascular diseases and COAD were identified as risk factors [24, 31, 33, 36, 37].

The patterns of tumour recurrence were as follows: 3 patients (6.38%) in the TTE group experienced recurrence (2 local and 1 distant) and 6 patients (15%) in the THE group experienced recurrence (5 local and 1 distant) (*P* = 0.291). Although statistically non-significant in our series, this higher rate of recurrence has been reported in the literature and is the point of controversy among authors. Some believe that TTE allows better access to the posterior mediastinum, with extended en bloc dissection of all peritumoural tissue and lymphadenectomy, hence reducing the rate of loco-regional recurrence [19], while others consider mediastinal lymph node involvement as systemic micro-metastatic disease and, thus, extended resection will not change the outcome [38, 39].

Colvin et al. conducted a meta-analysis from 1950 to 2010 (five randomized controlled trials and one meta-analysis) and concluded that TTE may offer a superior 5-year survival rate in patients with limited positive lymph nodes. However, other authors reported no significant difference (Boshier et al.: TTE 26.6% versus THE 25.8, *P* = 0.84 [11]; Kawoosa et al.: TTE 32.76% versus THE 30.24%, *P* = 0.596 [39]; and Rindani et al.: TTE 26% versus THE 24% [33]). The Kaplan-Meier survival curve (Fig. 1) shows 5-year survival in both the TTE and THE groups. The mean survival duration was higher in group A (TTE) (65.56 months) than in group B (THE) (45.01 months), with *P* = 0.146 (log-rank test).

Overall, there is no high level of evidence to date to demonstrate the superiority of one surgical approach over another, and there are several concerns and advantages with each surgical approach (TTE and THE) that remain controversial. The decision to perform oesophagectomy with either technique depends on the preference and experience of the operating surgeon and baseline physiological characteristics such as comorbidities and level and stage of the tumour [40, 41].

Our study was conducted on a relatively small sample and was non-randomized. The duration of follow-up was relatively acceptable for most patients. A larger study with randomization is required for a stronger level of evidence.

Conclusions

Oesophageal carcinoma is a rapidly increasing cancer worldwide, with a distinct geographical distribution. Surgery remains the cornerstone for curative treatment in the early stages of oesophageal carcinoma, although long-term survival is poor. Considerable debate exists over the best surgical approach based on perioperative morbidity and mortality and long-term survival. Transhiatal oesophagectomy is associated with a longer hospital stay, a higher rate of respiratory complications, post-operative anastomotic leaks, recurrent laryngeal nerve injury, post-operative strictures, subsequent dysphagia and recurrence. Long-term survival is higher with TTE.

Abbreviations

EC: Oesophageal carcinoma; TTE: Trans-thoracic oesophagectomy; THE: Trans-hiatal oesophagectomy; MIE: Minimally invasive oesophagectomy; STROCSS: Strengthening the Reporting of Cohort Studies in Surgery; US: Ultrasound; CT: Computed tomography; PFT: Pulmonary function test; EGD: Oesophagogastroduodenoscopy; EUS: Endoscopic ultrasound; TNM: Tumour, node and metastasis; SPSS: Statistical Package for the Social Sciences; COAD: Chronic obstructive airway disease; LN: Lymph node; AF: Atrial fibrillation; LRLN: Left recurrent laryngeal nerve paresis

Acknowledgements

We would like to acknowledge all our personnel who assisted in serving our patients.

Authors' contributions

All authors have read and approved the manuscript. AB: Surgeon in charge, study design, follow-up, data collection, manuscript revision and statistical analysis. HS: Assisted in surgeries, follow-up, study design, data collection and drafting

Author details

[1]Department of Surgery, School of Medicine, Faculty of Medical Sciences, University of Sulaimani, François Mitterrand Street, Sulaymaniyah 46001, Iraq. [2]Department of Thoracic and Cardiovascular Surgery, Sulaimani Teaching Hospital, Al Sulaymaniyah, Kurdistan Region 46001, Iraq. [3]Kurdistan Board for Medical Specialization/Cardiothoracic and Vascular Surgery, Sulaimani DOH, Al Sulaymaniyah, Kurdistan Region, Iraq.

References

1. Zhang Y (2013) Epidemiology of esophageal cancer. World J Gastroenterol 19(34):5598–5606. https://doi.org/10.3748/wjg.v19.i34.5598
2. Napier KJ, Scheerer M, Misra S (2014) Esophageal cancer: a review of epidemiology, pathogenesis, staging workup and treatment modalities. World J Gastrointest Oncol 6(5):112–120. https://doi.org/10.4251/wjgo.v6.i5.112
3. Bray F, Ferlay J, Soerjomataram I, Siegel RL, Torre LA, Jemal A (2018) Global cancer statistics 2018: GLOBOCAN estimates of incidence and mortality worldwide for 36 cancers in 185 countries. CA Cancer J Clin 68(6):394–424. https://doi.org/10.3322/caac.21492
4. Siegel RL, Miller KD, Jemal A (2020) Cancer statistics, 2020. CA A Cancer J Clin 70:7–30. https://doi.org/10.3322/caac.21590
5. Torre LA, Bray F, Siegel RL, Ferlay J, Lortet-Tieulent J, Jemal A (2015) Global cancer statistics, 2012. CA Cancer J Clin 65(2):87–108. https://doi.org/10.3322/caac.21262
6. Pennathur A, Gibson MK, Jobe BA, Luketich JD (2013) Oesophageal carcinoma. Lancet 381(9864):400–412. https://doi.org/10.1016/S0140-6736(12)60643-6
7. Klingelhöfer D, Zhu Y, Braun M et al (2019) A world map of esophagus cancer research: a critical accounting. J Transl Med 17:150. https://doi.org/10.1186/s12967-019-1902-7
8. Arnold M, Soerjomataram I, Ferlay J, Forman D (2015) Global incidence of oesophageal cancer by histological subtype in 2012. Gut. 64(3):381–387. https://doi.org/10.1136/gutjnl-2014-308124
9. Enzinger PC, Mayer RJ (2003) Esophageal cancer. N Engl J Med 349(23):2241–2252. https://doi.org/10.1056/NEJMra035010
10. Gao H, Li L, Zhang C et al (2019) Systematic review with meta-analysis: association of *Helicobacter pylori* infection with esophageal cancer. Gastroenterol Res Pract 2019:1953497. https://doi.org/10.1155/2019/1953497
11. Boshier PR, Anderson O, Hanna GB et al (2011) Ann Surg 254(6):894–906. https://doi.org/10.1097/SLA.0b013e3182263781
12. Chang AC, Ji H, Birkmeyer NJ, Orringer MB, Birkmeyer JD (2008) Outcomes after transhiatal and transthoracic esophagectomy for cancer. Ann Thorac Surg 85(2):424–429. https://doi.org/10.1016/j.athoracsur.2007.10.007
13. Ewis I (1946) The surgical treatment of carcinoma of the oesophagus; with special reference to a new operation for growths of the middle third. Br J Surg 34:18–31. https://doi.org/10.1002/bjs.18003413304
14. Orringer MB, Sloan H. Esophagectomy without thoracotomy. J Thorac Cardiovasc Surg. 1978;76(5):643-654.
15. McKeown KC. Trends in oesophageal resection for carcinoma with special reference to total oesophagectomy. Ann R Coll Surg Engl. 1972;51(4):213-239. PMID 5083864
16. Cuschieri A, Shimi S, Banting S. Endoscopic oesophagectomy through a right thoracoscopic approach. Journal of the Royal College of Surgeons of Edinburgh. 1992 Feb;37(1):7-11. PMID 1573620
17. Colvin H, Dunning J, Khan OA (2011) Transthoracic versus transhiatal esophagectomy for distal esophageal cancer: which is superior? Interact Cardiovasc Thorac Surg 12(2):265–269. https://doi.org/10.1510/icvts.2010.252148
18. Yang K, Chen HN, Chen XZ et al (2012) Transthoracic resection versus non-transthoracic resection for gastroesophageal junction cancer: a meta-analysis. PLoS One 7(6):e37698. https://doi.org/10.1371/journal.pone.0037698
19. Hulscher JB, van Sandick JW, de Boer AG et al (2002) Extended transthoracic resection compared with limited transhiatal resection for adenocarcinoma of the esophagus. N Engl J Med 347(21):1662–1669. https://doi.org/10.1056/nejmoa022343
20. Hulscher JB, Tijssen JG, Obertop H, van Lanschot JJ (2001) Transthoracic versus transhiatal resection for carcinoma of the esophagus: a meta-analysis. Ann Thorac Surg 72(1):306–313. https://doi.org/10.1016/s0003-4975(00)02570-4
21. Patel S, Petrov R, Abbas A, Bakhos C. Robotic-assisted McKeown esophagectomy. J Vis Surg. 2019;5:43. doi https://doi.org/10.21037/jovs.2019.03.14
22. D'Amico TA. Mckeown esophagogastrectomy. J Thorac Dis. 2014;6 Suppl 3(Suppl 3):S322-S324. doi https://doi.org/10.3978/j.issn.2072-1439.2014.03.28
23. Smithers BM (2010) Minimally invasive esophagectomy: an overview. Expert Rev Gastroenterol Hepatol 4(1):91–99. https://doi.org/10.1586/egh.09.62
24. McK Manson J, Beasley WD (2014) A personal perspective on controversies in the surgical management of oesophageal cancer. Ann R Coll Surg Engl 96(8):575–578. https://doi.org/10.1308/003588414x13946184901605
25. Agha R, Abdall-Razak A, Crossley E, Dowlut N, Iosifidis C, Mathew G, for the STROCSS Group (2019) The STROCSS 2019 Guideline: Strengthening the Reporting of Cohort Studies in Surgery. Int J Surg. 72:156–65. https://doi.org/10.1016/j.ijsu.2019.11.002. Epub 2019 Nov 6.

26. Khoshnaw N, Mohammed HA, Abdullah DA (2015) Patterns of cancer in Kurdistan - results of eight years cancer registration in Sulaymaniyah Province-Kurdistan-Iraq. Asian Pac J Cancer Prev 16(18):8525–8531. https://doi.org/10.7314/apjcp.2015.16.18.8525
27. Decker G, Coosemans W, De Leyn P et al (2009) Minimally invasive esophagectomy for cancer. Eur J Cardiothorac Surg 35(1):13–21. https://doi.org/10.1016/j.ejcts.2008.09.024
28. Barreto JC, Posner MC (2010) Transhiatal versus transthoracic esophagectomy for esophageal cancer. World J Gastroenterol 16(30):3804–3810. https://doi.org/10.3748/wjg.v16.i30.3804
29. Mitchell H (2014 Jan) Rosner, Alan C Dalkin. Electrolyte disorders associated with cancer. Adv Chronic Kidney Dis 21(1):7–17. https://doi.org/10.1053/j.ackd.2013.05.005
30. Wu G, Yin M, Zhao YS et al (2017) Novel esophageal stent for treatment of cervical anastomotic leakage after esophagectomy. Surg Endosc 31(12): 5024–5031. https://doi.org/10.1007/s00464-017-5545-6
31. Gooszen JAH, Goense L, Gisbertz SS, Ruurda JP, van Hillegersberg R, van Berge Henegouwen MI (2018) Intrathoracic versus cervical anastomosis and predictors of anastomotic leakage after oesophagectomy for cancer. Br J Surg 105(5):552–560. https://doi.org/10.1002/bjs.10728
32. Jauch KW, Bacha EA, Denecke H, Anthuber M, Schildberg FW. Esophageal carcinoma: prognostic features and comparison between blunt transhiatal dissection and transthoracic resection. Eur J Surg Oncol. 1992;18(6):553-562. PMID 1478287
33. Urschel JD. Esophagogastrostomy anastomotic leaks complicating esophagectomy: a review. Am J Surg. 1995;169(6):634-640.doi https://doi.org/10.1016/s0002-9610(99)80238-4
34. Blewett CJ, Miller JD, Young JE, Bennett WF, Urschel JD. Anastomotic leaks after esophagectomy for esophageal cancer: a comparison of thoracic and cervical anastomoses. Ann Thorac Cardiovasc Surg. 2001;7(2):75-78.PMID 11371275
35. Rindani R, Martin CJ, Cox MR. Transhiatal versus Ivor-Lewis oesophagectomy: is there a difference?. Aust N Z J Surg. 1999;69(3):187-194. doi https://doi.org/10.1046/j.1440-1622.1999.01520.x
36. Law S, Fok M, Chu KM, Wong J (1997) Comparison of hand-sewn and stapled esophagogastric anastomosis after esophageal resection for cancer: a prospective randomized controlled trial. Ann Surg 226(2):169–173. https://doi.org/10.1097/00000658-199708000-00008
37. van Heijl M, Gooszen JA, Fockens P, Busch OR, van Lanschot JJ, van Berge Henegouwen MI (2010) Risk factors for development of benign cervical strictures after esophagectomy. Ann Surg 251(6):1064–1069. https://doi.org/10.1097/sla.0b013e3181deb4b7
38. Davies AR, Forshaw MJ, Khan AA et al (2008) Transhiatal esophagectomy in a high volume institution. World J Surg Oncol 6:88. https://doi.org/10.1186/1477-7819-6-88
39. Kawoosa NU, Dar AM, Sharma ML et al (2011) Transthoracic versus transhiatal esophagectomy for esophageal carcinoma: experience from a single tertiary care institution. World J Surg 35(6):1296–1302. https://doi.org/10.1007/s00268-011-1020-z
40. Eslick GD (2009) Epidemiology of esophageal cancer. Gastroenterol Clin N Am 38(1):17–vii. https://doi.org/10.1016/j.gtc.2009.01.008
41. Liu YJ, Fan J, He HH, Zhu SS, Chen QL, Cao RH (2018) Anastomotic leakage after intrathoracic versus cervical oesophagogastric anastomosis for oesophageal carcinoma in Chinese population: a retrospective cohort study. BMJ Open. 8(9):e021025.doi https://doi.org/10.1136/bmjopen-2017-021025

10

Ministernotomy approach for modified Blalock-Taussig shunts in neonates

Ashraf A. H. El Midany[*] and Ayman A. Doghish

Abstract

Background: The original approach to performing a modified Blalock-Taussig (MBT) shunt is via a left thoracotomy. However, the median sternotomy has become the preferred approach of many surgeons. We think that the upper ministernotomy approach provides several advantages and avoids the disadvantages of both the sternotomy and thoracotomy approaches. Here, we describe our experience in constructing neonatal MBT shunts via upper ministernotomy.

Methods: A prospective study was conducted on 50 neonates who underwent modified Blalock-Taussig shunt performed through upper ministernotomy between March 2011 and December 2016. Preoperative characteristics, mortality, and morbidity were recorded.

Results: Mean age was 16.9 ± 10.4 days, and weight was 3.5 ± 0.5 kg. All patients received grafts of size 3.5 mm. The mean oxygen saturation increased from 59.5 ± 7.3% preoperatively to 84.8 ± 4.2% postoperatively. There were three cases of mortality (6%). One patient suffered from an unstable sternum (2%). No patients required conversion to full sternotomy. Superficial wound infection occurred in three cases (6%), and there were no cases of mediastinitis. Mean duration of ventilation was 55.64 ± 37.5 h, mean ICU stay was 5.44 ± 3.9 days, and mean hospital stay was 14.7 ± 7.2 days.

Conclusion: Upper ministernotomy is a safe approach with good early results. It provides adequate exposure with limited surgical trauma. Emergency conversion to full sternotomy and initiation of cardiopulmonary bypass can be achieved easily. It avoids lung compression and respiratory compromise. Additional costs for specific instruments are not necessary.

Keywords: Modified Blalock-Taussig shunt, Neonatal Blalock shunt, Surgical approach, Ministernotomy, Congenital cyanotic heart disease

Background

In the current era, biventricular corrective surgery is the preferred approach for neonates or young infants, whenever possible. However, palliative systemic-pulmonary arterial shunt is still needed in cases of single ventricle physiology, reduced pulmonary blood flow with vital instability, and in resource-limited regions where funding for open heart procedures, especially in such high-risk patient groups, is not available.

The modified Blalock-Taussig (MBT) shunt was introduced as one of many options for connecting the systemic and pulmonary circulations and involves a polytetrafluorethylene (PTFE) tube graft being inserted between the subclavian and pulmonary arteries. It has become a widely accepted palliative procedure due to the low morbidity and mortality rates associated with the procedure [1–3].

The original approach for the MBT shunt, as described by de Leval and co-workers, was via a left thoracotomy [4]. However, in recent times, the median sternotomy has evolved to become the preferred approach of many surgeons. Some of the reasons for this include the following:

* Correspondence: ashelmidany@gmail.com
Department of Cardiovascular & Thoracic Surgery, Faculty of Medicine, Ain Shams University Hospital, Cairo 11588, Egypt

it is a less demanding operation, it provides greater control of the blood vessels without the risk of respiratory compromise due to lung compression, and it enables construction of the anastomosis at the side of the superior vena cava for possible correction of pulmonary artery distortion during later conversion to the bidirectional Glenn [5]. However, subsequent procedures require repeat sternotomy, which is more time consuming and carries greater risk due to sternal adhesions.

The upper ministernotomy approach to MBT shunt construction has not been described in the literature. We believe that it can provide adequate exposure and easy construction of an anastomosis and carries less risk for subsequent sternal re-entry. In this report, we study the feasibility of MBT shunt construction in neonates via upper ministernotomy. Our endpoints include mortality and morbidity in terms of sternal stability, pulmonary mechanics reflected by the presence of lung collapse and duration of mechanical ventilation, and superficial and deep wound infections.

Methods

Preoperative characteristics

After receiving approval from the local ethics committee in Faculty of Medicine at Ain Shams University, a prospective study was conducted on 50 successive neonate patients between March 2011 and December 2016. All neonates who presented with desaturation due to decreased pulmonary blood flow and scheduled for an MBT shunt were included in the study. Patients who required cardiopulmonary bypass for other concomitant procedures, such as pulmonary artery reconstruction, unifocalisation of collaterals, and Norwood, were excluded from the study. However, off-pump pulmonary artery reconstruction was not an exclusion criterion.

Preoperative diagnoses are summarised in Table 1.

Table 1 Preoperative patient characteristics

Variable	Number (percentage) (Total number = 50)
Demographics	
Male	21 (42%)
Female	29 (58%)
Preoperative diagnosis	
PA-IVS	18 (36%)
PA-VSD	15 (30%)
TGA, VSD, PS	5 (10%)
Tricuspid atresia	9 (18%)
TOF/DORV	3 (6%)

PA pulmonary atresia, *IVS* intact interventricular septum, *VSD* ventricular septal defect, *TGA* transposition of great arteries, *PS* pulmonary stenosis, *TOF* tetralogy of Fallot, *DORV* double outlet right ventricle

All patients underwent regular preoperative medical examination and laboratory investigations. Informed written consent was obtained from each patient's guardian(s).

Diagnosis was achieved via echocardiographic and multislice computed tomography (MSCT) examinations to establish the intracardiac anatomy, the systemic and pulmonary vessel distribution and dimensions, and the presence, site, and size of patent-ductus arteriosus (PDA).

Operative procedure

All patients received intramuscular ketamine (3 mg/kg) for sedation and stress-free separation from their parents. In the operating room, patients were monitored using five-lead ECG, pulse oximetry (SpO_2), capnography for end-tidal carbon dioxide (Drager PM 8040-CATO, lübeck, Germany), planter surface temperature, and invasive blood pressure. Central venous catheters and arterial catheters were inserted after induction of general anaesthesia. Mechanical ventilation was provided by a Narkomed anaesthesia machine (North American Drager, Telford, PA) with fractional inspiratory oxygen concentration (fiO_2) maintained 0.9 and 1.0. The end-tidal carbon dioxide (CO_2) was maintained between 35 and 40 mmHg, using a tidal volume of 10 mL/kg and respiratory rate adjusted according to age. Positive end-expiratory pressure of 2–5 cmH_2o and inspiratory to expiratory ratio (I:E ratio) of 1:1.5–1:2 were used.

All MBT shunt procedures were performed via upper ministernotomy. A small skin incision was made from 0.5 cm below the suprasternal notch to 1 cm below the sternal angle. Then, the manubrium and the sternum were divided longitudinally in a J-shaped manner, using Mayo scissors up to the level of the third right intercostal space. After opening the sternum, the right lobe of the thymus was excised; the innominate artery was dissected up to its branches, with dissection of the right subclavian artery. The pericardium was opened above the aorta and stay sutures were inserted. The right pulmonary artery, between the ascending aorta and the superior vena cava up to the upper lobar branch, was dissected.

The systemic site of the shunt insertion was either the innominate or right subclavian artery, and the site of the distal anastomosis was the right pulmonary artery as close to the middle line as possible.

The systemic artery was partially clamped with a Cooley clamp, and a longitudinal arteriotomy was performed at the undersurface of the artery. A transversely cut polytetrafluoroethylene (Gore-Tex) tube graft (W. L. Gore & Associates, Inc., USA) was sutured end-to-side to the arteriotomy. The clamp was then released in situ to ensure good shunt flow and a competent anastomosis. The systemic artery was clamped again, and the shunt was flushed by heparinised saline to flush any thrombi, then the shunt was trimmed to the appropriate length.

The right pulmonary artery was partially clamped with a Cooley clamp, and an end-to-side distal anastomosis was performed in the same way (Figs. 1, 2, and 3).

All neonates in this series received 3.5-mm grafts, and the ductus was not ligated.

Before closure, haemostasis was secured, and a retrosternal drain was inserted

Postoperative events

Postoperatively, all neonates were ventilated. After haemostasis was ascertained, heparin was administered as a continuous infusion at 10–20 units/kg/h and was later changed to an oral low dose of aspirin (5 mg/kg/day). All patients received a postoperative echocardiographic examination to check the patency of the shunt

Study endpoints

Study endpoints were in-hospital mortality, reoperation for immediate shunt-related complications (thrombosis or anastomotic stenosis), conversion to full sternotomy, duration of ventilation, intensive care unit (ICU) stay, hospital stay, postoperative peripheral oxygen saturation (SaO_2) at discharge, and postoperative complications in terms of respiratory failure, re-exploration for bleeding, unstable sternum, superficial wound infections, and mediastinitis.

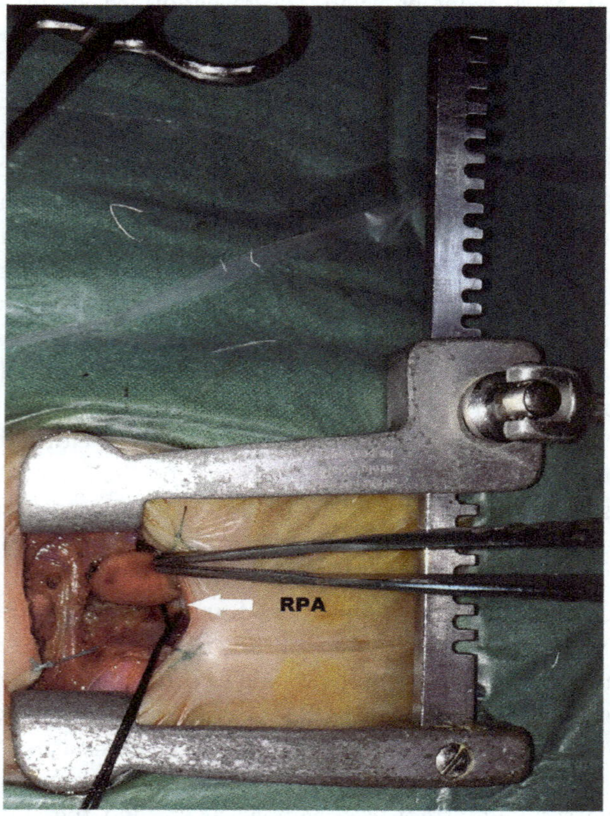

Fig. 1 Operative view showing the right pulmonary artery via the ministernotomy approach. RPA right pulmonary artery

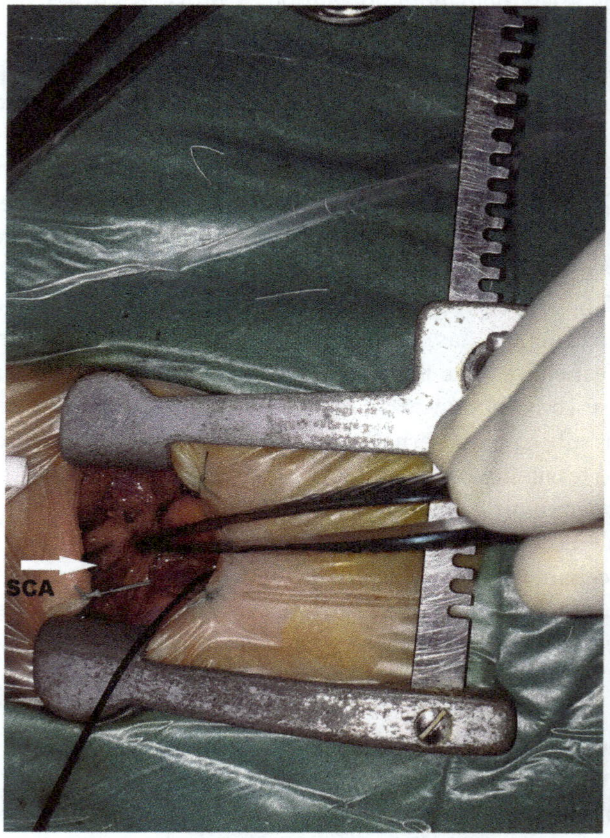

Fig. 2 Operative view showing the right subclavian artery via the ministernotomy approach. SCA subclavian artery

Statistical analysis

The collected data were revised, tabulated, and analysed using Statistical package for Social Science (SPSS) version 25 (SPSS, Inc., Chicago, IL, USA). Statistical data were expressed as mean ± standard deviation (SD) for continuous variable or as value and percentage for categorical data.

Results

All 50 patients were enrolled in the study. No patient required conversion to full sternotomy or emergency cardiopulmonary bypass. The mean age of the patients was 16.9 ± 10.4 days, and the mean weight was 3.5 ± 0.5 kg.

Mortality

There were three in-hospital deaths (6%). The causes of death were low cardiac output, sepsis, and acute respiratory distress syndrome (ARDS).

Outcomes

The mean preoperative SaO_2 was 59.5 ± 7.3 %, and the postoperative saturation was 84.8 ± 4.2%. The mean duration of ventilation was 55.64 ± 37.5 h, mean ICU stay was 5.44 ± 3.9 days, and the mean hospital stay was 14.7 ± 7.2 days.

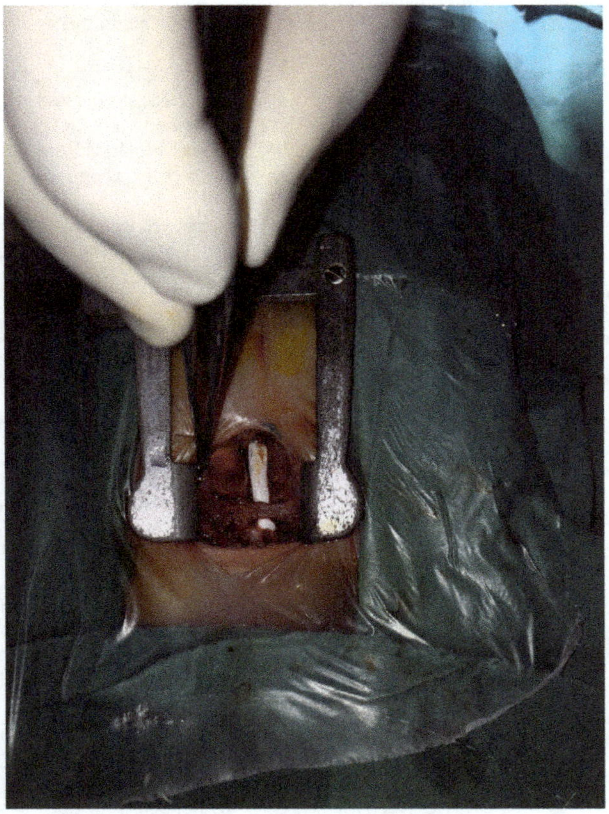

Fig. 3 Operative view of the MBT shunt constructed via upper ministernotomy in a neonate patient

Morbidity

Shunt thrombosis occurred in two (4%) patients who needed shunt revision and the graft was replaced with one of the same size. Shunt overflow was reported in five cases (10%), and there were no cases of shunt failure due to small shunt size. One case had an unstable sternum after re-exploration for shunt revision. The stainless wires were broken, and re-exploration was required for sternal fixation. No cases required re-exploration for bleeding. Superficial wound infection occurred in three patients (6%), which were all treated properly by repeated dressing changes and antibiotics. There were no cases of mediastinitis (Table 2).

Discussion

Minimal-access approaches have become more popular and widely used in paediatric cardiac surgery in recent times. They reduce surgical trauma, morbidity, and length of hospital stay. They have been reported to be associated with less blood transfusion and less postoperative pain [6–8]. There are several incision options for different minimally invasive approaches, based on the operation needed, including the parasternal incision, lateral thoracotomy, and upper or lower partial ministernotomy. The main concepts for all approaches are to provide adequate surgical exposure and the certain safety of the procedure [9]. MBT shunt was classically performed via the thoracotomy approach. Although it is a minimal access incision that gives good surgical exposure and adhesion-free mediastinum on subsequent sternotomy, it does not provide complete safety of the procedure in terms of overlooking some cardiac anomalies that may be missed in the preoperative diagnosis. In addition, it lacks the cosmetic advantage by making a second scar on the chest. It also has potential disadvantages, such as chylothorax, pulmonary artery distortion, and preferential pulmonary blood flow [1]. Many authors have reported the advantages of the sternotomy approach for MBT shunt; it provides good exposure of the vessels, easy control of patent ductus arteriosus, initiation of cardiopulmonary bypass if necessary, and easy takedown of the shunt and reconstruction of the pulmonary artery during later procedures. Moreover, it avoids lung compression, respiratory compromise, late scoliosis, and a second chest scar [1, 3, 10, 11].

Table 2 Mortality and morbidity

Outcome	Number (percentage %) (Total number = 50)
Mortality	3 (6%)
Morbidity	
Shunt overflow	5 (10%)
In-hospital shunt thrombosis	2 (4%)
Unstable sternum	1 (2%)
Superficial wound infection	3 (6%)

We aimed to provide the advantages but avoid the disadvantages of both sternotomy and thoracotomy approaches, via a minimal access upper ministernotomy approach. We found adequate exposure for construction of the MBT shunt, and we did not need any special instruments or devices. Thorough exploration of other cardiac defects, pulmonary artery branch size and distribution, and patent ductus arteriosus was easily carried out. Conversion to full sternotomy and initiation of cardiopulmonary bypass is also possible; however, it was not needed in our study.

Many authors have reported advantages of ministernotomy compared to median sternotomy, including less surgical trauma, less blood transfusion, less postoperative pain, better recovery, and shorter hospital stay [6, 7, 9, 12]. Nevertheless, others disagree and have reported contrary results, for example, Aris et al. [13] reported that ministernotomy did not reduce the length of hospital stay, postoperative pain, or bleeding, and Laussen and colleagues [14] failed to demonstrate better patient recovery in minimally invasive incisions.

We did not objectively assess postoperative pain or pulmonary function because they are difficult to measure in this age group. However, diminished surgical trauma and nearly intact chest cage resulted in good patient recovery and respiratory mechanics. This can be noticed in the average results for mechanical ventilation, ICU stay, and length of hospital stay.

All MBT shunt patients will require a second procedure for biventricular repair or Fontan operation. Therefore, the ministernotomy approach in such patients has a peculiar advantage as it exposes only a limited portion of the great vessels, thereby saving the cardiac chambers, especially the right ventricle. Therefore, it results in fewer sternal adhesions, minimising the risks of cardiac injury and blood loss on sternal re-entry. Moreover, subsequent operation(s) with a single scar on the chest provide a cosmetic advantage. The smaller surgical incision results in limited soft tissue dissection with reduced risk of postoperative soft tissue infections and mediastinitis [15], and this explains our results that show a low incidence of superficial soft tissue infection and no cases of mediastinitis.

Study limitations and future prospective

This was a prospective feasibility study to show that the procedure is possible with no major complications. The number of patients in the study was limited, and the study focused on only the short-term outcomes. Further studies are needed to compare this approach with others and to report the long-term follow-up and the potential advantages of the ministernotomy approach in the second stage operations.

Conclusion

Upper ministernotomy is a safe alternative approach for MBT shunt in neonates. It provides the advantages of adequate exposure with less surgical trauma. It avoids lung compression and respiratory compromise, and there is no technical compromise in the construction of the anastomosis. In addition, extra costs for specific instruments are not necessary. Further comparative studies with long-term follow-ups are essential.

Acknowledgements
Not applicable

Authors' contributions
AAH created the idea of the operations and performed most of them, collected the data, participated in the design of the study, and drafted the manuscript. AD performed some of the operations, participated in the collection of data, participated in the sequence alignment, performed the statistical analysis, and helped to draft the manuscript. Both authors read and approved the final manuscript.

References

1. Shauq A, Agarwal V, Karunaratne A, Gladman G, Pozzi M, Kaarne M et al (2010) Surgical approaches to the Blalock shunt: does the approach matter? Heart Lung Circ 19:460–464
2. Ahmad U, Fatimi SH, Naqvi I, Atiq M, Moizuddin SS, Sheikh KB et al (2008) Modified Blalock-Taussig shunt: immediate and short-term follow-up results in neonates. Heart Lung Circ. 17:54–58
3. Odim J, Portzky M, Zurakowski D, Wernovsky G, Burke RP, Mayer JE Jr et al (1995) Sternotomy approach for the modified Blalock-Taussig shunt. Circulation. 92(9 Suppl):II256–II261
4. de Leval MR, McKay R, Jones M, Stark J, Macartney FJ (1981) Modified Blalock-Taussig shunt. Use of subclavian artery orifice as flow regulator in prosthetic systemic-pulmonary artery shunts. J Thorac Cardiovasc Surg. 81:112–119
5. Alkhulaifi AM, Lacour-Gayet F, Serraf A, Belli E, Planche C (2000) Systemic pulmonary shunts in neonates: early clinical outcome and choice of surgical approach. Ann Thorac Surg. 69:1499–1504
6. Mihaljevic T, Cohn LH, Unic D, Aranki SF, Couper GS, Byrne JG (2004) One thousand minimally invasive valve operations: early and late results. Ann Surg 240:529e34
7. Grossi EA, Galloway AC, LaPietra A, Ribakove GH, Ursomanno P, Delianides J et al (2002) Minimally invasive mitral valve surgery: a 6-year experience with 714 patients. Ann Thorac Surg 74:660e4
8. Svensson LG, Atik FA, Cosgrove DM, Blackstone EH, Rajeswaran J, Krishnaswamy G et al (2010) Minimally invasive versus conventional mitral valve surgery: a propensity-matched comparison. J Thorac Cardiovasc Surg 139:926e32
9. Hsiao CY, Ou-Yang CP, Huang CH (2012) Less invasive cardiac surgery via partial sternotomy. J Chin Med Assoc. 75(12):630–634
10. Dirks V, Prêtre R, Knirsch W, Valsangiacomo Buechel ER, Seifert B, Schweiger M, Hübler M, Dave H (2013) Modified Blalock Taussig shunt: a not-so-simple palliative procedure. Eur J Cardiothorac Surg. 44(6):1096–1102
11. Amato JJ, Marbey ML, Bush C, Galdieri RJ, Cotrone JV, Bushong J (1988) Systemic-pulmonary polytetrafluoroethylene shunts in palliative operations for congenital heart disease. J Thorac Cardiovasc Surg 95:62–69
12. Bonacchi M, Prifti E, Giunti G, Frati G, Sani G (2002) Does ministernotomy improve postoperative outcome in aortic valve operation? A prospective randomized study. Ann Thorac Surg 73:460–465; discussion 465- 466
13. Aris A, Cámara ML, Montiel J, Delgado LJ, Galán J, Litvan H (1999) Ministernotomy versus median sternotomy for aortic valve replacement: a prospective, randomized study. Ann Thorac Surg 67:1583–1587; discussion 1587–1588
14. Laussen PC, Bichell DP, McGowan FX, Zurakowski D, DeMaso DR, del Nido PJ (2000) Postoperative recovery in children after minimum versus full length sternotomy. Ann Thorac Surg 69:591–596
15. Perrotta S, Lentini S (2009) Ministernotomy approach for surgery of the aortic root and ascending aorta. Interact Cardiovasc Thorac Surg. 9(5):849–858

11

Feasibility and outcome of mitral valve repair in patients with infective endocarditis

Valentina Scheggi[1*], Iacopo Olivotto[2], Stefano Del Pace[2], Nicola Zoppetti[3], Alterini Brunetto[1], Niccolò Marchionni[2], Alfredo Cerillo[4] and Pier Luigi Stefàno[4]

Abstract

Background: Valve repair is the treatment of choice for native mitral valve regurgitation. The feasibility of repair when the defect is caused by acute infective endocarditis (IE) is debated. This study aims to compare the outcome of repair and replacement procedures, to report the rate of repair in a single surgical center, and to review the literature on this topic.

Results: We retrospectively analyzed 108 patients with native mitral IE, potentially eligible for surgical repair. Of these 108, 90 (83%) underwent surgery, and 18 were treated conservatively. Among the 90 surgical patients, 57 (63%) underwent valve replacement and 33 valve repair (37%). The mean follow-up duration was 3 years. The two primary endpoints were mortality and freedom from recurrent endocarditis. Secondary endpoints were the post-operative incidence of major adverse events (hospitalization for any cause, pacemaker implantation, new onset of atrial fibrillation, sternal dehiscence), left ventricular systolic function (LVSF), and valvular function at 1-year echocardiographic follow-up. All-cause mortality was lower for valve repair, although not significantly ($p = 0.86$), as well as nonfatal adverse events ($p = 0.92$) and relapse rate ($p = 0.20$) at 3 years. We did not find differences between the two groups at echocardiographic follow-up, neither for left ventricular systolic function ($p = 0.22$), nor for valvular continence ($p = 0.28$).

Conclusions: In our experience, the mid-term outcome of repair in IE is comparable to valve replacement and should be considered whenever possible, as in degenerative valve disease. The review of the literature supports this strategy.

Keywords: Infective endocarditis, Valve repair, Valve replacement, Outcome

* Correspondence: scheggiv@aou-careggi.toscana.it; valentina.scheggi@gmail.com
All authors take responsibility for all aspects of the reliability and freedom from bias of the data presented and their discussed interpretation.
[1]Division of Cardiovascular and Perioperative Medicine, Cardiothoracovascular Department, Azienda Ospedaliero-Universitaria Careggi and University of Florence, Largo Brambilla 3, 50133 Florence, Italy
Full list of author information is available at the end of the article

Background

Treatment of infective endocarditis (IE) is surgical in patients with complications: heart failure, a paravalvular extension of the infection, sepsis unresponsive to antibiotics, systemic embolism despite appropriate antibiotic therapy, and occasionally for large vegetation. While the treatment of choice for degenerative mitral valve regurgitation is valve repair, this is often challenging in IE because of structural damage and concerns regarding durability. For eradication of infection, all grossly infected tissue must be removed, limiting the possibility of repair. In expert hands, however, it can be approached by different techniques.

In patients undergoing surgery for mitral, several studies and meta-analyses have suggested a more favorable survival following valve repair, compared to replacement [1–8]. These data derive from small, retrospective observational studies, and a selection process triaging milder patients for repair represents a likely bias. On the other hand, randomized trials appear scarcely feasible in this setting, owing to the rarity of IE and different clinical profiles of candidates for the two procedures. Thus, there is still a need for further single-center investigation in this field that is the base for future meta-analyses. We assessed the feasibility and outcomes of valve repair in a consecutive series of IE patients seen in a surgical center in Florence and provided 1-year echocardiographic follow-up.

Methods

Patient selection

During the last 3 years, we have collected all the cases admitted to our department between January 2013 and December 2019 with a definite diagnosis of IE, according to modified Duke University criteria [9]. In this way, we have generated a single-center registry of IE, consisting now of 363 patients and 294 variables. Among these 363 cases, we retrospectively selected 108 consecutive patients with a definite diagnosis of native mitral valve IE. Of these 108, 90 were treated surgically and constituted our study cohort: 57 underwent valve replacement (63%) and 33 valve repair (37%) (Fig. 1). Of these 90 patients, 20 also had a second infected valve (19 aortic and one tricuspid): aortic valves were replaced in all cases, while the tricuspid one was repaired (Fig. 2).

Data collection method, diagnostic work-up, and surgical indications are reported in another study conducted on the same registry, focusing on embolic risk stratification in patients with IE [10].

Operative technique

Surgical planning was re-evaluated intraoperatively, based on direct valve inspection. Underlying valve disease in patients treated with valve repair and replacement is reported in Table 1 and the surgical procedures for valve repair for each specific lesion are listed in Table 2. An example of mitral repair is reported in Fig. 3.

Follow-up and study endpoints

The follow-up duration was calculated from the time of IE diagnosis to the final contact. A structured phone interview was implemented to update the follow-up of all patients to December 2019. In a subset of 32 patients, 1-year

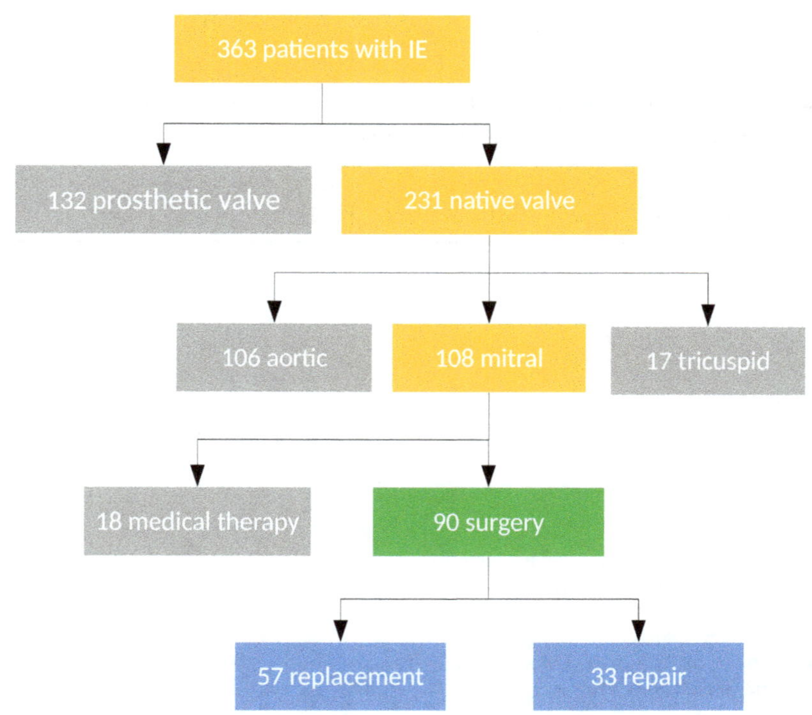

Fig. 1 Study flow chart

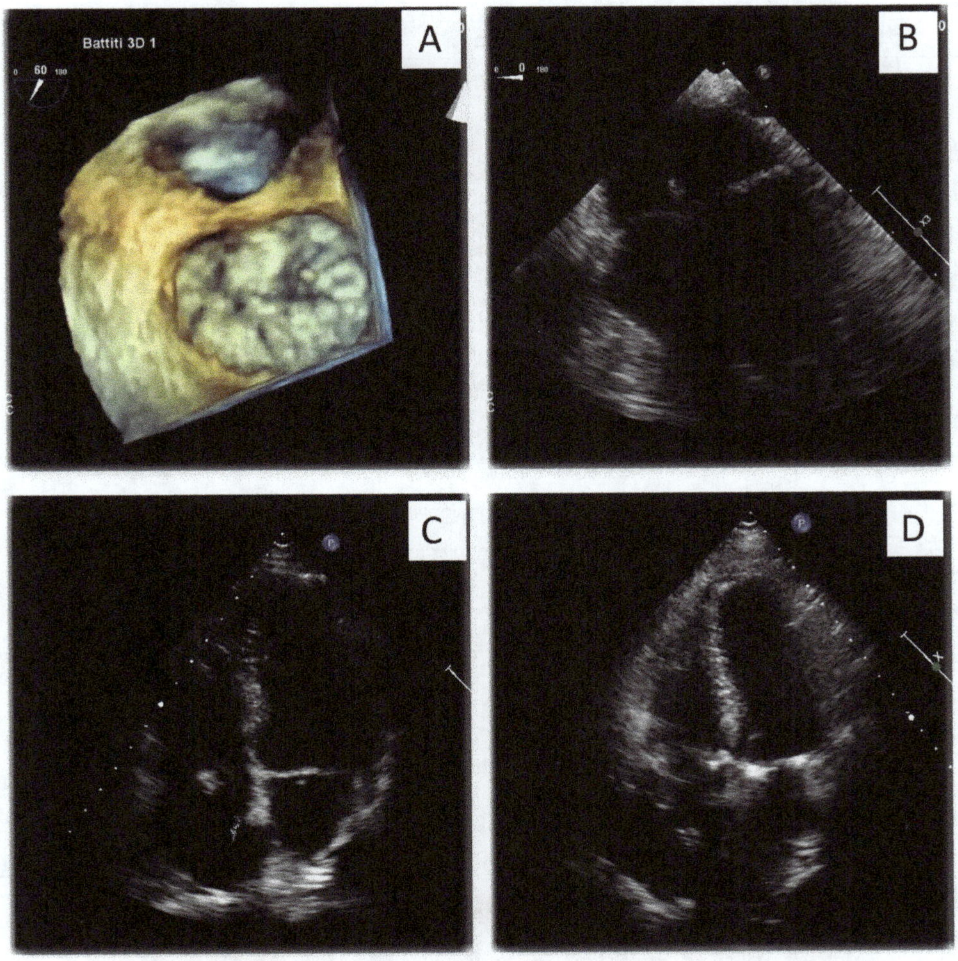

Fig. 2 Echocardiographic images of the patient with mitral and tricuspid IE. **a** 3D transesophageal view of mitral valve. **b** 2D transesophageal view of mitral valve. **c** Transthoracic four chamber view before surgery. **d** Transthoracic four chamber view after surgery. Vegetation is marked with arrows in each view

echocardiographic follow-up was performed (13 repairs, 19 replacements). The two primary endpoints were mortality and freedom from recurrent endocarditis, comparing repair and replacement procedures. Secondary endpoints were the post-operative incidence of major adverse events (hospitalization for any cause, pacemaker implantation, new onset of atrial fibrillation, sternal dehiscence), left ventricular systolic function (LVSF), and valvular function at 1-year echocardiographic follow-up of the two procedures. LVSF was measured through left ventricular ejection fraction (LVEF) at 1-year follow-up and normalized for pre-operative EF; the logarithm of the ratio of LVEF at follow-up and LVEF had a normal distribution. Valvular regurgitation was estimated by the PISA method (Proximal Isovelocity hemispheric Surface Area).

Table 1 Underlying valve disease in patients treated with valve repair and replacement

Pathology (mitral)	Valve repair, *n* = 33	Valve replacement, *n* = 57	*p*
Vegetation—anterior leaflet, *n* (%)	4 (12)	8 (14)	0.49
Vegetation—posterior leaflet, *n* (%)	10 (30)	19 (33)	0.22
Bileaflet vegetation, *n* (%)	7 (21)	21 (37)	0.12
Ruptured chordae/leaflet prolaps, *n* (%)	7 (21)	7 (12)	0.26
Leaflets' erosion/retraction, *n* (%)	3 (9)	2 (3)	0.26
Perforation, anterior leaflet, *n* (%)	4 (12)	6 (10)	0.81
Perforation, posterior leaflet, *n* (%)	2 (6)	10 (30)	0.12
Bileaflet perforation, *n* (%)	1 (3)	4 (7)	0.42
Annular abscess, *n* (%)	2 (6)	8 (24)	0.24

Table 2 Surgical procedures for valve repair

Mitral lesion (*n*)	Repair procedure	*N* (%)
Vegetation (21)	Quadrangular/triangular resection	8 (38)
	Vegetectomy	7 (33)
	Peeling	6 (28)
	Associated ring annuloplasty	19 (90)
Perforation (7)	Patch repair of perforations	4 (57)
	Direct suture repair of perforations (anterior leaflet)	3 (42)
	Associated ring annuloplasty	6 (86)
Abscess (2)	Patch repair of perforations	2 (100)
	Associated ring annuloplasty	1 (50)
Chordal rupture (7)	Quadrangular/triangular resection	6 (86)
	Neochordae implantation	1 (14)
	Associated ring annuloplasty	7 (100)
Erosion/retraction (3)	Quadrangular/triangular resection	2 (67)
	Neochordae implantation	1 (33)
	Associated ring annuloplasty	3 (100)

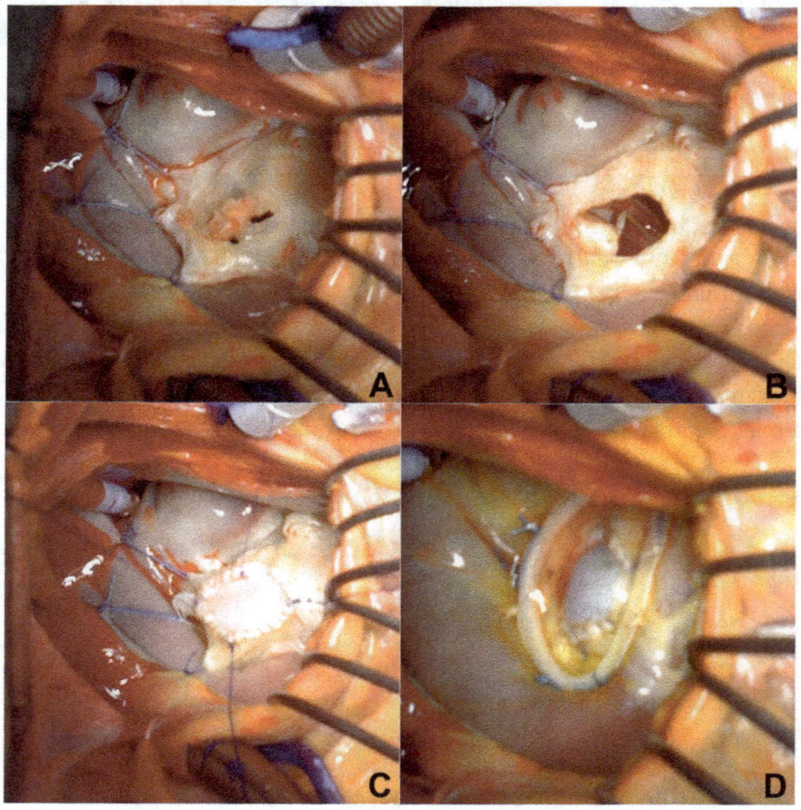

Fig. 3 Mitral endocarditis with perforation of the anterior leaflet. **a**, **b** After careful debridement and removal of the infected tissue, a large hole is left in the body of the anterior mitral leaflet. The perforation is repaired with an appropriate size fresh autologous pericardial patch (**c**). The final test with saline demonstrates a perfectly competent mitral valve (**d**)

Statistical analysis

We used the chi-square test to compare proportions, the Mann-Whitney test to compare continuous variables with non-normal distribution, and the two-tailed Student's t test for continuous variables with normal distribution. We performed univariable and multivariable analyses using logistic regression and general linear models. We used the Kaplan-Meier method to estimate the univariate cumulative incidence of events and event-free survival. All tests were 2-sided, and statistical significance was defined as a p value < 0.05. Analyses were performed with SPSS 23.0 package.

Results

The mean age at the time of surgery was 63.6 ± 13.5 years. Of 90 operated patients, seven had undergone previous surgical valve repair. The mean vegetation length was 11.6 ± 7.7 mm. Blood cultures were positive in 81% of cases (*Streptococci* 31%, *Staphylococcus aureus* 19%, negative coagulase staphylococci 11%, enterococci 13%, Gram-negative, fungi, and other Gram-positive 6%). IE was at its first occurrence in 83 patients (92%) and relapse in seven (8%). Embolic events were reported at the time of admission in 45 patients (50%), in 23 of whom involving the central nervous system. Early surgery (within 2 weeks of diagnosis) was performed in 70 patients (78%), with valve replacement in 57 (63%) and valve repair in 33 (37%). The repair was performed more frequently in patients with IE involving two valves (12/33 vs. 8/57, p = 0.014), in patients with a first episode of IE (33/33 vs 50/57, p = 0.036), and in patients affected by spondylodiscitis (7/33 vs 4/57, p = 0.048). Moreover, vegetation length was significantly smaller in patients undergoing repair (p = 0.001; best predictive threshold for replacement at ROC analysis 8.5 mm, AUC 0.78; Fig. 4). The presence of endocarditis involving two valves, the combination of endocarditis and spondylodiscitis, having a first episode of IE rather than a relapse, and the vegetation length were not associated with a higher mortality at Kaplan-Meyer survival analysis nor with a higher relapse rate.

The other baseline clinical characteristics were similar in the repair and replacement groups (Table 3).

At multivariable analysis, variables independently associated with repair procedure were vegetation length (OR 0.78, 95% CI 0.69–0.87, p = 0.000), male gender (OR 5.0, 95% CI 1.2–20.7, p = 0.025), and severe valvular dysfunction (OR 0.10, 95% CI 0.02–0.48, p = 0.004).

At echocardiographic follow-up, the logarithm of the ratio of LVEF at follow-up and basal was not statistically different between the two groups (p = 0.22). Severe valvular regurgitation was reported only in 1 patient that

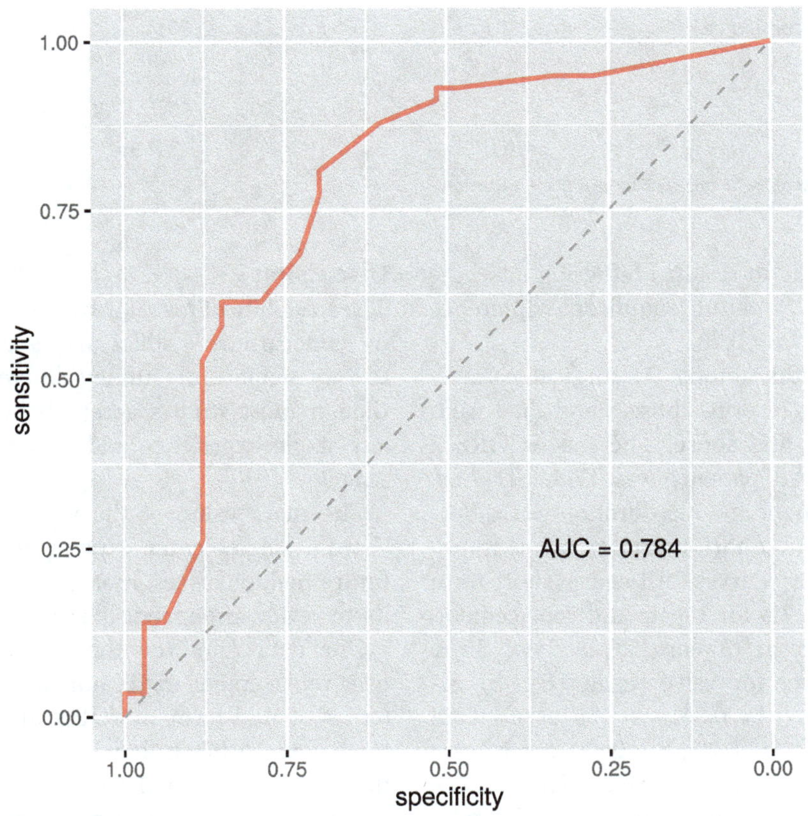

Fig. 4 ROC curve of vegetation dimension for replacement; AUC 0.78, p = 0.001

Table 3 Demographic, clinical, echocardiographic, and microbiological characteristics in 90 surgical patients affected by IE on native mitral valve treated with valve repair or replacement

Variable	Repair (*n* = 33)	Replacement (*n* = 57)	*p* value
Second valve infection	12 (36%)	8 (14%)	0.014
Vegetation length (mm), mean ± SD	6.99 ± 7.14	14.35 ± 6.78	0.001
Spondylodiscitis, *n* (%)	7 (21)	4 (7)	0.048
Gender (women), *n* (%)	6 (18)	20 (35)	0.088
First episode of IE, *n* (%)	33 (100)	50 (88)	0.036
Age (years), mean ± SD	63.7 ± 13.1	63.6 ± 13.9	0.96
BMI, mean ± SD	24.1 ± 4.4	25.5 ± 4.5	0.33
Diabetes, *n* (%)	4 (12)	16 (28)	0.079
Chronic kidney disease, *n* (%)	4 (12)	17 (30)	0.056
Arterial hypertension, *n* (%)	13 (39)	33 (58)	0.091
Previous malignancies, *n* (%)	5 (15)	10 (17)	0.76
Dyslipidemia, *n* (%)	7 (23)	18 (33)	0.29
Pacemaker, *n* (%)	1 (3)	5 (9)	0.58
Drug abuse, *n* (%)	3 (9)	5 (9)	0.29
Paravalvular extension, *n* (%)	3 (9)	7 (12)	0.63
Severe valvular dysfunction, *n* (%)	20 (61)	41 (59)	0.26
LVEF (%), mean ± SD	58.5 ± 9.0	60.0 ± 10.5	0.48
TAPSE (mm), mean ± SD	22.3 ± 5.0	23.1 ± 6.0	0.67
EuroScore-II	9.4 ± 28.8	9.8 ± 13.7	0.93
Early surgery, *n* (%)	28 (85)	42 (74)	0.22
***Streptococcus* spp./, *n* (%)**	13 (40)	15 (26)	0.19
***Staphylococcus aureus*, *n* (%)**	6 (18)	11 (19)	0.89
Negative coagulase staphylococci, *n* (%)	2 (6)	8 (14)	0.36
Enterococci, *n* (%)	5 (15)	6 (10)	0.51
Other, *n* (%)	1 (3)	4 (7)	0.60
Negative cultures, *n* (%)	6 (18)	13 (23)	0.57

LVEF left ventricular ejection fraction, *TAPSE* tricuspid annular plane excursion

had undergone repair, due to residual tethering in severe ventricular dysfunction, without significant difference between the two groups (p = 0.28).

We registered 19 deaths among 90 surgical patients (21%). Three of them were drug abusers and died from complications related to the abuse. The EuroSCORE 2 of the remaining 16 dead patients was 17.3 (SD 13.9, maximum 56.2). Since the follow-up duration was different among patients of our cohort, mortality was extrapolated from Kaplan-Meyer curves. All-cause short-term (30 days, 3 ± 3% vs 4 ± 2% for repair and replacement, respectively) and long-term (3 years, 26 ± 9 vs. 36 ± 11%) mortality was lower for valve repair (Fig. 5), although not significantly (p = 0.86), as well as nonfatal adverse events (15 ± 4 vs. 20 ± 2%, p = 0.92) and relapse rate (1 ± 1% vs. 3 ± 1%, p = 0.20) at 3 years. The absence of statistical significance probably depends on the relatively small size of the sample.

Discussion

The feasibility of mitral valve repair in patients with infective endocarditis is still a matter of debate, since it seems to vary significantly among different centers [11–22]. Although most studies agree about the benefits of repair, any single experience adds strength to recommend this strategy.

The main value of the present study is therefore to share a single-center experience that can be useful for future meta-analyses; moreover, we seized the opportunity to review the recent literature about this topic.

Our data reinforce the preference for mitral repair over replacement in IE, not only for the good results in terms of mid-term mortality and relapse rate, but also for 1-year echocardiographic results. More than one third of patients with native mitral valve IE could be managed (in most cases early after diagnosis) with valve repair, with mid-term outcomes (3 years) similar to

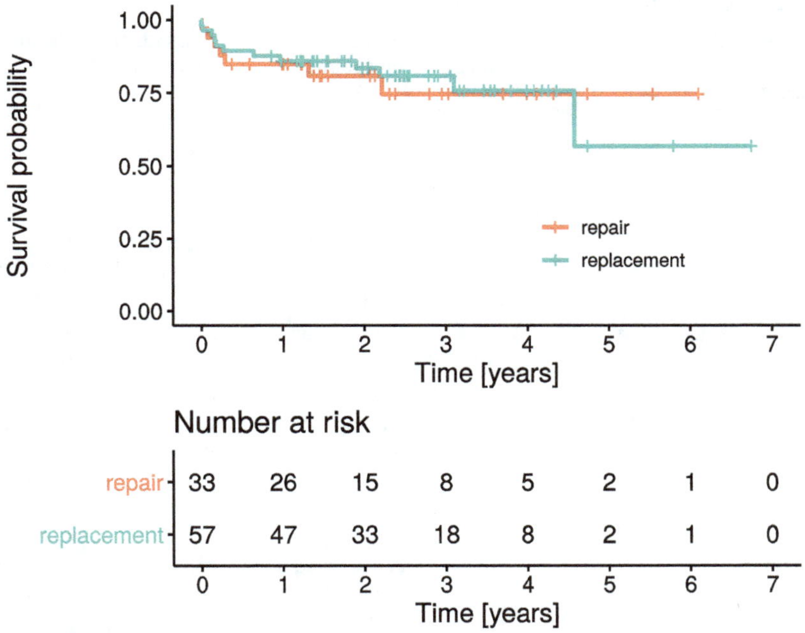

Fig. 5 Survival probability (± 95% CI) after repair and replacement procedure in IE

those obtained with replacement, but with potentially better long-term results. LVEF and valvular continence at follow-up are surrogate endpoints that reflect long-term durability and safety of valve repair.

In our experience, selection for repair was largely based on the qualitative assessment of valvular damage by experienced cardiologists and surgeons.

The repair was particularly favored in the presence of spondylodiscitis to lower the risk of relapse in a subset of patients with an active infective focus. The presence of spondylodiscitis, which may act as a persisting infective focus, should be considered one further reason to attempt at valve repair in IE whenever anatomically feasible, in order to possibly reduce the risk of early relapse.

Notably, most of the baseline features were similar in repair and replacement cohorts.

At multivariable analysis, the main independent predictors of the feasibility of repair were vegetation dimension that was significantly smaller in the repair group, and the entity of mitral regurgitation, where severe regurgitation was inversely associated with the procedure of repair, so we can conclude that the ultimate decision could not be foreseen a priori. While guidelines and algorithms are desirable for IE, these findings suggest that there is no real substitute for direct clinical experience in IE management.

During the last 20 years, many attempts have been undertaken to repair the mitral valve in IE, avoiding the insertion of prosthetic material in infected tissue; the review of the literature shows that an ever-increasing percentage of mitral IE has been judged amenable to valve repair worldwide in the last years, especially if surgery was performed in an early stage (Table 4).

Reconstructive surgery in inflammatory tissue may be hard, and the feasibility of repairing infected mitral valves for acute IE has been reported to vary considerably [11–18]. In a systematic review of 24 studies on this issue, Feringa et al. [3] observed that valve repair was possible in approximately 39% of patients presenting with mitral valve IE, but some recent experiences report a higher feasibility rate, even over 80% [19–21].

The repair rate in our study was similar to that reported in the review of Feringa et al., but clearly lower than the feasibility reported by Defauw et al. of 66% [21] or by de Kerchove et al. of 80% [22]; on the other hand, we registered a lower in-hospital mortality (4%) than the latter two, who reported 15.4% and 16%, respectively. We favored safety, at the price of a lower rate of complex repair procedures, with similar long-term survival rate.

Similar to the degenerative MR experience, valve repair recently became the procedure of choice in IE, as confirmed by several studies [18–22]. Patients who undergo mitral valve repair need significantly fewer reinterventions during the early post-operative period and long-term follow-up and have less long-term IE relapses and cerebrovascular events.

The hard task of the surgeon is to balance the risks connected with repair failure with the numerous advantages of a successful repair. This challenge probably gives the reason for the high variability of repair feasibility in the literature.

Table 4 Review of the literature concerning mitral valve repair in IE

First author, year	Study design	Number of patients	Repair	Replacement	Infected valve	Primary endpoints	Secondary endpoints	Results
Hendren W.G. et al., 1992 [1]	Retrospective single-center cohort study	22	22	0	Mitral	Clinical results of repair	In-hospital mortality	Mitral repair had a low mortality and no reinfections.
Podesser B.K. et al., 2000 [2]	Retrospective single-center cohort study	22	22	0	Mitral	Survival rate at 1–5 years	In-hospital mortality	Mitral valve repair in IE had a low incidence of complications and a good medium-term survival.
Feringa H.H. et al., 2007 [3]	Systematic review	1194	470	724	Mitral	Morbidity and mortality		Repair had lower early and late mortality, less reoperations, lower rate of adverse events.
Ishikawa S. et al., 2008	Retrospective single-center cohort study	40	4	31	Mitral and aortic valves	Intra-operative results	In-hospital mortality	Good operative results after infective sites resection.
Huang X.S. et al., 2009 [5]	Retrospective observational study	40	39	1	Mitral	Clinical and echocardiographic results of repair	In-hospital mortality	Good clinical results of mitral repair with favorable atrial and ventricular remodeling and valvular function.
Omoto T. et al., 2011 [6]	Retrospective single-center cohort study	22	15	7	Mitral	In-hospital mortality	Survival rate at 1–5 years	Mitral valve repair in IE is feasible and is associated with a larger reduction of end diastolic ventricular volume. Concerns about durability of large resection.
Evans C.F. et al., 2011 [7]	Systematic review						Event-free survival	Repair was associated with lower mortality (< 10%), better survival rate (> 80% at 5 years), lower relapse rate, and neurologic complications.
De Kerchove et al., 2012 [22]	Retrospective single-center cohort study	137	109	28	Mitral	Hospital mortality	Freedom from mitral valve repair failure	Hospital mortality was 16%. At 8 years, overall survival was 62% ± 10% with no differences between patients with or without patch repair (p = .5). Freedom from mitral valve repair failure was 81% ± 14% in patients with patch repair and 90% ± 10% in patients without patch repair (p = .09).
Chang H.W. et al., 2014 [8]	Retrospective single-center cohort study	26	11	6			In-hospital mortality	No patients had residual regurgitation post-operatively nor at follow-up. None in-hospital death.
Zhao D. et al., 2014 [11]	Systematic review				Mitral and aortic valves	Morbidity and mortality	Event-free survival	Repair had a better overall survival and event-free survival.
Mick S.L. et al., 2015 [12]	Systematic review				Mitral	Mortality		Valve repair had a lower in-hospital and long-term mortality and lower risk of neurological events and relapse.
Rostagno C. et al., 2017 [13]	Retrospective single-center cohort study	34	34	0	Mitral	Survival rate at 1–5 years	Event-free survival rate	Repair was associated with good long-term results.
Toyoda et al., 2017 [23]	Retrospective multicentric study	1979	367	1603	Mitral	Long-term survival	Recurrent endocarditis and mitral reoperation	Repair is associated with better survival and lower risk of recurrent infection.
Hu Y.N. et al., 2018 [14]	Systematic review	779	779	0	Mitral	Mortality		Short-term mortality after mitral repair in IE was 6%; freedom from reintervention was > 90% at 5 years and > 85% at 10 years. Long-term results support adequate durability of

Table 4 Review of the literature concerning mitral valve repair in IE *(Continued)*

First author, year	Study design	Number of patients	Repair	Replacement	Infected valve	Primary endpoints	Secondary endpoints	Results
								repair.
Liu J.Z. et al., 2018 [15]	Meta-analysis	633	265	368	Mitral	Operative mortality. Survival rate at 1–5 years	Post-operative results	Good post-operative results and survival.
Solari S. et al., 2018 [17]	Retrospective single-center cohort study	192	155	37	Mitral	Overall survival. Event-free survival		Repair had a good durability and low rate of IE relapse.
Harky A. et al., 2018 [18]	Meta-analysis	8978	2906	6072	Mitral	Morbidity and mortality		Repair had lower relapse rate, better event-free survival, and overall survival at 1–5 years.
Lee HA et al., 2018 [19]	Retrospective multicenter study	1999	424	1575	Mitral	Morbidity and mortality		Mitral repair for IE has better perioperative and late outcomes than mitral replacement.
Okada y et al., 2020 [20]	Retrospective single-center study	171	147	24	Mitral	Survival, freedom from reoperation, and event-free survival		Mitral valve repair was highly successful using autologous pericardium, chordal reconstruction, and ring annuloplasty if required. Long-term results were acceptable.
Defauw RJ et al., 2020 [21]	Retrospective single-center study	149	97	52	Mitral	Survival	Recurrence, reintervention	Beyond 1 year post-surgery, replacement was associated with decreased survival.

Okada et al. [20] reported even 86% rate of mitral valve repair, with an in-hospital mortality of 0.7%. However, 67% of patients undergoing valve repair had healed at the time of surgery, and only 33% had active infective endocarditis. For this reason, their valuable experience does not fully answer the query of the feasibility of valve repair in IE. Moreover, in order to prevent embolic events, early surgery is generally preferred over delayed surgery, which is recommended only for conditions that may increase operative mortality, such as large volume (> 2 cm) intracranial hemorrhage.

Solari et al. [17] recently showed that an early repair-oriented surgical approach can achieve high repair rates with a good long-term durability of the repair and a very low rate of recurrence of endocarditis.

In a recent multicentric study in New York and California states, Toyoda et al. [23] reported a mitral repair rate of 19% in 1970 patients with IE; this percentage is probably more representative of the real world. Consistently with the literature, their experience confirmed that repair was associated with better survival and lower risk of recurrent infection compared with valve replacement. Radical removal of all infected material and inflamed tissue is a key issue for successful operative technique, using the broad spectrum of surgical armamentarium to recreate a normal-functioning valve with the available vital tissue. Patching of perforations, vegetectomy, and resection of the involved leaflet and leaflet patching with an autologous or bovine pericardium, commissural debridement, and reconstruction, left ventricular abscess debridement with annular patch reconstruction and leaflet re-suspension with artificial chordae, sliding plasty, flip-over technique, and ring annuloplasty can all be employed to obtain a perfect functional result [22]. Finally, when a repair is not possible and replacement becomes mandatory, the choice between mechanical and bioprosthetic valves should be made based on usual clinical considerations.

The main limitations to be acknowledged for our study are its retrospective nature, based on a single-center experience, and consequently on a relatively small cohort. However, since our hospital is the referral center, our population covers the entire spectrum of IE in the region and is, therefore, representative of real-world experience. As discussed, criteria for repair are largely based on expert consensus and operative strategy has to be confirmed or changed after direct inspection by an expert surgeon, and no pre-specified criteria exist. This may limit the generalizability of our results to other centers and populations, but we all are aware that prospective studies would be useful but hardly feasible due to practical considerations.

Conclusions

Outcome of repair in IE guarantees a more favorable outcome than valve replacement and should be considered whenever possible in IE as in degenerative valve disease. Identifying patients who will benefit from surgery, operating them timely and following technically individualized surgical approach may decrease the mortality and morbidity of mitral valve IE.

Abbreviations
IE: Infective endocarditis; LVSF: Left ventricular systolic function; LVEF: Left ventricular ejection fraction; PISA: Proximal Isovelocity hemispheric Surface Area; ROC: Receiver operating characteristic; AUC: Area under the curve

Acknowledgements
Not applicable

Authors' contributions
VS projected the study, analyzed and interpreted the data, and wrote the manuscript. NZ carried out the statistical analysis. PLS performed the surgical interventions and was a major contributor in writing the manuscript. NM and IO revised the final version of the manuscript. SDP and BA performed clinical follow-up and contributed to collecting the data for analysis. All authors read and approved the final manuscript.

Author details
[1]Division of Cardiovascular and Perioperative Medicine, Cardiothoracovascular Department, Azienda Ospedaliero-Universitaria Careggi and University of Florence, Largo Brambilla 3, 50133 Florence, Italy. [2]Division of General Cardiology, Cardiothoracovascular Department, Azienda Ospedaliero-Universitaria Careggi and University of Florence, Florence, Italy. [3]IFAC-CNR Institute of Applied Physics "Nello Carrara" of the National Research Council, Sesto Fiorentino, Florence, Italy. [4]Division of Cardiac Surgery, Cardiothoracovascular Department, Azienda Ospedaliero-Universitaria Careggi and University of Florence, Florence, Italy.

References
1. Hendren WG, Morris AS, Rosenkranz ER, Lytle BW, Taylor PC, Stewart WJ, Loop FD, Cosgrove DM Mitral valve repair for bacterial endocarditis. J Thorac Cardiovasc Surg 1992 103(1):124–128 discussion 128-129
2. Podesser BK, Rodler S, Hahn R, Eigenbauer E, Vodrážka M, Moritz A, Laufer G, Simon P, Wolner E (2000) Mid-term follow up of mitral valve reconstruction due to active infective endocarditis. J Heart Valve Dis 9(3):335–340
3. Feringa H, Shaw LJ, Poldermans D, Hoeks S, Van der Wall E, Dion R, Bax J (2007) Mitral valve repair and replacement in endocarditis: a systematic review of literature. Ann Thorac Surg 83(2):564–570
4. Ishikawa S, Kawasaki A, Neya K, Abe K, Suzuki H, Koizumi S, Shibuya H, Horikawa M, Ueda K (2009) Surgical treatments for infective endocarditis involving valve annulus. Ann Thorac Cardiovasc Surg 15(6):378–381
5. Huang XS, Xie JS, You B, Gu CX, Wang SY, Zhang JQ Clinical outcome of mitral valve repair in primary infective endocarditis with mitral insufficiency. Zhonghua Wai Ke Za Zhi 2009 47(16):1236–1238
6. Omoto T, Tedoriya T, Oi M, Nagai N, Miyauchi T, Ishikawa N (2011) Significance of mitral valve repair for active-phase infective endocarditis. Asian Cardiovasc Thorac Ann 19(2):149–153
7. Evans CF, Gammie JS (2011) Surgical management of mitral valve infective endocarditis. Semin Thorac Cardiovasc Surg 23(3):232–240
8. Chang HW, Kim KH, Hwang HY, Kim JS (2014) Role of mitral valve repair in infective endocarditis. J Heart Valve Dis 23(3):350–359
9. Habib G, Lancellotti P, Antunes MJ, Bongiorni MG, Casalta JP, Del Zotti F, Delgheru R, El Khoury G, Erba PA, Iung B, Miro JM, Mulder BJ, Plonska-Gosciniak B, Price S, Roos-Hesselink J, Snygg-Martin U, Thuny F, Mas PT, Vilacosta I, Zamorano JL (2015) ESC guidelines for the management of infective endocarditis: the task force for the management of infective endocarditis of the European Society of Cardiology (ESC). Eur Heart J 36: 3075–3128
10. Scheggi V, Alterini B, Olivotto I, Del Pace S, Zoppetti N, Tomberli B, Bartalesi F, Brandi L, Ceschia N, Andrei V, Suardi LR, Marchionni N, Stefàno PL. Embolic risk stratification and prognostic impact of early surgery in left-sided infective endocarditis. Eur J Intern Med. 2020;78:82–87
11. Zhao D, Zhang B (2014) Are valve repairs associated with better outcomes than replacements in patients with native active valve endocarditis? Interact Cardiovasc Thorac Surg 19(6):1036–1039
12. Mick SL, Keshavamurthy S, Gillinov M (2015) Mitral valve repair versus replacement. Ann Cardiothorac Surg 4(3):230–237
13. Rostagno C, Carone E, Stefàno PL (2017) Role of mitral valve repair in active infective endocarditis: long term results. J Cardiothorac Surg 12(1):29
14. Hu YN, Wan S (2018) Repair of infected mitral valves: what have we learned? Surg Today 48(10):899–908
15. Liu JZ, Li XF, Miao Q, Zhang CJ (2018) Surgical treatment of active native mitral infective endocarditis: a meta-analysis of current evidence. J Chin Med Assoc 81(2):147–154
16. Thitipong T, Chartaroon R, Apichat T, Noppon T, Surin W, Suphachai C, Weerachai N (2019) Comparison between mitral valve repair and replacement in active infective endocarditis. Gen Thorac Cardiovasc Surg 67(12):1030–1037
17. Solari S, De Kerchove L, Tamer S, Aphram G, Baert J, Borsellino S, Mastrobuoni S, Navarra E, Noirhomme P, Astarci P, Rubay J, El Khoury G (2019) Active infective mitral valve endocarditis: is a repair-oriented surgery safe and durable? Eur J Cardiothorac Surg 55(2):256–262
18. Harky A, Hof A, Garner M, Froghi S, Bashir M Mitral valve repair or replacement in native valve endocarditis? Systematic review and meta-analysis. J Card Surg 2018 33(7):364–371
19. Lee HA, Cheng YT, Wu VC, Chou AH, Chu PH, Tsai FC, Chen SW. Nationwide cohort study of mitral valve repair versus replacement for infective endocarditis. J Thorac Cardiovasc Surg. 2018 Oct;156(4):1473-1483.e2.
20. Okada Y, Nakai T, Muro T, Ito H, Shomura Y (2020) Mitral valve repair for infective endocarditis: Kobe experience. Asian Cardiovasc Thorac Ann 28:384
21. Defauw RJ, Tomšič A, van Brakel TJ, Marsan NA, Klautz RJM, Palmen M (2020) A structured approach to native mitral valve infective endocarditis: is repair better than replacement? Eur J Cardiothorac Surg 58(3):544–550
22. De Kerchove L, Price J, Tamer S, Glineur D, Momeni M, Noirhomme P, ElKhoury G (2012) Extending the scope of mitral valve repair in active endocarditis. J Thorac Cardiovasc Surg 143(4 Suppl):S91–S95
23. Toyoda N, Itagaki S, Egorova NN, Tannous H, Anyanwu AC, El-Eshmawi A, Adams DH, Chikwe J. Real-world outcomes of surgery for native mitral valve endocarditis. J Thorac Cardiovasc Surg. 2017 Dec;154(6):1906-1912.e9.

12

Gastrointestinal presentation of COVID-19 in a pediatric heart transplant recipient

Abdelmonem Helal[1,2], Ahmed F. Elmahrouk[3,4*], Ahmed A. Jamjoom[3] and Jameel A. Al-Ata[1,5]

Abstract

Background: Severe acute respiratory syndrome coronavirus 2 (SARS-CoV-2)-associated coronavirus disease 2019 (COVID-19) most commonly causes a mild respiratory illness; however, there are wide ranges of presenting symptoms and disease severity. It has a mortality rate around 7%.

Case presentation: We present a case of a 9-year-old female patient with hypoplastic left heart syndrome status post heart transplantation at age of 7 days. She presented to our emergency room complaining of intermittent fever, chills, fatigue, poor appetite, and diarrhea.
A throat swab nucleic acid test was positive for severe acute respiratory syndrome coronavirus 2 (SARS-CoV-2). Intravenous fluids therapy was used for correction of hydration status. To the best of our knowledge this is the first reported case of non-pulmonary presentation of coronavirus disease-2019 (COVID-19) in a pediatric heart transplant recipient, which was successfully managed conservatively.

Conclusions: Gastrointestinal manifestations can be the only presenting symptom in pediatric heart transplant recipients with COVID-19. Conservative treatment could be used successfully. Immunomodulatory medications that are used in heart transplant recipients may have protective value in SARS-CoV-2 infection.

Keywords: SARS-CoV-2, Pediatric heart transplant recipient, Gastrointestinal presentation

Background

Severe acute respiratory syndrome coronavirus 2 (SARS-CoV-2)-associated coronavirus disease 2019 (COVID-19) most commonly causes a mild respiratory illness, however, there are wide ranges of presenting symptoms and disease severity [1]. It has a mortality rate around 7% [2].

Serious and fatal cases of COVID-19 have been recorded in children; however, most pediatric groups tend to have asymptomatic, mild, or moderate presentations. Most of them recover within 1 to 2 weeks of the onset of illness [3].

* Correspondence: Ael-Mahrouk@kfshrc.edu.sa; A_marouky@hotmail.com; Ahmed.elmahrouki1@med.tanta.edu.eg
[3]Division of Cardiac Surgery, Cardiovascular Department, King Faisal Specialist Hospital and Research Center, MBC J-16, P.O. Box: 40047, Jeddah 21499, Saudi Arabia
[4]Cardiothoracic Surgery Department, Tanta University, Tanta, Egypt
Full list of author information is available at the end of the article

Case presentation

A 9-year-old female patient was presented to our emergency room complaining of intermittent fever, chills, fatigue, poor appetite, and diarrhea. On examination, she was afebrile, (however, her family reported a tympanic temperature of 37.8 °C at home), oxygen saturation was 99% on room air, her respiratory rate was 20 breaths per minute with a heart rate of 90 beats/min, and her blood pressure measurement was 100/75 mmHg. The patient's residential area is known to be a hotspot for SARS-CoV-2 infection. She had no history of similar manifestations in her family members.

Past medical history

The child was born with hypoplastic left heart syndrome; she underwent a heart transplant operation at the age of 7 days. She had regular follow-up appointments in our pediatric cardiology clinic. Three years back, she was admitted to our facility with severe gastroenteritis attacks that required intensive care unit admission and intravenous inotropic support. After 10 days, she was discharged with stable hemodynamic conditions and normal cardiac functions. Last year, she was complaining about frequent attacks of eczema flare-up, which was treated successfully by a 5-day course of topical hydrocortisone 1% cream. Her current medications are aspirin 81 mg daily, immunosuppressive therapy in the form of tacrolimus 7 mg once daily, and mycophenolate mofetil 0.3 g three times a week. The last recorded blood concentration of tacrolimus 1 month before admission was 6 ng/ml, and cardiac allograft function was normal with an elevated baseline creatinine level of 70 umol/L and cyclic leucopenia with measured white blood cell count of 3.2×10^9 cells/l and 5.3×10^9 cells/l 4 and 2 months prior to this admission respectively (Fig. 1a). Absolute neutrophilic count was low on admission (0.3×10^9 cells/l) and continue to rise to reach 2.5×10^9 cells/l on follow-up (Fig. 1b).

Differential diagnosis

The differential diagnosis included bacterial gastroenteritis, viral gastroenteritis, and coronavirus disease-2019 (COVID-19).

Investigations

Laboratory tests showed a leucopenia (white blood cell count of 2.86×10^9 cells/l) hemoglobin 9.2 g/dl, creatinine level 120 umol/l, renal Co2 12 mmol/l, procalcitonin level 8.4 ng/mL (normal range up to 2 ng/mL), D dimer 1.555 mg/l (normal range up to 0.555 mg/L), ferritin 229 μg/l,

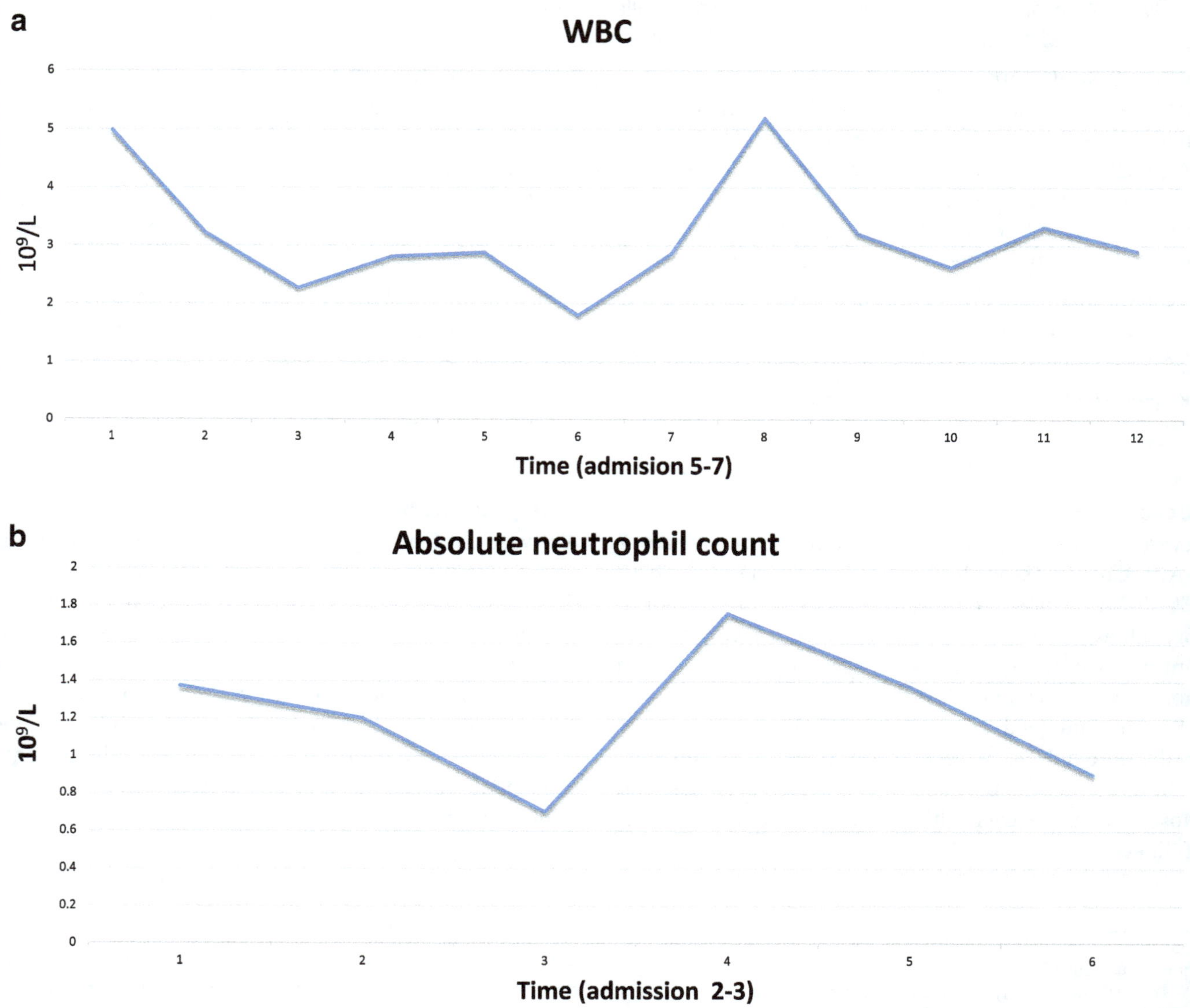

Fig. 1 a A flow chart for leucocytic count (WBC) showing cyclic leucopenia prior COVID-19 infection, and a leucocytic count lower than her usual baseline during this admission, which started to recover by discharge. **b** A flow chart for absolute neutrophilic count showing neutropenia during COVID-19 infection, which started to recover by discharge

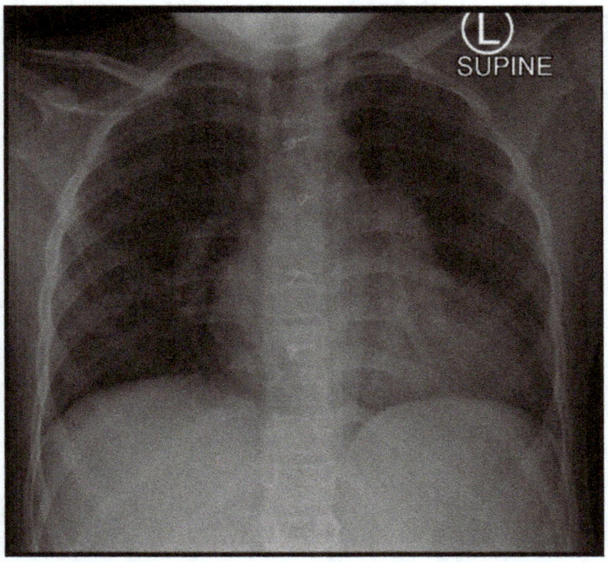

Fig. 2 Chest X-ray showing that the cardiac silhouette is enlarged with the prominence of the left pulmonary artery. The lung fields and the costophrenic angles are clear

and ProBNP 680 pg/ml (normal range up to 450 pg/ml). Chest X-ray showed clear both lung fields and costophrenic angles. (Fig. 2).

A throat swab nucleic acid test was positive for SARS-CoV-2. Vancomycin-resistant enterococci swab and methicillin-resistant Staphylococcus aureus swab screening were negative. Blood, urine, and stool cultures were negative for bacterial infection, and rapid antigen stool test was negative. Echocardiography study showed normal systolic and diastolic function with no pericardial effusion (Fig. 3).

Management

Immunosuppressive drugs were adjusted in the form of tacrolimus 5 mg as tacrolimus trough level concentration on admission was 11 ng/ml (Fig. 4) and continued on the same dose of mycophenolate mofetil and aspirin. Since the child condition was stable, a decision was made in a multi-disciplinary meeting between pediatric cardiology, cardiac surgery, pediatric infectious disease, and immunology to proceed with conservative management, and we did not start any antiviral medications for SARS-CoV-2 virus infection. Intravenous fluids therapy was used for the correction of hydration status. Body temperature was normal during the admission period (Fig. 5), gastrointestinal symptoms were gradually improving over three days, and she resumed her normal oral intake. On the 7th day of admission, laboratory tests showed creatinine level 70 umol/l, renal Co2 19 mmol/l. The patient was discharged after two consecutive negative reverse transcriptase–polymerase chain reaction throat swabs for SARS-CoV-2 on the 12th and 18th days from admission.

Follow-up

The patient remained hospitalized for 15 days of isolation as per the ministry of health guidelines. She was scheduled for a follow-up appointment in the pediatric cardiology clinic.

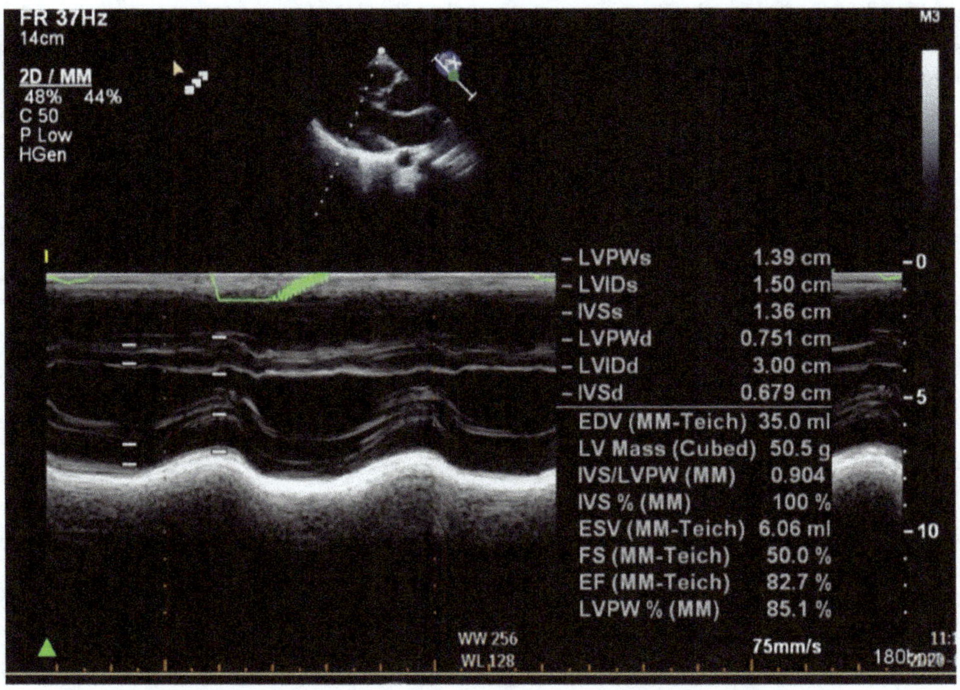

Fig. 3 Echocardiography study showed normal systolic and diastolic function with no pericardial effusion

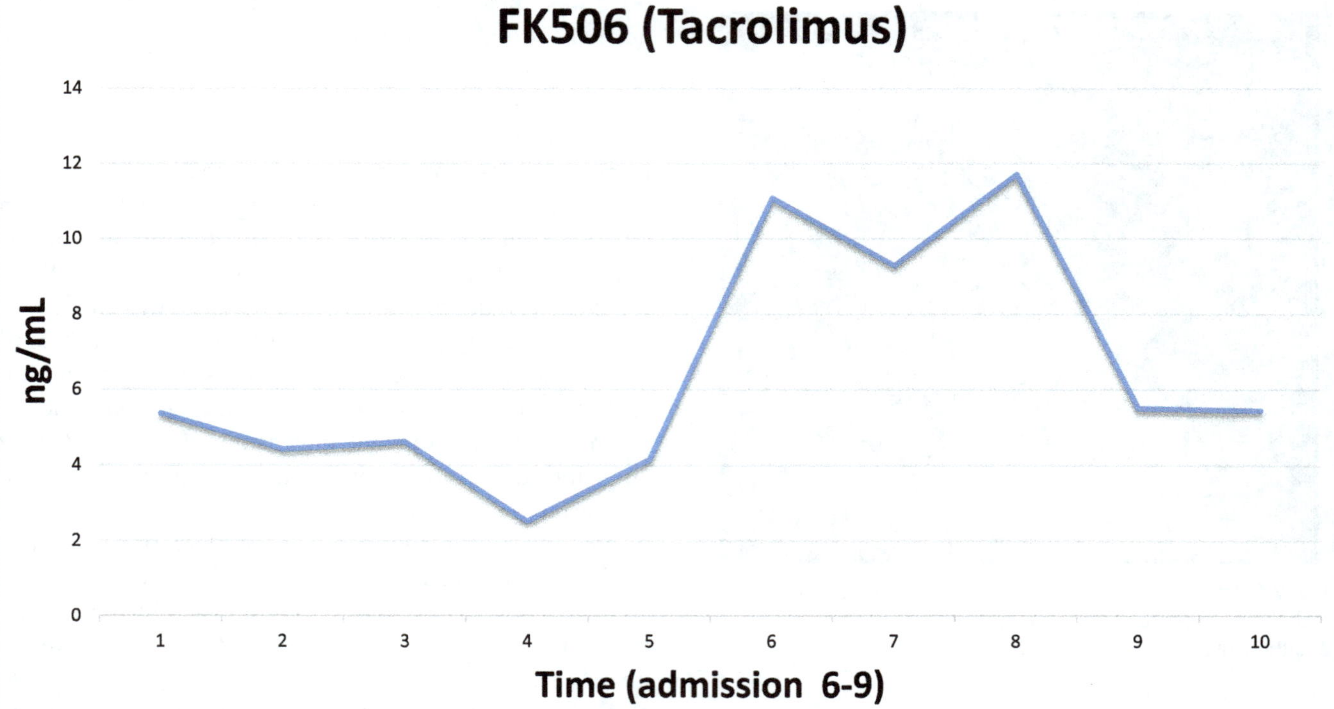

Fig. 4 A flow chart of tacrolimus trough level showing an elevated level during the initial presentation of the disease, and the decrease of the level in response to dose adjustment

Discussion

Multiple reports suggested that pediatric COVID-19 patients experience not only less severe but different symptoms than adults. Their rate of hospitalization was 5.7% with less than 0.6% needed ICU admission, with mortality rate of 0.11% [4].

The severity of COVID-19 tends to be caused not only by viral invasion and proliferation but also by an extreme immune response characterized by cytokine storm, myocardial injury, and coagulopathy [5]. Questions were raised about whether heart transplant recipients may be at elevated risk of adverse outcomes with SARS-CoV-2 infection due to several specific comorbidities following cardiac transplantation, including hypertension and cardiac allograft vasculopathy [6]. In addition, while maintaining immunosuppression predisposes recipients to a higher risk of infection, immunosuppression has also been theorized as being protective against cytokine storms [7]. Moreover, an earlier study demonstrated that FK506 (Tacrolimus) inhibited the growth and replication of

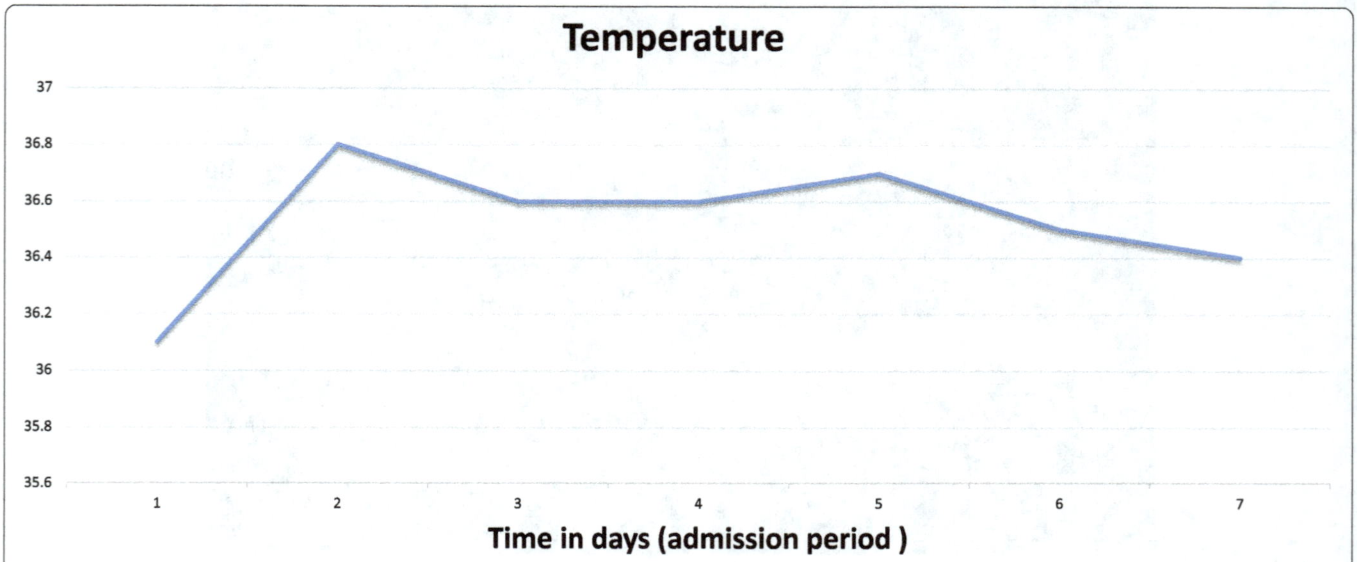

Fig. 5 A temprature chart for recorded values throughout the admission period showing a highest recorded value of 37.5 °C

human coronaviruses SARS-CoV, at low, non-cytotoxic concentrations in cell culture [8]. Our patient was receiving tacrolimus at the time of infection; therefore, she may have a more efficient immune response than if she had received corticosteroid.

There have been conflicting reports about mortality among recipients of a heart transplant with COVID-19. While one report did not find any increase in mortality [1], another article showed 25% mortality in an adult cohort of 22 transplant recipients with SARS-CoV-2 infection [9].

In the case report by Russell MR et al. [10], the patient was admitted to receive intravenous immunoglobulin 1 week after surveillance laboratory studies showed anti-human leukocyte antigen antibody. Because of the history of cough, SARS-CoV-2 reverse transcriptase polymerase chain reaction test was performed and returned positive. They suggested that careful measurement of donor-specific antibodies be undertaken in heart transplant survivors of COVID-19 [10].

Our child had a good immunosuppressive balance, with no signs of rejection. Moreover, echocardiography study showed normal systolic and diastolic function with no pericardial effusion. For that, we did not feel the need to perform donor specific antibodies test.

Our patient had an acceptable course over the last 9 years. Although laboratory investigation showed increased levels of inflammatory markers, the clinical presentation was in a mild form with no significant signs of systemic viral manifestations or cytokine storm. With all previous factors, we decided not to start antiviral medication. Monitoring hemodynamic parameters and correction of hydration status were the main line of management. The patient improved slowly on this conservative treatment.

Conclusions

Gastrointestinal manifestations can be the only presenting symptom in pediatric heart transplant recipients with COVID-19. Conservative treatment could be used successfully. Immunomodulatory medications that are used in heart transplant recipients may have protective value in SARS-CoV-2 infection. More studies are needed to evaluate the difference in clinical course and outcome between pediatric and adult heart transplant recipients with COVID-19.

Abbreviations

SARS-CoV-2: Severe acute respiratory syndrome coronavirus 2; COVID-19: Coronavirus disease-2019

Acknowledgements

None.

Authors' contributions

AH have conducted a literature search; data acquisition; data interpretation and drafted the manuscript, AE have also conducted a literature review; data acquisition; data interpretation; data analysis and drafted the manuscript, AJ have made a substantial contribution to the conception, the acquisition and the interpretation of data; he also substantively revised the manuscript. JA have conducted a literature review; analysis and interpretation of data; he also critically revised the manuscript. All authors have read and approved the final manuscript.

Author details

[1]Pediatric Cardiology Section, Department of Pediatrics, King Faisal Specialist Hospital & Research Center, Jeddah, Kingdom of Saudi Arabia. [2]Department of Pediatrics and Pediatric Cardiology, Cairo University, Cairo, Egypt. [3]Division of Cardiac Surgery, Cardiovascular Department, King Faisal Specialist Hospital and Research Center, MBC J-16, P.O. Box: 40047, Jeddah 21499, Saudi Arabia. [4]Cardiothoracic Surgery Department, Tanta University, Tanta, Egypt. [5]Section of Pediatric Cardiology, Department of Pediatrics, King Abdulaziz University, Jeddah, Saudi Arabia.

References

1. Li F, Cai J, Dong N (2020) First cases of COVID-19 in heart transplantation from China. J Heart Lung Transplant 39(5):496–497. https://doi.org/10.1016/j.healun.2020.03.006 Epub 2020 Mar 17. PMID: 32362394; PMCID: PMC7156127
2. Dong E, Du H, Gardner L. An interactive web-based dashboard to track COVID-19 in real time. Lancet Infect Dis. 2020; 20(5): 533-534. doi: https://doi.org/10.1016/S1473-3099(20)30120-1. Epub 2020 Feb 19. Erratum in: Lancet Infect Dis. 2020 Sep;20(9):e215. PMID: 32087114; PMCID: PMC7159018.
3. Chang TH, Wu JL, Chang LY (2020) Clinical characteristics and diagnostic challenges of pediatric COVID-19: A systematic review and meta-analysis. J Formos Med Assoc 119(5):982–989. https://doi.org/10.1016/j.jfma.2020.04.007 Epub 2020 Apr 16. PMID: 32307322; PMCID: PMC7161491
4. CDC COVID-19 Response Team (2020) Coronavirus Disease 2019 in Children - United States, February 12-April 2, 2020. MMWR Morb Mortal Wkly Rep 69(14):422–426. https://doi.org/10.15585/mmwr.mm6914e4 PMID: 32271728; PMCID: PMC7147903
5. Guzik TJ, Mohiddin SA, Dimarco A, Patel V, Savvatis K, Marelli-Berg FM, Madhur MS, Tomaszewski M, Maffia P, D'Acquisto F, Nicklin SA, Marian AJ, Nosalski R, Murray EC, Guzik B, Berry C, Touyz RM, Kreutz R, Wang DW, Bhella D, Sagliocco O, Crea F, Thomson EC, McInnes IB (2020) COVID-19 and the cardiovascular system: implications for risk assessment, diagnosis, and treatment options. Cardiovasc Res 116(10):1666–1687. https://doi.org/10.1093/cvr/cvaa106 PMID: 32352535; PMCID: PMC7197627
6. Ketcham SW, Adie SK, Malliett A, Abdul-Aziz AA, Bitar A, Grafton G, Konerman MC (2020) Coronavirus Disease-2019 in Heart Transplant Recipients in Southeastern Michigan: A Case Series. J Card Fail 26(6):457–461. https://doi.org/10.1016/j.cardfail.2020.05.008 Epub 2020 May 14. PMID: 32417380; PMCID: PMC7224667
7. Alijotas-Reig J, Esteve-Valverde E, Belizna C, Selva-O'Callaghan A, Pardos-Gea J, Quintana A, Mekinian A, Anunciacion-Llunell A, Miró-Mur F (2020) Immunomodulatory therapy for the management of severe COVID-19. Beyond the anti-viral therapy: A comprehensive review. Autoimmun Rev 19(7):102569. https://doi.org/10.1016/j.autrev.2020.102569 Epub 2020 May 3. PMID: 32376394; PMCID: PMC7252146
8. Carbajo-Lozoya J, Müller MA, Kallies S, Thiel V, Drosten C, von Brunn A (2012) Replication of human coronaviruses SARS-CoV, HCoV-NL63 and HCoV-229E is inhibited by the drug FK506. Virus Res 165(1):112–117. https://doi.org/10.1016/j.virusres.2012.02.002 Epub 2012 Feb 10. PMID: 22349148; PMCID: PMC7114512
9. Latif F, Farr MA, Clerkin KJ, Habal MV, Takeda K, Naka Y, Restaino S, Sayer G, Uriel N (2020) Characteristics and Outcomes of Recipients of Heart Transplant With Coronavirus Disease 2019. JAMA Cardiol:e202159. https://doi.org/10.1001/jamacardio.2020.2159 Epub ahead of print. PMID: 32402056; PMCID: PMC7221850
10. Russell MR, Halnon NJ, Alejos JC, Salem MM, Reardon LC (2020) COVID-19 in a pediatric heart transplant recipient: Emergence of donor-specific antibodies. J Heart Lung Transplant 39(7):732–733. https://doi.org/10.1016/j.healun.2020.04.021 Epub 2020 Apr 29. PMID: 32430156; PMCID: PMC7189188

13

Urgent surgical repair is pivotal in the management of major airway injury due to blunt trauma

Hysam Abdelmohty[1], Mohamed A. Elanwar[2] and Basem M. Abdelgawad[3*]

Abstract

Background: Blunt traumatic airway injury is a life-threatening injury in which urgent management is pivotal and this would come through improving our clinical management and diagnostic tools. Our objective was to emphasize the importance of early referral and urgent surgical repair of major airway injury.

Results: Records of 42 patients with major airway injury out of 17,520 registered thoracic trauma cases were reviewed over the past 15 years. Twenty-eight cases documented to have major tracheobronchial injuries due to blunt trauma underwent surgical repair either urgent (21 cases) or late (7 cases). The age ranged from 8 to 43 years old with a mean age of 22.3 ± 0.8. The most common presenting symptom was shortness of breath in 22 (78.6%) cases and the most frequent sign was subcutaneous emphysema which was seen in 22 (78.6%) cases. The postoperative morbidity and mortality rates were significantly higher in the delayed repair group (p value < 0.001).

Conclusion: The urgent surgical repair is the treatment of choice for major airway injury which is facilitated by early recognition and referral. It is pivotal to avoid respiratory and systemic complications and related mortality.

Keywords: Airway injury, Tracheobronchial tear, Surgical emphysema, Air leak

Background

Acute posttraumatic tracheobronchial injuries (TBI) are rare but potentially life-threatening events. It is responsible for nearly 30% of deaths at the scene [1]. The increasing incidence may be due to modernization, increased number of motor car accidents, work environment-related, or lately with the growing youth population competing in all sorts of sports. Rapid diagnosis and management are essential together with the proper assessment of associated injuries to set up the priorities in the ladder of management. Urgent surgical management of airway injuries prevents both early and late sequelae such as mediastinitis, airway stenosis, lobe collapse, and empyema.

The historical observation confirms that thoracic surgeons were aware of the airway injury as a swift killer, a century ago, and more. Despite that, the airway injuries still represent a difficult diagnostic and curative situation but fortunately, these injuries are rare. Some authors have reported that fatality is because of respiratory distress, difficulties in establishing an intact airway, and tension pneumothorax together with the high frequency of associated multiple precious organ injuries (head, spine, vascular, or parenchymal injuries) [2].

It is crucial to highlight the importance and the increasing incidence of major airway injury, and how to identify them among the great number of trauma patients. Furthermore, we emphasize the importance of early referral and urgent surgical repair of such injuries.

Methods

Research design

A retrospective comparative study reviewing records from the emergency hospital database over 15 years from January 2004 to January 2019. Data of 28 patients with

* Correspondence: bassem.abdelgawad@fmed.bu.edu.eg
[3]Cardiothoracic Surgery Department, Faculty of Medicine, Benha University, 15 Hasan Muwafi St., Hi Elrawdah, New Benha, Qalyobia 13518, Egypt
Full list of author information is available at the end of the article

major airway injury due to blunt thoracic trauma who underwent surgical repair were studied. These patients were divided into two groups: the first group offered the urgent repair strategy and included 21 patients, and the second group was surgical repair was delayed and included seven patients.

Inclusion and exclusion criteria

The injuries involving the airway from below the cricoid cartilage until the secondary bronchial bifurcations were included. We have excluded injuries caused by penetrating trauma like stab wounds and also those caused by iatrogenic trauma such as rigid bronchoscope injuries. This decision was based on the higher trauma severity and multiple associated injuries accounting for the higher mortality in blunt trauma group compared to penetrating or iatrogenic groups thus making the results biased if the latter two groups were included in the study.

Data management

Details of demographic data, mode of injury, associated injuries, diagnostic modalities, management strategy, and outcomes were collected and retrospectively analyzed. We have collected the presenting symptoms and signs suggestive of airways injury. In stable cases, chest x-ray (CXR), abdominal ultrasound (US), and computed tomography (CT) of the chest; then, bronchoscopy of the airways were performed whenever possible. In hemodynamically unstable patients with shock or respiratory distress, resuscitation was performed according to the advanced trauma life support (ATLS) protocol; then, they were approached in the same manner as the stable patients or rushed to the operative theater for an exploratory thoracotomy.

The protocol of management

1. *Indications for bronchoscopy.* These were based on any clinical suspicion of significant airway injury like persistent pneumothorax with ineffective intercostal tube (ICT) drainage as witnessed by persistent high grade of air leak, presence of traumatic hemoptysis, progressive surgical or emphysema, and CT evidence of tracheal or bronchial discontinuity.
2. *Resuscitation.* Treating patients in shock, restoration of the reasonable airway, and alleviating pain
3. *Monitoring.* Continuous ECG monitoring, noninvasive blood pressure measurement, and obtaining peripheral oxygen saturation coupled with arterial baseline blood gasses
4. *Anesthesia.* Close co-operation between the anesthetist and the surgeon especially at the introduction of the endotracheal tube (ETT) that might need to be inserted with fiber-optic bronchoscopy. We have used a double-lumen ETT to facilitate healthy lung ventilation and to prevent blood spillover from the injured site. However, a single lumen tube was satisfactory in tracheal injuries.
5. *Indications for surgery.* The indications were evident significant (> 2 cm) tear of the trachea or bronchi—detected bronchoscopically—as well as observing massive and persistent high degrees of air leakage from the thoracostomy tube and/or persistent acute respiratory distress.
6. *Operative procedure*

(1) Most of our patients had been explored via a classical posterolateral thoracotomy passing through the fourth intercostal space

(2) Careful inspection of the hemithorax was done with removing of collected blood, identifying the disturbed anatomy, and repairing any bleeding points.

(3) Identification of the tear edges and looking for any associated injuries

(4) Raw interrupted stitches were used to get the torn edges together after gentle debridement and reenforcement—when possible—by pleural or intercostals muscle flap.

(5) Testing for the integrity of the suture line and hemostasis. Then, two chest drains were inserted and thoracotomy was closed in layers.

7. *Postoperative care.* Our principle was to perform on-table or early extubation and encouraging self-ventilation and self-exhaling of secretions together with proper physiotherapy. Early ambulation with strict physiotherapy was continued and a follow-up chest x-ray was performed before discharge, and CT chest and/or bronchoscopy were done when the residual injury was suspected.

Statistical analysis

Statistical analysis data were statistically described in terms of mean, standard deviation (± SD), frequencies (number of cases), and relative frequencies (percentages) when appropriate. A comparison of quantitative variables between the groups was done using the Mann-Whitney *U* test, Chi-square (χ^2) test was performed for qualitative variables. A probability value (*P* value) less than 0.05 was considered statistically significant. All statistical calculations were done using computer programs Microsoft Excel version 7 and SPSS version 23 statistical program.

Results

Forty-two out of 17,520 registered thoracic trauma patients (0.24%) reported having major airway injuries.

Among those 42 patients, blunt trauma was the cause of injury in 31 (73.8%) patients, while seven (16.6%) injuries were due to iatrogenic causes, and only four (9.52%) penetrating injuries.

Twenty-eight out of the 31 cases documented to have major TBI due to blunt trauma underwent surgical repair either early (21 cases) or late (seven cases). In our cohort, males were 22 and females six with a ratio of 3.7: 1. The age ranged from 8 to 43 years old with a mean age of 22.3 ± 0.8.

The most common mode of injury in blunt trauma was the motor car accidents that were seen in 16 cases (57.1%). While falling from height principally among working men was seen in four cases with a ratio of 14.3%. Also falling of heavy objects on the chest either on-front or on-behind in four cases (14.3%), raising concerns about their working environment. In our community, it is not uncommon to face animal attacks where a 17-year-old male received a kick by a calf to the front of the chest (3.6%). Hit and run over a pedestrian by tricycle or motorbike was recorded in two cases (7.1%) and one case (3.6%) was registered sports injury.

Most of our cases arrived at the emergency room (ER) conscious but we did receive five cases (17.9%) with a disturbed level of consciousness with the Glasgow coma scale between 9 and 13. Two of them (7.1%) were admitted to our hospital already intubated by their referring hospitals, and three (10.7%) were intubated in the ER. The most frequent presenting symptom and signs are shown in Table 1.

Chest radiographs were obtained in anteroposterior position, due to hemodynamic instability, disturbed level of consciousness, presence of masking surgical emphysema, and as a precaution for the possible cervical spine or orthopedic injuries, CT was done in almost all patients. The radiological findings as complete loss of the tracheal wall contour, displacement of the ETT, the air within the pericardium, mediastinal emphysema, pneumothorax, and lung collapse were detailed in Table 2 with examples in Figs. 1 and 2.

Tube thoracostomy was inserted in most cases at the primary hospital and a few of them at our ER. The unilateral tube was required in 18 (64.3%) cases, a second apical tube was inserted in 4 (14.3%) cases due to massive air leak and 6 (21.4%) cases offered bilateral chest tubes. Bronchoscopy was diagnostic with the view of disrupted or lacerated tissues, continuous bleeding, and the presence of clots. Bronchoscopy was also useful in detecting the level of injury. We used primarily the rigid bronchoscopy except when its use becomes contraindicated in the presence of cervical spine injury. Bronchoscopy was not used in the six cases of upper tracheal injury where the neck tear was clear by the naked eye examination. Moreover, three cases with main stem bronchus injury were diagnosed by radiological findings (see Table 3).

Extra-thoracic injuries were common in severely traumatized patients. No significant injuries were collected and data are shown in Table 4. During surgical repair of the airways, two patients of the urgent group underwent evacuation of extradural hematoma and one patient underwent laparotomy for intra-abdominal collection.

We have used the previous data to suggest the criteria suspecting major TBI and indicating the use of bronchoscopy to confirm the diagnosis and to proceed for urgent surgical repair as detailed in Table 5.

We have used right thoracotomy in 16 cases, left thoracotomy in six cases, and cervical approach in six cases, where we have done 23 airway repairs, three lobectomies (10.7%), and two pneumonectomies (7.1%). None of our patients had the chance of emergency thoracotomy at the scene as this service is only available in tertiary centers. We did direct suturing to all cases after debridement of the tear edges. We had to do lobectomy in three cases (10.7%) and pneumonectomy in two cases (7.1%) due to severely damaged lung tissues.

Our patients were followed-up for periods ranged from 1 to 3 years with a mean follow-up period of 10.7 ± 6.9 months with 7 (25%) patients who had missed data during the follow-up. The early outcome during the follow-up period is shown in Table 6.

Discussion

We had an incidence of 42 out of 17,520 registered thoracic trauma patients (0.24%) reported having major airway injuries. The worldwide reported incidence in many works of literature is between 0.35 and 5.3%. We can explain our incidence as cases that might be diagnosed as

Table 1 Clinical presentations

Presenting symptoms	Total cases (28)	Urgent repair (21)	Delayed repair (7)	*P* value
Subcutaneous emphysema	22 (78.6%)	17 (81%)	5 (71.4%)	0.34
Dyspnea	22 (78.6%)	15 (71.4%)	7 (100%)	0.010
Hemoptysis	9 (32%)	9 (42.8%)	0	0.023
Desaturation/cyanosis	16 (57.1%)	14 (66.6%)	2 (28.6%)	0.027
Hoarseness of voice	7 (25%)	6 (28.6%)	1 (14.3%)	0.045
Shock	17 (60.7%)	15 (71.4%)	2 (28.6%)	0.039

Table 2 Radiological findings and associated injuries

Radiological findings:	Total cases (28)	Urgent repair (21)	Delayed repair (7)	*P* value
Surgical emphysema	27 (96.4%)	20 (95.2%)	7 (100%)	0.147
Pneumomediastinum	23 (82.1%)	16 (76.2%)	7 (100%)	0.06
Lung contusion	22 (78.6%)	18 (85.7%)	4 (57.1%)	0.019
Pneumothorax	15 (53.6%)	11 (52.4%)	4 (57.1%)	0.049
Hemopneumothorax	9 (32.1%)	7 (33.3%)	2 (28.6%)	0.499
Clavicle fracture	9 (32.1%)	7 (33.3%)	2 (28.6%)	0.499
Flail chest	8 (28.6%)	7 (33.3%)	1 (14.3%)	0.025
Fallen lung sign	6 (21.4%)	4 (19%)	2 (28.6%)	0.419

a major airway injury but dies before surgery is conducted. Besides, the cases that passed unregistered or undiagnosed by the trauma team were not obvious and required a high degree of suspicion.

Most studies report that the most common cause of TBI is blunt trauma. In the present study, TBI was caused by blunt trauma in 73.8% of trauma cases. Approximate figures were reported by many authors such as Richardson [3], Scaglione et al, [4], and Koletsis et al. [5] who had found, respectively, that 76.7%, 67%, and 66.7% of injuries were due to blunt trauma. However, few authors reported their cases to be caused mainly by penetrating trauma such as Fatimi et al. [6] and Saad et al. [7]. We think that the accuracy of these figures was biased by the small sample size in most of the studies.

In our study, the age ranged from 8 to 43 years old with a mean age of 22.3 ± 0.8 and 11 patients (39.3%) were under 18 years old. Similar results were reported by Balci et al. [8] and Saad et al. [7] as they had a mean age of 22.3 years (range 4–53) and 26 years (range 17–38), respectively.

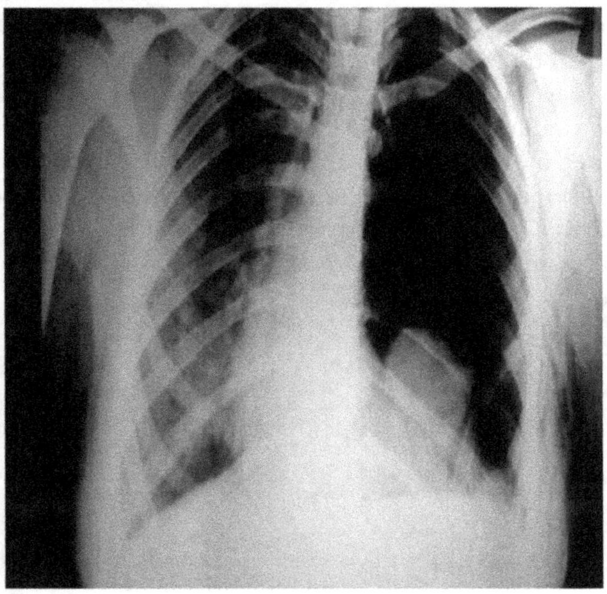

Fig. 1 Fallen lung sign of kumpe

Several mechanisms causing tracheal injury have been suggested: tracheal compression between the sternum and the vertebral column or abrupt increase in intraluminal pressure due to forced expiration against a closed glottis [9]. Direct trauma to the cervical trachea also causes tracheal injury [10]. Tracheobronchial injuries involve mostly the main bronchus within 2 cm close to the carina; the right bronchus is more commonly affected [11]. Chest compression squeezes the right main bronchus that is seated in front of the vertebral bodies and increases the risk of tear during blunt incidents, while the left main bronchus gets protection by the arch riding above it. Also, the longer air column with the left bronchus buffers the increasing intraluminal pressure and reduces the tear incidence [10].

In our cohort, the injuries were more common at the upper airways especially the cervical part of the trachea and this finding was consistent with almost all previous reports. Some authors like Farzanegan et al. who studied 35 patients with major airway injury and included 16 (45%) of them with a laryngeal injury [12]. We have excluded such patients as they are out of our scope of care being managed by the ENT surgeons.

Injuries ranged from contusion, a small laceration, to complete avulsion of the airways. Once the injury violates the integrity of the mediastinal pleura, it will produce persistent air leak and desaturation, but if it remains intact, it might go unnoticed as both ends are connected by the peribronchial tissues but later on stenosis endures and patients come with dyspnea at rest [9].

In our population, surgical emphysema was the most frequent presentation followed by dyspnea. Many authors reported the same findings even with more distress in the form of tachypnea and stridor [8, 13, 12, 5]. The incidence of hemodynamic instability and shock was 60.7% which is higher than those documented in many studies as we included only cases of blunt trauma that commonly involved other systems.

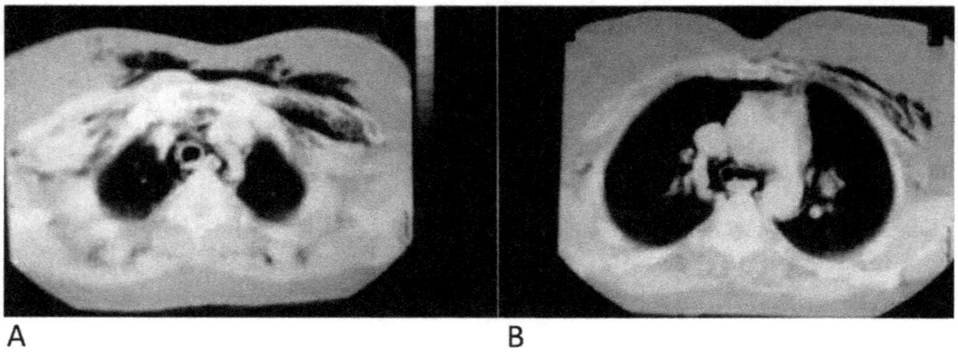

Fig. 2 a, b Air encircling the trachea till carina and around vessels, pneumomediastinum, and surgical emphysema

In our study, pneumothorax was present in 24 (85.7%) of cases and lung contusion was reported in 22 (78.6%) of them. Few patients displayed no signs or symptoms until one or 2 days post-injury [10[. Serious associated other injuries included multiple ribs fracture, flail chest, and head or abdominal injuries; they occur in more than 50% of patients as similarly reported by others [14].

The chest CT is able to detect the site of blunt tracheobronchial injuries in more than 90% of cases. However, bronchoscopic examination remains the standard tool for diagnosing TBI not only to detect but also to define the site and the extent of any tear or laceration [15]. Bronchoscopic findings may be in the form of single transverse (between the rings) or longitudinal along the membranous segment or maybe complex with rupture in more than one site or form [16].

Immediate surgical repair was chosen in most cases to avoid airway and pulmonary complications. In a few selected cases, surgical intervention was postponed if the patient did not have major injury suspicious criteria or did not have a large tracheobronchial tear by bronchoscopic examination. The latest ATLS guidelines recommended the immediate operative intervention in such injuries except for more stable patients; operative treatment of TBI may be delayed until the acute inflammation and edema resolve [2]. Although conservative treatment may be an option in selected patients, it is crucial to bear in mind that it may be a one-way choice, as the success of subsequent surgical treatment in case of failure may be limited by the progression of sepsis, reduced vascularization of the margins of the airway laceration, and the development of adhesions [17].

The following is a decision-making flow chart for managing chest trauma with keeping major TBI in mind:

A cervical tracheal tear can be approached by collar cervical incision while right posterolateral thoracotomy provides good access to the intrathoracic trachea, right main bronchus, and proximal part of the left main bronchus [17]. Some authors reported a high rate of pneumonectomy, 23%, and referred that to the high rate of gun-shot injuries [3].

All cases were managed by direct repair after trimming of tear edges without much dissection to keep reasonable blood supply to the suture lines. We have used absorbable 3/0 interrupted sutures with ties outside and in few cases; we covered the suture line with mediastinal pleura. Using of absorbable sutures in repairing of the tracheal tear is best with less chance for the formation of granulation tissue than the non-absorbable suture. Also, it is liable to cause abscess, infection, or dehiscence. Interrupted sutures with knots outside are commonly performed than the continuous technique. The suture line can be supported by Teflon or a pleural flap [18].

Postoperative use of bronchoscopic examination, nasotracheal suction, or forced coughing is important, and the patients should be reassessed by bronchoscope 3 months after repair [18, 19]. Tracheal stenosis is

Table 3 The site of the tracheobronchial tear

Site of the tear	Total cases (28)	Urgent repair (21)	Delayed repair (7)	*P* value
Upper half of trachea	6 (21.4%)	6 (28.6%)	0	0.04
Main stem bronchus	8 (28.6%)	5 (17.9%)	3 (42.8%)	0.071
Lower trachea extending to Rt main bronchus	7 (25%)	4 (19.1%)	3 (42.8%)	0.218
Lower trachea extending to Lt main bronchus	4 (14.3%)	3 (14.3%)	1 (14.3%)	0.982
Complex injury	3 (10.7%)	3 (14.3%)	0	0.019

Table 4 Extra-thoracic injuries

Extra-thoracic injuries	Total cases (28)	Urgent repair (21)	Delayed repair (7)	*P* value
Severe head trauma*	8 (28.6%)	6 (28.6%)	2 (28.6%)	0.98
Abdominal organs injury with Intra-abdominal collection or capsular hematoma	8 (28.6%)	5 (17.9%)	3 (42.8%)	0.071
Long bones fracture	14 (50%)	10 (47.6%)	4 (57.1%)	0.037
Pelvic fracture	3 (10.7%)	3 (14.3%)	0	0.019
Spinal cord injury	2 (7.1%)	2 (9.5%)	0	0.03

*Severe head trauma: associated with intracranial hemorrhage, fracture base, or post-concussion symptoms with disturbed consciousness

diagnosed if the diameter decreased to 50% and clinically it does dyspnea only on exertion but if it reaches below one quarter, stridor and dyspnea will occur at rest especially if little secretions or inflammatory swelling was seated inside [17].

In our patients, the postoperative morbidity and mortality rates were significantly higher in the delayed repair group (*p* value < 0.001). These rates were affected by the longer time of lung collapse, lung and surgical site infection, and presence of retained hemothorax. We had three cases of tracheal stenosis; one of them responded to multiple bronchoscopic dilatations, and the other two needed surgery for disabling dyspnea. The two empyema cases in the urgent repair group managed by tube thoracostomy drainage and medical treatment and showed a complete cure. The only case of empyema in the delayed repair group died after developing septic shock. One case with massive air leakage with significant lung collapse underwent early thoracoscopic repair. The other two cases required no further intervention rather than physiotherapy and observation. They improved and discharged after 2 weeks. Local granulation appeared over the anastomosis in two patients and was successfully removed with the bronchoscope.

Table 5 Criteria raising suspicion of major tracheobronchial injury

A. Criteria in the early presentation or during conservative treatment	
History	Severe chest trauma especially to the upper part, neck trauma
Symptoms	Severe dyspnea, voice change
Signs	Progressive surgical emphysema, cyanosis, shock
X-ray	Mediastinal emphysema, fallen lung
CT findings	Endotracheal cuff herniation, tracheal wall discontinuity, bronchus discontinuity, displacement of the ETT, overdistension of the endotracheal cuff
After ICT	Massive air leakage with the failure of lung re-expansion
B. Criteria in late presentation	
History of severe chest trauma with continuing dyspnea, recurrent chest infection, lung consolidation or collapse	

There were non-comparable reasons for mortality in both groups. In the urgent repair group, the mortality of three cases was attributed to the involvement of other organ damage; two cases died because of brain injury, one case because of increased abdominal bleeding and shock after thoracic surgery and the fourth one died after adult respiratory distress syndrome (ARDS). In the delayed group, one patient developed complicated acute renal failure and the other two patients died after septic shock; one of them due to pneumonia after surgical airway repair and the other patient due to prolonged empyema.

The mortality varied according to the anatomical location of the airway injury, studies show a higher rate of fatality if the thoracic portion of the trachea was injured compared to the cervical part and higher mortality if injury with lower bronchus is injured [4]. Because it is difficult to ventilate/oxygenate, even after tracheal intubation and mechanical ventilation, and even get worsened [18]. Thus, those who survive the accident were those with upper injuries while those who die at the scene were those with lower injuries [19].

Conclusion

Bronchoscopic examination remains the standard tool for diagnosing major tracheobronchial injuries. We recommend urgent surgical repair for the treatment of major airway injury to avoid infections and other complications. The conservative management must be reserved for smaller tears in stable patients and should be reverted to surgery upon the worsening of clinical or radiological findings.

Study limitation

Our limitations included the retrospective nature of the study depending on the available amount of data contained in the computer database. Missing data like

Table 6 Outcome of surgical repair

	Total cases (28)	Urgent repair (21)	Delayed repair (7)	*P* value
Suture line dehiscence/prolonged air leakage*	3 (10.7%)	1 (4.8%)	2 (28.6%)	< 0.001
Empyema	3 (10.7%)	2 (9.5%)	1 (14.3%)	
Airway stenosis	3 (10.7%)	1 (4.8%)	2 (28.6%)	
Endobroncheal granulation tissue	2 (7.1%)	1 (4.8%)	1 (14.3%)	
Mortality	7 (25%)	4 (19.1%)	3 (42.8%)	

*Prolonged air leakage: more than seven days of air leakage

airway management at the scene and the follow-up data were not complete with short-term follow-up period. The co-relation of death and the airway injury was determined subjectively as usually there are no detailed nor clear statements in our patients' files on the exact scenario of death.

Abbreviations
TBI: Tracheobronchial injuries; CXR: Chest x-ray; US: Ultrasound; CT: Computed tomography; ATLS: Advanced trauma life support; ICT: Intercostal tube; ETT: Endotracheal tube; ER: Emergency room; ARDS: Adult respiratory distress syndrome

Acknowledgements
Not applicable.

Authors' contributions
-HEA, MAE, and BMA: (1) Substantial contributions to conception and design, acquisition of data, or analysis and interpretation of data; (2) drafting the article or revising it critically for important intellectual content; and (3) final approval of the version to be published. HEA and BMA: Data collection and analysis, methodology development, and manuscript writing.

Author details
[1]Cardiothoracic Surgery Department, Faculty of Medicine, Mansoura University, Mansoura, Egypt. [2]Cardiothoracic Surgery Department, Faculty of Medicine, Cairo University, Cairo, Egypt. [3]Cardiothoracic Surgery Department, Faculty of Medicine, Benha University, 15 Hasan Muwafi St., Hi Elrawdah, New Benha, Qalyobia 13518, Egypt.

References
1. Schneider T, Volz K, Dienemann H, Hoffmann H (2009) Incidence and treatment modalities of tracheobronchial injuries in Germany. Interact Cardiovasc Thorac Surg. 8:571–576
2. Henry S, Brasel K, Stewart RM (2018) Advanced trauma life support, student course manual Tenth edition. American College of Surgeons. 65
3. Richardson JD (2004) Outcome of tracheobronchial injuries: a long term perspective. J Trauma. 56:30–36
4. Scaglione M, Romano S, Pinto A, Sparano A, Scialpi M, Rotondo A (2006) Acute tracheobronchial injuries: impact of imaging on diagnosis and management implications. Eur J Radiol. 59:336–343
5. Koletsis E, Prokakis C, Baltayiannis N, Apostolakis E, Chatzimichalis A, Dougenis D (2012) Surgical decision making on the basis of clinical evidences and the injury's anatomical setting. Injury. 43:1437–1441
6. Fatimi SH, Hanif HM, Ahmed A, Shamsi G, Muzaffar M (2011) Outcomes of surgical management of tracheobronchial injuries - a case series from a developing country. Chinese J Traumatol. 14(3):161–164
7. Saad R Jr, Gonçalves R, Perlingeiro JA DNVG, Rivaben JH, Botter M et al (2017) Tracheobronchial injuries in chest trauma: a 17-year experience. Rev. Col. Bras.Cir. 44(2):194–201
8. Balci AE, Eren N, Eren S, Ulku R (2002) Surgical treatment of post-traumatic tracheobronchial injuries: 14-year experience. European Journal of Cardio-thoracic Surgery. 22:984–989
9. Milner A (2008) The airway in face, head, and neck injury. SAJAA. 14:52–57
10. Nelson LA (2007) Airway trauma. Int Anesthesiol Clin. 45:99–118
11. Kummer C, Netto FS, Rizoli S, Yee D (2007) A review of traumatic airway injuries: potential implications for airway assessment and management. Injury. 38:27–33
12. Farzanegan R, Alijanipour P, Akbarshahi H, Abbasidezfouli A, Pejhan S, Daneshvar A et al (2011) Major airways trauma, management and long term results. Ann Thorac Cardiovasc Surg. 17:544–551
13. Rossbach MM, Johnson SB, Gomez MA, Sako EY, Miller OL, Calhoon JH (1998) Management of major tracheobronchial injuries: a 28 year experience. Ann Thorac Surg. 65:182–186
14. Savas R, Alper H (2008) Fallen lung sign: radiographic findings. Diagn Interv Radiol. 14:120–121
15. Scaglione M, Romano S, Pinto A et al (2006) Acute tracheobronchial injuries: impact of imaging on diagnosis and management implications. Eur J Radiol. 59:336–343
16. Iwasaki M, Kaga K, Ogawa J, Inoue H, Shohtsu A (1994) Bronchoscopy findings and early treatment of patients with blunt tracheo-bronchial trauma. J Cardiovasc Surg. 35:269–271
17. Carretta A, Melloni G, Bandiera A, Negri G, Voci C, Zannini P (2011) Conservative and surgical treatment of acute posttraumatic tracheobronchial injuries. World J Surg. 35:2568–2574
18. Glazer ES, Meyerson SL (2008) Delayed presentation and treatment of tracheobronchial injuries due to blunt trauma. J Surg Educ. 65:302–308
19. Hurford WE, Peralta R (2003) Management of tracheal trauma. Can J Anesth. 50(suppl):R1–R6

14

Uniportal video-assisted thoracoscopic drainless sympathectomy for palmar and palmo-plantar hyperhidrosis: an institutional experience

Mohammed Ahmed El-Hag-Aly[1], Rafik Fekry Soliman[1], Nehad Abdo Zaid[2], Mahmoud Said Eldesouky[2], Mohamed Mordy Bakoush[1] and Mohamed Gamal Hagag[1*]

Abstract

Background: Primary hyperhidrosis (PH) still impacts negatively the patient's quality of life (QoL). Progressively, it leads to poorer QoL regardless of gender. The endoscopic thoracic sympathectomy has been used safely and effectively for control of palmar hyperhidrosis, but it is still questionable in palmo-plantar type. We assessed the benefits of uniportal drainless thoracoscopic sympathectomy (UDTS) for palmo-plantar hyperhidrosis patients compared to palmar ones.

This prospective study comprised 213 consecutive patients with PH. They underwent bilateral simultaneous UDTS. We used the Hyperhidrosis Disease Severity Scale (HDSS) scoring system for assessment of QoL pre- and postoperatively. Follow-up was continued for 1-year that was aiming to detect the QoL improvement, recurrence, and compensatory hyperhidrosis (CH).

Results: All patients experienced immediate complete resolution of hyperhidrosis postoperatively. Recurrence was encountered in one patient during the first 6 months. All patients had improved QoL postoperatively, but at the end of 1-year follow-up, 2.8% of patients were still suffering moderate to severe impaired QoL. Mean hospital stay was 31.79 ± 17.5 h. We found significant longer hospital stay in palmar group than palmo-plantar group. There was no significant difference between both groups in neither operative time, recurrence, nor CH.

Conclusions: UDTS offers better QoL for patients with PH even the palmo-plantar type. The palmo-plantar type benefits similarly to the palmar type in terms of comparable postoperative QoL and CH incidence.

Keywords: Hyperhidrosis, Sympathectomy, Thoracoscopy, Thoracic surgery, Video assisted

Background

Hyperhidrosis is a sweat glands' benign functional disorder. Usually, the hyperhidrosis patient presents by heat or emotional stimulated excessive sweating beyond the physiological needs. Moreover, it causes psycho-social and professional embracement that negatively impacts the quality of life (QoL) [1–3].

* Correspondence: mohamedhagag@med.menofia.edu.eg
[1]Cardiothoracic Surgery Department, Faculty of Medicine, Menoufia University, Yassin Abdel Ghaffar Street, Shebin El-Kom, Menoufia, Egypt
Full list of author information is available at the end of the article

Hyperhidrosis may be primary or secondary. The etiology of primary hyperhidrosis (PH) is still unknown. It affects about 0.6 to 1% in the general population. The most usual sites or domains of hyperhidrosis are the hands in 25% of cases, armpit in 20%, both in 55%, and plantar hyperhidrosis in 45% of cases [2, 4].

Management of those patients includes many medications as topical medication and botulinum toxin injection [5]. In 1920s, the trans-thoracotomy surgical treatment started to appear in medical practice with significant patient morbidity. It failed to generate widespread acceptance [6]. Evolving thoracoscopy approach enhanced the thoracoscopic sympathectomy to become the surgical technique of choice for treating PH. This minimally invasive procedure is simple and safe, with a high success rate with low morbidity and short hospital stay [7]. Although, being an effective method for management of PH, it has some complications such as compensatory hyperhidrosis (CH), pneumothorax, Horner's syndrome, postoperative pain, and recurrence [8, 9].

We assessed the benefits of uniportal drainless thoracoscopic sympathectomy (UDTS) for palmo-plantar hyperhidrosis patients compared to palmar ones.

Methods

From April 2018 to August 2019, we enrolled in a prospective observational study 213 consecutive patients with a diagnosis of PH. They underwent bilateral UDTS. Inclusion criteria were as follows: patients had bilateral PH, no hormonal or electrolyte imbalances, failed medical treatment with different topical medication for 3 months, failed or refused botulinum toxin injection, and patients with Hyperhidrosis Disease Severity Scale (HDSS) [10] score of 3 or 4. Exclusion criteria included secondary hyperhidrosis and previous thoracic surgeries. Primary surgical outcome was set as improved HDSS score of 2° at 1-year follow-up, while secondary surgical outcomes were postoperative pain score, complications, hospital stay, residual pneumothorax, patients needing chest tube placement, and CH severely affecting QoL.

We managed the patients in the Cardiothoracic Surgery and Vascular Surgery departments in our institution. Our Institutional ethical committee approved data collection and waived the need for patient consent.

We used The HDSS scoring system (Table 1) to evaluate patient's QoL throughout the study. We included patients with severe QoL impairment; those are patients who scored 3 or 4 in the scale. They were managed by bilateral simultaneous UDTS. We operated the right side at first then the left one in the same session.

Anesthesiologist used general inhalational anesthesia through double lumen endotracheal tube. The latter allowed for single lung ventilation during the operation. The patients were positioned in 45° anti-Trendelenburg supine position with both arms abducted at 90°; this enhanced that both sides could be operated on the same session without repositioning. It ended up with saving more time.

We operated through one skin incision (12–15 mm). In males, the incision was placed in the 3rd or 4th space at anterior axillary line; while in females, it was placed under mammary crease for cosmetic purpose. Through this single opening, we introduced 10-mm camera (Karl Storz, Germany) and electrocautery endoscopic spatula (Karl Storz, Germany); no insufflator was required. We preferred the 10-mm camera as its shaft is rigid enough to retract the lung in comparison to the 5-mm camera which will be more fragile and may be scratched or spoiled during introduction of spatula with the 5-mm camera through the same opening.

Parietal pleura, overlying the chain, was incised using electrocautery surgical unit (EMED "es350", Poland). The electrocautery unit was set at 40 degrees level of soft dissecting coagulation mode. Then, the sympathetic chain was divided by 5-s continuous cautery at top and bottom of R2, R3, and R4 levels. The lateral aspect of each rib was cauterized for 1–2 cm to ensure a complete cut of any Kuntz's inter-neuronal connections. If the

Table 1 HDSS scoring system [10]

Hyperhidrosis Disease Severity Scale
'How would you rate the severity of your hyperhidrosis?'
□ 1. My sweating is never noticeable and never interferes with my daily activities.
□ 2. My sweating is tolerable but sometimes interferes with my daily activities
□ 3. My sweating is barely tolerable and frequently interferes with my daily activities
□ 4. My sweating is intolerable and always interferes with my daily activities
HDSS Score of 1: mild; HDSS Score of 2: moderate; HDSS Score of 3–4: severe.

Kuntz Fibers were left uncut, it may cause failure of the sympathetic denervation.

At the end of the procedure, the anesthesiologist resumed the continuous positive pressure ventilation for both lungs. We observed the lung re-expansion again. One or two stitches were applied to close the port site; the other side was operated afterwards using the same technique.

All patients were extubated and transferred to the recovery room till achieving full recovery from anesthesia. Discharge criteria to ward were normal equality of air entry on both sides and normal oxygen saturation. We used either paracetamol or non-steroidal anti-inflammatory drugs (NSAIDS) for pain control. We performed a chest x-ray film to detect postoperative hemothorax or pneumothorax. We recorded neurological problems (as: Horner's syndrome) and hospital stay (in hours).

Follow-up in the outpatient clinic was at 1-week, 6-month, and 1-year intervals after discharge. Every visit, we checked for improvement of QoL (using HDSS score), recurrence, CH (site and severity), and wound infection.

Table 2 Patient preoperative characteristics

Variable	*n* = 213
Age, mean ± SD	20.83 ± 4.12
Sex, *n* (%)	
Male	82 (38.5%)
Female	131 (61.5%)
BMI, mean ± SD	23.1 ± 2.9
Area/domain affected, *n* (%)	
Palmar	213 (100%)
Axillary	101 (47.4%)
Plantar	79 (37.1%)
Preoperative HDSS, *n* (%)	
3	118 (55.4%)
4	95 (44.6%)

BMI body mass index, *HDSS* Hyperhidrosis Disease Severity Scale

Statistical analysis

Collected data was expressed as mean and standard deviation (M ± SD) or number and percent (*n*, %). Comparison between the two groups was performed using *t* test, chi-square analysis (χ^2), or Fischer's exact test when appropriate. The data were considered significant if *P* value was less than 0.05. Statistical analysis was performed using IBM Statistical Package for Social Science (SPSS) version 20 (IBM corporation, Chicago, IL, USA).

Results

We operated 213 patients (61.5% females) using UDTS. They were 20.83 ± 4.12 years old. Seventy-nine (37.1%) patients had plantar domain of hyperhidrosis. Patient's characteristics are enlisted in Table 2.

Average overall hospital stay was 31.79 ± 17.5 h entailing the whole patient's stay within the hospital from admission till discharge. Unfortunately, some patients suffered few complications (Table 3) as pneumothorax in 6 (2.8%) patients from which 2 (0.9%) patients only required intercostal chest tube (ICT) insertion. No Horner's syndrome cases, wound infection, nor mortality were encountered in our series. The mean follow-up period for the overall cohort was 13.56 ± 1.11 months.

Starting from the 6-month follow-up visit, our patients began to complain of CH; the overall incidence was 35.7% of patients. Domains and percentages are grouped in Table 3. Moreover, we had one patient (0.5%) presented with recurrence. He refused to undergo a redo procedure again because it was affecting his left non-dominant limb, so according to his words "it is not affecting my daily life to force me for surgery again."

All patients experienced immediate complete resolution of hyperhidrosis postoperatively; however, 1 (0.5%) patient was still suffering severe impaired QoL at 6 months in comparison to 6 (2.8%) patients at 1-year interval (Table 3).

Table 3 Procedure data

Variable	*n* = 213
Operative time (minutes), mean ± SD	35.03 ± 4.1
Hospital stay (hours), mean ± SD	31.79 ± 17.5
Postoperative pneumothorax, *n* (%)	6 (2.8%)
Postoperative ICT, *n* (%)	2 (0.9%)
Duration of follow-up (months), mean ± SD	13.56 ± 1.11
Compensatory hyperhidrosis (CH), *n* (%)	76 (35.7%)
Areas/domains affected by CH, *n* (%)	
Palmar	1 (0.5%)
Axillary	1 (0.5%)
Plantar	30 (14.1%)
Facial	1 (0.5%)
Trunkal	75 (35.2%)
Recurrence	1 (0.5%)
Postoperative HDSS score at 6 months	
1	212 (99.5%)
3	1 (0.5%)
Postoperative HDSS score at 1 year	
1	200 (93.9%)
2	7 (3.3%)
3	4 (1.9%)
4	2 (0.9%)

ICT intercostal chest tube, *HDSS* Hyperhidrosis Disease Severity Scale

Ten (4.7%) patients did not achieve the primary outcome, and their QoL did not improve 2° at 1-year follow-up; consequently, they were excluded from further analysis.

On comparing the 75 (36.95%) patients with plantar domain (palmo-plantar group) to the remaining patients (palmar group) in the study group (Table 4), we detect significant longer hospital stay in palmar group. On the other side, we got no significant difference between both groups in operative time, recurrence, CH (percent and domains), nor postoperative HDSS score at 6-month and 1-year intervals.

Discussion

Currently, the endoscopic thoracic sympathectomy is accepted as a standard treatment technique for PH. This minimally invasive approach has many benefits as reducing postoperative pain, shorter hospitalization, earlier recovery and return to work, and fewer complications. Both sides can be treated in the same sitting, thus avoiding readmission for a second procedure for the opposite side [11].

This thoracoscopic approach allows clear delineation of the sympathetic chain and the ganglia including the collateral branches (Kuntz's nerves). Also, it allows for better visualization of the stellate ganglion and its preservation to avoid development of postoperative Horner's syndrome [12].

The initial history of the uniportal video-assisted thoracoscopic surgery had started from the results of the first prospective trial reporting the method to perform several thoracic procedures via 2-cm uniportal technique; it was initiated in 1998 and published in 2000 [13], 2001 [14], and 2003 [15]. The two most common limitations for the 2-cm uniportal technique are the crowding of surgical instruments that collide with one another and the optic that gets dirty easily [16].

The more cosmetic and interesting needlescopic sympathectomy, which was reported 20 years ago by Yamamoto et al. [17], did not gain popularity in practice or publications. Yamamoto et al., in their next publication in 2017, noted that "Only one article, which was authored by us, reported on the needlescopic technique through a single skin incision. The appliance had to be pulled out to enable use of a different shape. With the

Table 4 Palmar versus palmo-plantar outcome

Variable	Palmar (n = 128)	Palmo-plantar (n = 75)	P value
Age, mean ± SD	21.16 ± 3.79	20.6 ± 4.53	0.34
Sex, n (%)			
Male	50 (39.1%)	30 (40%)	1
Female	78 (60.9%)	45 (60%)	
BMI, mean ± SD	23.65 ± 3.29	22.21 ± 2	0.001
Preoperative HDSS score, n (%)			
3	68 (53.1%)	42 (56%)	0.77
4	60 (46.9%)	33 (44%)	
Operation time, mean ± SD	35.59 ± 3.99	34.35 ± 4.02	0.03
Hospital stay, mean ± SD	35.38 ± 21.26	26.07 ± 4.55	0.001
Pneumothorax, n (%)	6 (4.7%)	0	0.08
ICT, n (%)	2 (1.6%)	0	0.53
Compensatory hyperhidrosis (CH), n (%)	41 (32%)	26 (34.7%)	0.76
Areas affected by CH, n (%)			
Palmar	0	0	
Axillary	0	0	
Plantar	12 (9.4%)	9 (12%)	0.63
Facial	0	0	
Trunkal	40 (31.3%)	26 (34.7%)	0.64
Post-operative HDSS score at 6 months, n (%)			
1	128 (100%)	75 (100%)	
Post-operative HDSS score at 1 year, n (%)			
1	127 (99.2%)	73 (97.3%)	0.56
2	1 (0.8%)	2 (2.7%)	

BMI body mass index, *ICT* intercostal chest tube, *HDSS* Hyperhidrosis Disease Severity Scale previous technique, a sharp tip device could not be inserted. Mobilization, separation, and extraction were not possible with the previous technique." Furthermore, they expected that the new 2017 device would not be popular also; they reported that "some difficulties in the use of the new device include shortage of strength and unsuitability for complicated structures because of its joints and limited diameter. Parts of the appliance falling off might become a serious medical accident" [18].

Our study included 213 patients diagnosed as PH and managed by UDTS. They had immediate improvement of hyperhidrosis without any mortality. There was no need for the placement of any additional ports. We had no conversions to open thoracotomy in our series.

Mean BMI in our study was 23.1 ± 2.9. This is going similarly with Woloske et al.'s [19] study who reported mean BMI of 20.6 ± 3 and 21.9 ± 2.55 for their adolescent and adult groups. Miller et al. [20], in their study of 282 patients, found that increased BMI was associated with increased CH. Patients with higher BMI have more difficulty with their thermoregulation.

Using the HDSS scoring for selecting patients, the patients who scored 3 were 55.4% of study patients and those who scored 4 were 44.6%. Postoperatively, at 1-year follow-up, dramatic improvement of patients' QoL was achieved. Our patients' HDSS score was changed to 93.9% mild and 6.1% moderate to severe. This was quite the same as Kuijpers et al. [21]; in their study including 100 patients with bilateral thoracoscopic sympathectomy, they reported significant improvement of HDSS score with mean preoperative HDSS score of 3.69 ± 0.47 and mean postoperative HDSS of 1.06 ± 0.34. This emphasizes that UDTS is an effective line in management of PH with improved QoL.

Despite that dramatic improvement in QoL, we noticed the occurrence of CH. It manifests as excessive sweating in different areas of body appearing later after completely free interval of any excessive sweating. In our study, most of them were after 6 months; its overall incidence was 35.7% of patients. This is still the most common late complication, although its mechanism is still unclear.

CH after thoracoscopic sympathectomy has been previously explained as a thermoregulatory response to the anhidrosis induced by the sympathectomy. It is doubtful, however, that the large quantity of sweat observed in CH aids in body temperature control. There is vast evidence to indicate that there is a nerve system emitting a large quantity of sudomotor signaling to the skin where CH appears. Interrupting one of the nerve circuits related to CH could result in CH being ameliorated; however, it has proved difficult to detect precisely where the nerve circuitry is located [22].

The incidence of CH in our study was lower than that of Prasad et al.'s [23] study. They had CH incidence of 63% postoperatively after R3 resection. Ibrahim et al. [24], who resected from R2 to R4, reported that 19% of their patients got CH and showed a gradually decreasing intensity over the follow-up period.

Our lower incidence of CH may be due to adding the cauterization of R2 with lateral extension of cauterization for 2 cm at every level that ensured good control of early migrating fibers of Kuntz nerves. The latter is usually claimed for the CH. The other contributing factor to lower CH incidence may be the cauterization at upper and lower margins of every level.

The UDTS procedure required an operative time of 20–45 min with mean of 35.03 ± 4.1 min. Nearly, Ibrahim et al. [24], who operated 260 patients with single-stage bilateral thoracoscopic sympathectomy, reported a mean operating time of 38 ± 5.0 min. On the other side, Kuijpers et al. [21] got a mean operative time of 74 ± 12 min for a bilateral sympathectomy. Kuijpers et al. [21] used to perform their operation in lateral decubitus position, so more time was consumed in patient repositioning. When they changed the patient's positioning to beach chair position, they could perform the surgery on both sides without the need for repositioning. This modification saved more time and showed significant reduction in their operation time to 47 ± 18 min ($p < 0.001$).

Post-UDTS pain was tolerable; it required only oral paracetamol or NSAIDs. No patient needed morphine. The UDTS approach causes less postoperative pain as post-thoracoscopic pain is usually related to the trauma of the thoracic wall caused by introducing the trocars into the intercostal space and periosteal injury.

Concerning the importance of the palmo-plantar type, the plantar domain affects considerable part (about 45%) of those patients with PH [4]. Other studies reported incidence of plantar domain of 70 to 100% in patients with PH; the latter researchers used extended technique of ablation from R3 to R12 to manage those cases [25]. In the Society of Thoracic Surgeons 2011 Expert Consensus for the Surgical Treatment of Hyperhidrosis [26], no recommendations for plantar domain management were noted. All the previous reasons aroused us to study the plantar type of hyperhidrosis patients using a less invasive technique and searching for acceptable outcome.

On comparing the palmo-plantar patients to palmar ones, we found comparable groups with no significant difference regarding age, sex distribution, preoperative HDSS score, pneumothorax, or recurrence.

Mean hospital stay was 35.38 ± 21.26 h in palmar group. It was significantly longer than the mean hospital stay in palmo-plantar group that was 26.07 ± 4.55 h (p = 0.001). That longer stay may be due to higher rate of pneumothorax (4.7%) and intercostal tube insertion (1.6%) in the palmar group.

Regarding CH incidence, it was not significant between the two groups (32% in palmar group and 34.7% in palmo-plantar group). Moreover, its distribution was not significant; the most common site was trunkal region followed by plantar region. Precisely, the plantar CH incidence was 9.4% in palmar group. This was nearly like the CH incidence of 12% in palmo-plantar group. This similar incidence is enforcing the hypothesis that patients with palmo-plantar hyperhidrosis would benefit from UDTS.

At last, the overall outcome was satisfactory. The patients' HDSS score at 1-year follow-up was 1 (mild) in 99.2% of palmar group patients and 97.3% of palmo-plantar ones. Even with the suffering of CH, it still affects the QoL less than PH. The reported CH in our series was mild and much less affecting the professional or social life of our patients.

Overtime, the researchers are still trying to provide more options for managing the CH. This future solutions for CH will allow us to provide more UDTS procedures for PH patients. One of that promising trials is the use of intraoperative monitoring with laser speckle flowgraphy (LSFG) to indicate the causative ganglion of the CH. Ganglionectomy was then performed [22]. It is a very good technique but expensive. The cost of LSFG is about US$30,000.00. Weksler [27] commented to the report of LSFG technique saying that "the case report lacks some details that would be helpful to others attempting to duplicate the results. Specific parameters used for ganglia stimulation during laser speckle flow graphing, including voltage and duration, are not reported, and it is not clear what precautionary measures Yamamoto and Okada [22] took preoperatively and intraoperatively to ensure that the identified ganglia were, in fact, responsible for the CH. Yamamoto and Okada [22] also did not comment on the presence or absence of any undesirable side effects of the procedure. Larger studies are needed to define clearly the efficacy of this procedure and its reproducibility." Ongoing studies and researches everywhere keep on trying to help CH patients, and that provides the light at the end of the tunnel for those patients.

Conclusion

UDTS offers better QoL for patients with PH even the palmo-plantar type. The palmo-plantar type benefits similarly to the palmar type in terms of comparable postoperative QoL and CH incidence.

Abbreviations

CH: Compensatory hyperhidrosis; HDSS: Hyperhidrosis Disease Severity Scale; ICT: Intercostal chest tube; NSAIDS: Non-steroidal anti-inflammatory drugs; PH: Primary hyperhidrosis; QoL: Quality of life; UDTS: Uniportal drainless thoracoscopic sympathectomy

Acknowledgements

Not applicable.

Authors' contributions

All authors have read and approved the manuscript. They were all involved in conceptualization, investigation, methodology, resources, and visualization. RS and NZ were involved in project administration. MAE, RS, NZ, and MH were involved in supervision and review and editing of the writing. MAE, MSE, MB, and MH were involved in data curation, formal analysis, software, validation, and writing the original draft.

Author details

[1]Cardiothoracic Surgery Department, Faculty of Medicine, Menoufia University, Yassin Abdel Ghaffar Street, Shebin El-Kom, Menoufia, Egypt. [2]Vascular Surgery Department, Faculty of Medicine, Menoufia University, Yassin Abdel Ghaffar Street, Shebin El-Kom, Menoufia, Egypt.

References

1. Wolosker N, Munia MA, Kauffman P, Campos JR, Yazbek G, Puech-Leão P (2010) Is gender a predictive factor for satisfaction among patients undergoing sympathectomy to treat palmar hyperhidrosis? Clinics (Sao Paulo) 65(6):583–586. https://doi.org/10.1590/S1807-59322010000600004
2. Gossot D, Kabiri H, Caliandro R, Debrosse D, Girard P, Grunenwald D (2001) Early complications of thoracic endoscopic sympathectomy: a prospective study of 940 procedures. Ann Thorac Surg 71(4):1116–1119. https://doi.org/10.1016/S0003-4975(01)02422-5
3. Hajjar WM, Al-Nassar SA, Al-Sharif HM, Al-Olayet DM, Al-Otiebi WS, Al-Huqayl AA et al (2019) The quality of life and satisfaction rate of patients with upper limb hyperhidrosis before and after bilateral endoscopic thoracic sympathectomy. Saudi J Anaesth 13(1):16–22. https://doi.org/10.4103/sja.SJA_335_18
4. Karmota AG, Aboollo MF, Hafez BA, Shaker AA, Ghoneim B (2018) Prospective randomized study comparing video assisted thoracoscopic surgery (VATS) resection versus cautery for treatment of primary hyperhidrosis. J Egypt Soc Cardiothorac Surg 26:318–323. https://doi.org/10.1016/j.jescts.2018.11.005
5. Dumont P, Denoyer A, Robin P (2004) Long-term results of thoracoscopic sympathectomy for hyperhidrosis. Ann Thorac Surg 78(5):1801–1807. https://doi.org/10.1016/j.athoracsur.2004.03.012
6. Dewey TM, Herbert MA, Hill SL, Prince SL, Mack MJ (2006) One-year follow-up after thoracoscopic sympathectomy for hyperhidrosis: outcomes and consequences. Ann Thorac Surg 81(4):1227–1232; discussion 1232-3. https://doi.org/10.1016/j.athoracsur.2005.11.006
7. Chung IH, Oh CS, Koh KS, Kim HJ, Paik HC, Lee DY (2002) Anatomic variations of the T2 nerve root (including the nerve of Kuntz) and their implications for sympathectomy. J Thorac Cardiovasc Surg 123(3):498–501. https://doi.org/10.1067/mtc.2002.119340
8. Youssef T, Soliman M (2015) Unilateral sequential endoscopic thoracic sympathectomy for palmar hyperhidrosis: a proposed technique to overcome compensatory hyperhidrosis and improve plantar hyperhidrosis. J Laparoendosc Adv Surg Tech A 25(5):370–374. https://doi.org/10.1089/lap.2014.0620
9. Romero FR, Haddad GR, Miot HA, Cataneo DC (2016) Palmar hyperhidrosis: clinical, pathophysiological, diagnostic and therapeutic aspects. An Bras Dermatol 91(6):716–725. https://doi.org/10.1590/abd1806-4841.20165358
10. Schieman C, Gary J, Gelfand GJ, Grondin SC (2010) Hyperhidrosis: clinical presentation, evaluation and management. Expert Rev Dermatol 5(1):31–44. https://doi.org/10.1586/edm.09.61
11. Du X, Zhu X, Wang T et al (2018) Compensatory hyperhidrosis after different surgeries at the same sympathetic levels: a meta-analysis. Ann Transl Med 6(11):203. https://doi.org/10.21037/atm.2018.05.24
12. Vannucci F, Araújo JA (2017) Thoracic sympathectomy for hyperhidrosis: from surgical indications to clinical results. J Thorac Dis 9(Suppl 3):S178–S192. https://doi.org/10.21037/jtd.2017.04.04
13. Migliore M, Giuliano R, Deodato G (2000) Video assisted thoracic surgery through a single port. In: Thoracic surgery and interdisciplinary symposium on the threshold of the third millennium. An international continuing medical education programme, Naples, pp 29–30 Available online: http://xoomer.virgilio.it/naples2000/index1.html. Accessed 14 Aug 2020

14. Migliore M, Deodato G (2001) A single-trocar technique for minimally-invasive surgery of the chest. Surg Endosc 15:899–901. https://doi.org/10.1007/s004640090033
15. Migliore M (2003) Efficacy and safety of single-trocar technique for minimally invasive surgery of the chest in the treatment of noncomplex pleural disease. J Thorac Cardiovasc Surg 126:1618–1623. https://doi.org/10.1016/s0022-5223(03)00592-0
16. Migliore M, Calvo D, Criscione A, Borrata F (2015) Uniportal video assisted thoracic surgery: summary of experience, mini-review and perspectives. J Thorac Dis 7(9):E378–E380. https://doi.org/10.3978/j.issn.2072-1439.2015.07.35
17. Yamamoto H, Kanehira A, Kawamura M, Okada M, Ohkita Y (2000) Needlescopic surgery for palmar hyperhidrosis. J Thorac Cardiovasc Surg 120(2):276–279. https://doi.org/10.1067/mtc.2000.107830
18. Yamamoto H, Okada M (2017) A new device of needlescopic thoracic sympathectomy through a skin incision. Ann Thorac Surg 103:e465–e467. https://doi.org/10.1016/j.athoracsur.2016.11.068
19. Wolosker N, Faustino CB, de Campos JRM et al (2020) Comparative analysis of the results of videothoracoscopic sympathectomy in the treatment of hyperhidrosis in adolescent patients. J Pediatr Surg 55(3):418–424. https://doi.org/10.1016/j.jpedsurg.2019.11.004
20. Miller DL, Bryant AS, Force SD, Miller JI Jr (2009) Effect of sympathectomy level on the incidence of compensatory hyperhidrosis after sympathectomy for palmar hyperhidrosis. J Thorac Cardiovasc Surg 138(3):581–585. https://doi.org/10.1016/j.jtcvs.2009.03.059
21. Kuijpers M, Klinkenberg TJ, Bouma W, DeJongste MJ, Mariani MA (2013) Single-port one-stage bilateral thoracoscopic sympathicotomy for severe hyperhidrosis: prospective analysis of a standardized approach. J Cardiothorac Surg 8:216. https://doi.org/10.1186/1749-8090-8-216
22. Yamamoto H, Okada M (2019) The management of compensatory sweating after thoracic sympathectomy. J Thorac Cardiovasc Surg 158:1481–1488. https://doi.org/10.1016/j.jtcvs.2019.05.062
23. Prasad A, Ali M, Kaul S (2010) Endoscopic thoracic sympathectomy for primary palmar hyperidrosis. Surg Endosc 24(8):1952–1957. https://doi.org/10.1007/s00464-010-0885-5
24. Ibrahim M, Menna C, Andreetti C et al (2013) Bilateral single-port sympathectomy: long-term results and quality of life. Biomed Res Int 2013:348017. https://doi.org/10.1155/2013/348017
25. Elalfy K, Emile S, Elfeki H, Elmetwally A, Farag M, Gado W (2017) Sequential extended thoracoscopic sympathicotomy for palmo-axillo-plantar hyperhidrosis. Ann Thorac Surg 104(4):1200–1207. https://doi.org/10.1016/j.athoracsur.2017.04.035
26. Cerfolio RJ, De Campos JR, Bryant AS et al (2011) The Society of Thoracic Surgeons expert consensus for the surgical treatment of hyperhidrosis. Ann Thorac Surg 91(5):1642–1648. https://doi.org/10.1016/j.athoracsur.2011.01.105
27. Weksler B (2017) Is there light at the end of the tunnel for patients with severe compensatory hyperhidrosis? J Thorac Cardiovasc Surg 154(6):e117. https://doi.org/10.1016/j.jtcvs.2017.08.054

15

Primary versus staged repair of Fallot with borderline pulmonary artery anatomy

Basem M. Abdelgawad[1*], Mahmoud A. Elshafie[1], Suzan Bayoumy[2] and Elatafy E. Elatafy[3]

Abstract

Background: Surgical management of tetralogy of Fallot (TOF) can be either with a total primary repair or staged repair. The superiority of one technique over the other is still debatable, especially in developing countries with late presentation and limited resources. The objective of this study was to compare the outcome of patients with tetralogy of Fallot and borderline pulmonary anatomy defined as McGoon ratio between 1.2 and 1.6 who underwent primary versus staged repair.

Results: The patients were divided into two groups: group A included patients who underwent primary repair ($n = 120$) and group B included patients who underwent repair after previous modified Blalock-Taussig (MBT) shunt operation ($n = 100$). Patients in group B were significantly older (11 ± 2.6 vs. 7 ± 3.1 months; $p < 0.001$) and had higher McGoon ratio (1.61 ± 0.07 vs. 1.5 ± 0.08; $p < 0.001$). In group B, the total operative time (277 ± 21.3 vs. 232 ± 24.6 min; $p < 0.001$), cardiopulmonary bypass time (81 ± 13.7 vs. 60 ± 11.2 min; $p < 0.001$), and ischemic time (64 ± 12 vs. 53 ± 7.1 min; $p < 0.001$) were significantly higher. There was no difference in postoperative complications between both groups. In-hospital mortality was nine patients (7.5%) in group A and 6 (6%) in group B ($p = 0.791$).

Conclusion: Primary repair of tetralogy of Fallot in patients with borderline McGoon ratio is safe with low morbidity and mortality. It has the potential of decreasing hospital stay, cost, and resource utilization of the two-stage repair.

Keywords: Tetralogy of Fallot, McGoon ratio, Primary Fallot repair, Blalock-Taussig shunt

Background

Tetralogy of Fallot (TOF) is the most frequent cyanotic heart disease with an incidence of 3–6 per 10,000 live births. Significant advances in the surgical repair of TOF have been achieved, with more than 90% of patients surviving to adulthood [1].

The optimum timing and options for surgical repair of TOF is still the subject of ongoing research. Different surgical strategies are available according to the underlying anatomy, and the surgical approach can be either a single-stage or a two-stage repair. The latter consists of initial palliation with a modified Blalock–Taussig (MBT), followed by total repair at a later stage [2]. Opinions diverge from those who prefer neonatal repair in all symptomatic TOF patients to those preferring to postpone complete repair until later in life, depending on a temporary MBT shunt when necessary [3].

Two-stage repair avoids the risks of heart-lung machine in low-weight children. However, the early total correction has the benefits of avoiding MBT shunt complications, such as distortion of the pulmonary arteries, early relief of systemic hypoxia, which allows a normal rate of growth, preventing progressive right ventricle (RV) hypertrophy, and early normalization of cardiac chambers flow and pressure [4].

The objective of our study was to compare the outcomes of TOF patients with McGoon ratio between 1.2 and 1.6 who underwent primary repair versus those who underwent repair after a previous modified Blalock–Taussig (MBT) shunt.

Methods

Patients population

Our multicenter study included 220 consecutive TOF patients with McGoon ratio between 1.2 and 1.6 operated

* Correspondence: bassem.abdelgawad@fmed.bu.edu.eg
[1]Cardiothoracic Surgery Department, Faculty of Medicine, Benha University, 15 Hasan Muwafi St., Hi Elrawdah,, New Benha, Qalyobia 13518, Egypt
Full list of author information is available at the end of the article

between January 2014 and June 2019. Patients were divided into two groups: group A included 120 patients who underwent primary repair and group B included 100 patients who underwent the two-stage repair. Patients were assigned to each group according to the preference of the surgical team. Patients who had an associated absent pulmonary valve, atrioventricular canal defect, or pulmonary atresia were excluded. The choice of the patients into either group was based on surgical team preference and experience.

Preoperative parameters

Patient data were retrospectively collected from the data registry in the cardiac surgery unit of each hospital. Preoperative data included patients' characteristics, echocardiographic, and multi-slice CT details, especially right ventricular outflow tract (RVOT) pressure gradient, degree of aortic overriding, size of the pulmonary annulus, and McGoon ratio.

Surgical technique

Median sternotomy was performed, whether primary or redo sternotomy. At the second stage, dissection of MBT shunt was done before cardiopulmonary bypass (CPB) and then ligated and divided after starting bypass. Patent ductus arteriosus (PDA) was ligated and divided if present to free the pulmonary arteries. All operations were performed using aorto-bicaval cannulation with intermittent doses of cold blood cardioplegia for myocardial protection. The trans-atrial approach was chosen for ventricular septal defect (VSD) closure using Gore-Tex® or Dacron® patch (Gore-Tex; W. L. Gore & Associates, Inc., Flagstaff, Ariz). Trans-atrial infundibular resection was then performed and completed through a pulmonary arteriotomy "trans-atrial-transpulmonary approach." Trans-ventricular resection was performed, especially when the trans-annular patch was indicated or with a narrow right ventricular outflow tract (RVOT), which was augmented by a pericardial patch. Pulmonary commissurotomy was performed in almost all patients, and when a small annulus was detected by not passing the calculated Hegar dilator size, our incision was extended few millimeters below the annulus. We have routinely augmented the main pulmonary artery using a pericardial patch. The patch was extended proximally across the annulus when indicated and distally to enlarge any existing branch pulmonary artery stenosis. The tricuspid valve was repaired if there was more than mild regurgitation with the saline test. After weaning from bypass, right ventricle and pulmonary artery (PA) pressures were directly measured, and pressure gradient less than 30 mmHg and RV/left ventricle (LV) pressure less than 60% were accepted.

Operative parameters

Total operative, cardiopulmonary bypass, and cross-clamp times, a gradient across RVOT, and RV/LV pressure after repair were collected.

Postoperative parameters

Duration of intensive care unit (ICU) stay, mechanical ventilation, and hospital stay, and complications including bleeding, arrhythmias, wound or chest infections, renal or hepatic dysfunction, and need of inotropic support were collected from medical charts.

Echocardiography was done before discharge to evaluate gradient across the RVOT, tricuspid insufficiency, pulmonary insufficiency, right and left ventricular functions, pericardial effusions, and any residual shunts.

Statistical analysis

Data interpretation and statistical analysis were performed using SPSS vs.25. (IBM, Armonk, New York, USA). Comparisons between the two groups were done using the independent t test for numerical data. Categorical data were compared using the Chi-squared test. p values less than 0.05 were considered significant.

Results

Two hundred and twenty TOF patients with McGoon ratio between 1.2 and 1.6 were divided into two groups according to the repair strategy.

Preoperative and operative data

Preoperative patients' data are presented in Table 1. There was a higher-pressure gradient across the RVOT in group B ($p = 0.008$). McGoon ratio was 1.4 ± 0.12 before shunt operation and was 1.61 ± 0.07 before the second stage in group B and was 1.5 ± 0.08 in group A.

Total operative, cardiopulmonary bypass, and ischemic times were higher in group B ($p < 0.001$). Post-bypass evaluation of repair using RV/PA pressure and RV/LV pressure was non-significant between the two groups (33 ± 6.3 vs. 34 ± 9 in groups A and B respectively, $p = 0.35$). All patients were weaned successfully from cardiopulmonary bypass with no intraoperative mortality (Table 2).

Postoperative data

Four patients, two in each group, were transferred to ICU with open-chest; three of them were exposed to longer bypass time with visible myocardial edema despite using hemofilter, and the 4th case had excessive oozing with an anticipated need for exploration. All the 4 cases were closed after 24–48 h. The ICU and hospital stay time were non-significant between both groups ($p = 0.116$ and 0.183, respectively). Arrhythmias were treated medically in all patients, and two patients in group A and one in group B required permanent pacemaker insertion. (Table 3).

Table 1 Preoperative patients' data (continuous variables are presented as mean, standard deviation and range and categorical data as number and percent) (*RVOT* right ventricular outflow tract)

	Group A (n = 120)	Group B (n = 100)	p value
Age (months)			
Range	3.5–9	8–14	
Mean ± SD	7 ± 3.1	11 ± 2.6	< 0.001
Weight (kg)			
Range	4–8.5	8.3–14	
Mean ± SD	6.8 ± 2.2	9 ± 3.1	< 0.001
Male	66 (55%)	60 (60%)	0.455
McGoon ratio	1.5 ± 0.08	1.61 ± 0.07	
Mean ± SD			< 0.001
O_2 saturation (%)			
Range	60–92	76–88	< 0.001
Mean ± SD	74 ± 12	82 ± 4.3	
Pressure gradient across RVOT (mmHg)			
Range	67–90	71–105	0.008
Mean ± SD	81.6 ± 6.3	84.5 ± 9.3	

Table 2 Operative data (continuous variables are presented as mean, standard deviation, and range and categorical data as number and percent) (*RVOT* right ventricular outflow tract, *RV* right ventricle, *PA* pulmonary artery)

	Group A (n = 120)	Group B (n = 100)	p value
Total operative time (minutes)			
Range	195–270	210–315	< 0.001
Mean ± SD	232 ± 24.6	277 ± 21.3	
Total bypass time (minutes)			
Range	52–110	67–130	< 0.001
Mean ± SD	60 ± 11.2	81 ± 13.7	
Ischemic time (minutes)			
Range	43–80	47–95	<0.001
Mean ± SD	53 ± 7.1	64 ± 12	
Approach for RVOT resection			
Trans-atrial- transpulmonary	38(31.7%)	40 (40%)	
Trans-ventricular	82 (68.3%)	60 (60%)	0.198
Pulmonary valve commissurotomy	48 (40%)	58 (58%)	0.008
Trans-annular patch	72 (60%)	42 (42%)	
Post bypass pressure RV/PA			
Range	18–46	24–44	0.35
Mean ± SD	33 ± 6.3	34 ± 9	

Table 3 Postoperative data.

	Group A (n = 120)	Group B (n = 100)	p value
Time of ventilation (hours)			
Range	18–280	14–248	0.037
Mean ± SD	44 ± 9.3	41 ± 11.5	
ICU stay (days)			
Range	3–22	3–23	0.116
Mean ± SD	5.3 ± 4.2	6.3 ± 5.2	
Hospital stay (days)			
Range	7–28	7–31	0.183
Mean ± SD	10 ± 4.8	11 ± 6.3	
Exploration for bleeding	4 (3.3%)	7 (7%)	0.233
Arrhythmia	46 (38.3%)	36 (36%)	0.806
SVT	22 (18.3%)	16 (16%)	
Nodal Rhythm	21 (17.5%)	18 (18%)	
CHB	3 (2.5%)	2 (2%)	
Deep Wound infection	2 (1.7%)	6 (6%)	0.145
Diaphragmatic paralysis	6 (5%)	3 (3%)	0.515
Operative mortality	9 (7.5%)	6 (6%)	0.791

(Continuous variables are presented as mean, standard deviation, and range and categorical data as number and percent) (*CHB* complete heart block, *ICU* intensive care unit, *SVT* supraventricular tachycardia)

Pre-discharge echocardiographic data

Pre-discharge echocardiographic data are presented in Table 4. Pericardial effusion was higher in group B but did not reach a significant value (11% vs. 6.7%; p = 0.336).

Discussion

The optimal surgical management of TOF has been the subject of ongoing debate, especially in the

Table 4 Pre-discharge echocardiographic data.

	Group A (n = 120)	Group B (n = 100)	p value
Pulmonary regurgitation			
No–mild	64 (53.3%)	50 (50%)	
Moderate	43 (35.8%)	40 (40%)	
Severe	13 (10.8%)	10 (10%)	0.835
PG across RVOT			
Range	15–40	10–40	
Mean ± SD	21 ± 3.3	22 ± 5.2	0.085
Residual VSD (< 3 mm)	7 (5.8%)	4 (4%)	0.758
Pericardial effusion Surgical evacuation of PE	8 (6.7%) 0	11 (11%) 3 (3%)	0.336 0.092

(Continuous variables are presented as mean, standard deviation, and range and categorical data as number and percent) (*PE* pericardial effusion, *PG* pressure gradient, *RVOT* right ventricular outflow tract, *VSD* ventricular septal defect)

developing countries with late presentation of TOF patients. Surgical management of TOF can be either with a total primary repair or staged repair. The superiority of one technique over the other is still debatable. Kanter and associates reported that primary repair or shunting of symptomatic neonates provides the same long-term outcome [5]. However, reports from other studies have shown superior results for primary total correction [4, 6–9].

The safety issue of CPB in small infants was argued. Hirsch and coworkers reported the rate of CPB-related complications in neonates who underwent primary total correction versus those who underwent palliative procedures in different types of congenital cardiac pathology. They have shown that CPB per se is not an independent determinant of survival and concluded that effective repair and proper pre- and postoperative management are the critical determinants of survival [9]. Several recent studies supported the early total correction of TOF irrespective of age and weight [1, 2, 4, 7].

The age of our patients at primary intervention was relatively higher compared to other series, which could be attributed to late referral for surgery and crowded waiting lists. Furthermore, all patients had McGoon ratio between 1.2 and 1.6, which had put them in the category of less favorable anatomy and consequently less favorable outcome for many centers. Many authors have published a low mortality rate for primary repair even at a younger age; however, they have not considered pulmonary artery anatomy as a risk factor.

McGoon ratio was higher in group B, which could be attributed to the growth of the pulmonary arteries after performing MBT shunt. Although the rate of trans-annular patch use was higher in group A, we did not find a statistical difference between the two groups in post-repair RV/PA and RV/LV pressure gradients. The difference in total operative, cardiopulmonary bypass, and ischemic times was significantly different, and this was related to the nature of the reoperation in group B, which required a lot of dissection under bypass support. There was no significant difference in postoperative complications between the two groups. These results were the same as reported by many other authors who showed that a previous systemic–pulmonary artery shunting palliation was not a significant risk factor for mortality and there was no significant difference in the duration of ICU or hospital stay in the group of patients who had staged repair versus those who had primary repair [2, 3, 5, 10, 11].

Our 30-day mortality was 7.5% in group A and 6% in group B. In group A, two patients developed intractable pulmonary hemorrhage, five patients developed progressive low cardiac output and heart failure, and two patients died after prolonged ventilation with respiratory and multi-organ failure. The causes of death in group B were refractory ventricular arrhythmia in one patient, low cardiac output and heart failure in four patients, and sudden cardiac arrest in one patient. Mulder and associates have published a multi-institutional report that included 938 patients, and they found that mortality for repair versus shunt group was similar (4.3% vs. 4.4%) [12].

In summary, this study showed that the outcome of primary TOF repair was comparable to that of staged repair. Operative times were prolonged with the staged repair; however, the primary repair was associated with longer ventilation time and more use of the trans-annular patch.

Study limitations

This study is a retrospective cohort study with its drawbacks of selection and referral biases. Another limitation is the short-term follow-up, and a longer follow-up study is recommended. Lastly, the study did not report the outcome of the shunt operations before offering a total repair in group B.

Conclusion

Primary repair of the tetralogy of Fallot in patients with borderline McGoon ratio is safe with low morbidity and mortality. It has the potential to decrease hospital stay, cost, and resource utilization compared to the two-stage repair.

Abbreviations

CHB: Complete heart block; CPB: Cardiopulmonary bypass; ICU: Intensive care unit; LV: Left ventricle; MBT: Modified Blalock-Taussig shunt; PA: Pulmonary artery; PG: Pressure gradient; RV: Right ventricle; RVOT: Right ventricular outflow tract; SVT: Supraventricular tachycardia; TOF: Tetralogy of Fallot; VSD: Ventricular septal defect

Acknowledgements

Not applicable.

Authors' contributions

BMA has made substantial contributions to the conception and design of the work, the acquisition, analysis, and interpretation of data, and the creation of new software used in the work, has drafted the work and substantively revised it, has approved the submitted version (and any substantially modified version that involves the author's contribution to the study), and has agreed both to be personally accountable for the author's own contributions and to ensure that questions related to the accuracy or integrity of any part of the work, even ones in which the author was not personally involved, are appropriately investigated, resolved, and the resolution documented in the literature. MAE, SB, and EEE have made substantial contributions to the conception, analysis, and interpretation of the data, substantively revised this work, has approved the submitted version (and any substantially modified version that involves the author's contribution to the study), and has agreed both to be personally accountable for the author's own contributions and to ensure that questions related to the accuracy or integrity of any part of the work, even ones in which the author was not personally involved, are appropriately investigated, resolved, and the resolution documented in the literature. All authors read and approved the final manuscript.

Author details
[1]Cardiothoracic Surgery Department, Faculty of Medicine, Benha University, 15 Hasan Muwafi St., Hi Elrawdah,, New Benha, Qalyobia 13518, Egypt.
[2]Cardiology Department, Faculty of Medicine, Tanta University, Tanta, Egypt.
[3]Cardiothoracic Surgery Department, Faculty of Medicine, Tanta University, Tanta, Egypt.

References

1. Gerrah R, Turner ME, Gottlieb D, Quaegebeur JM, Bacha E (2015) Repair of tetralogy of Fallot in children less than 4 kg body weight. Pediatr Cardiol 36: 1344–1349
2. Mimic B, Brown KL, Oswal N, Simmonds J, Hsia TY, Tsang VT (2014) Neither age at repair nor previous palliation affects outcome in tetralogy of Fallot repair. Eur J Cardiothorac Surg 45:92–99
3. Fraser CD, McKenzie ED, Cooley DA (2001) Tetralogy of Fallot: surgical management individualized to the patient. Ann Thorac Surg 71: 556–563
4. Menaissy Y, Omar E, Mofreh B, Alassal M (2019) Total correction of tetralogy of Fallot in the first 60 days of life in symptomatic infants: is it the gold standard? J Thorac Cardiovasc Surg 67(2). Georg Thieme Verlag KGDate: Feb 9, 2019 https://doi.org/10.1055/s-0039-1678698
5. Kanter KR, Kogon BE, Kirshbom PM, Carlock PR (2010) Symptomatic neonatal tetralogy of Fallot: repair or shunt? Ann Thorac Surg 89:858–863
6. Pigula FA, Khalil PN, Mayer JE, Del Nido P, Jonas RA (1999) Repair of tetralogy of Fallot in neonates and young infants. Circulation 100: 157–161
7. Ramakrishnan KV, Zurakowski D, Pastor W, Jonas RA, Sinha P (2018) Symptomatic tetralogy of Fallot in young infants: primary repair or shunt—pediatric health information system database analysis. World J Pediatr Congenital Heart Surg 9(5):539–554
8. Tamesberger MI, Lechner E, Mair R, Hofer A, Sames-Dolzer E, Tulzer G (2018) Early primary repair of tetralogy of Fallot in neonates and infants less than four months of age. Ann Thorac Surg 86:1928–1936
9. Hirsch JC, Mosca RS, Bove EL, EL. (2000) Complete repair of tetralogy of Fallot in the neonate results in the modern era. Ann Surg 232(4):508–514
10. Seddio F, Migliazza L, Borghi A, Crupi G (2007) Previous palliation in patients with tetralogy of Fallot does not influence the outcome of later repair. J Cardiovasc Med 8:119–122
11. Arafat AA, Elatafy EE, Elshedoudy S, Zalat M, Abdallah N, Elmahrouk A (2018) Surgical strategies protecting against right ventricular dilatation following tetralogy of Fallot repair. J Cardiothorac Surg 13(1):14. Published 2018 Jan 22. https://doi.org/10.1186/s13019-018-0702-0
12. Mulder TJ, Pyles LA, Stolfi A, Pickoff AS, Moller JH (2002) A multicenter analysis of the choice of initial surgical procedure in tetralogy of Fallot. Pediatr Cardiol 23:580–586

16

The effect of hyperlactatemia timing on the outcomes after cardiac surgery

Khaled D. Algarni[1,2]

Abstract

Background: Several studies linked postoperative hyperlactatemia to worse outcomes in adult patients undergoing cardiac surgery. However, data on the effect of timing of hyperlactatemia on outcomes are scarce. We sought to determine the prevalence of early hyperlactatemia (EHL) and its impact on clinical outcomes compared to late hyperlactatemia (LHL) in patients undergoing ACS procedures.

Results: We included 305 consecutive adult patients who underwent cardiac surgery procedures between July 2017 and Nov 2019 at a single institution. Lactate level was measured in the first 10 h after surgery and EHL was defined as lactate level > 3 mmol/L in the first hour after surgery. Logistic regression analysis was performed to determine predictors of EHL. Seventeen percent (n = 52) had EH while 83% (n = 253) did not. Patients with EHL had significantly longer cardiopulmonary bypass (P = 0.001) and cross-clamp (P = 0.001) times due to increased surgical complexity in this group. Early hyperlactatemia was associated with increased post-operative extracorporeal membrane oxygenation (ECMO) support (0% vs 5.7%, P < 0.001), longer intensive care unit stay (P = 0.004), and increased hospital mortality (0% vs. 3.8%, P = 0.009). Cardiopulmonary bypass time (OR 1.001; 95% CI 1.011–1.012, P = 0.02) and glucose level (OR 1.2; 95% CI 1.1–1.3, P = 0.003) were independently associated with increased rate of EHL. In contrast, diabetes mellitus (OR 0.26; 95% CI 0.12–0.55, P < 0.001) significantly attenuated the rate of EHL.

Conclusions: Early hyperlactatemia after cardiac surgery was associated with increased morbidity and mortality. Late hyperlactatemia was very common and had a self-limiting and benign course.

Keywords: Lactate, Cardiac surgery, Early hyperlactatemia, Late hyperlactatemia

Background

Lactate level is a robust biomarker and strong predictor of clinical outcomes in patients undergoing open-heart surgery and in critically ill patients [1–5]. Several studies confirmed the prognostic value of hyperlactatemia (HL) after cardiac surgery in predicting mortality and major morbidity [3, 6–12].

However, new evidence suggests that not all forms of HL are harmful after cardiac surgery [13, 14]. Maillet and colleagues found that the timing of HL plays a major role where patients with an immediate post-operative increased lactate level had worse outcomes compared to patients who developed hyperlactatemia late after surgery [13]. Therefore, the timing of hyperlactatemia (early versus late) may have different underlying mechanisms and different impacts on clinical outcomes after cardiac surgery. Indeed, conventional understanding suggests that stress-induced HL is due to anaerobic glycolysis as a result of tissue hypoperfusion, hypoxia, or both. However, recent studies linked some forms of stress HL to increased aerobic lactate production secondary to increased adrenergic stimulation, with or without decreased lactate clearance [1]. Thus, it seems that not all patterns of hyperlactatemia are harmful after cardiac surgery and that the timing of hyperlactatemia is one potential confounder of benign versus detrimental hyperlactatemia.

Correspondence: Khaledga999@hotmail.com
[1]Department of Cardiac Sciences, College of Medicine, King Saud University, P.O. Box 7805, Riyadh 11472, Saudi Arabia
[2]Department of Adult Cardiac Surgery, Prince Sultan Cardiac Center, Riyadh, Saudi Arabia

The purpose of the present study is to bridge this gap in knowledge by shedding light on the prevalence, predictors, and clinical consequences of early compared to late hyperlactatemia in adult patients undergoing cardiac surgery.

Methods

Patient population, study design, and outcomes

This is a retrospective observational study. Clinical, operative, and outcome data were collected prospectively in a computerized database, and all consecutive adult patients (July 2017 to November 2019) undergoing open cardiac surgery procedures by one surgeon (KDA) were selected from the database and included in this study (N = 305). Data that were not included in the prospective database were collected retrospectively from electronic charts which include data about lactate levels (mmol/L) during the first 12 h after arrival to the intensive care unit (ICU) as well as the glucose (mmol/L) and arterial PH level upon arrival to the ICU. Procedures included isolated coronary artery bypass grafting (CABG); isolated single, double, and triple valve surgery; combined CABG and valve(s) procedures; and other procedures such as aortic dissection, aortic root replacement, and surgery for mechanical complications of myocardial infarction. Both first time and redo procedures (including multiple redo procedures) were included.

The study was approved by our institutional Research Ethics Board and the individual's consent for the study was waived. Early hyperlactatemia (EHL) was defined as a lactate level > 3 mmol/L during the first hour upon arrival to the intensive care unit. Late hyperlactatemia (LHL) was defined as lactate level > 3 mmol/L that develops after 1 h of arrival to the intensive care unit. The lactate cut-off value of 3 mmol/L for defining HL was based on previous literature that suggested a range of 3–5 mmol/L to define significant hyperlactatemia after cardiac surgery [14]. In addition, we determined this cut-off value based on receiver operating characteristic (ROC) curve analysis for postoperative lactate level in our study during the first hour after surgery and its association with postoperative mortality and major adverse cardiac and cerebrovascular events.

The primary outcome was hospital mortality which was defined as any postoperative death in hospital.

Anesthetics, cardiopulmonary bypass, and operative management

Details of anesthesia, cardiopulmonary bypass, cardioplegia, and operative management are provided in the Supplement (Sections 1 and 2).

Lactate level measurement (mmol/L)

To evaluate trends of lactate level, data on lactate levels were retrospectively collected for all patients for the first 12 h after arrival to the ICU. Lactate data beyond 10 h had large percentage of missing data (> 30%) as it was not consistently measured beyond 10 h. Therefore, lactate data for hours 11 and 12 were excluded. Missing values for other lactate data during the first 10 h after surgery were low (2.9%). Missing data analysis was performed using multiple imputations as detailed below.

Statistical analysis

Statistical analyses were performed with SPSS version 25 (SPSS, IBM, Armonk, NY, USA). The two groups were compared for statistical significance based on chi-square or Fisher's exact test for categorical variables which are expressed as percentages. All continuous variables were explored for normality using normality diagnostics (histograms, skewness, and kurtosis). Student's t test was used to analyze continuous variables that were normally distributed, and the Mann-Whitney U test was used for variables that had non-normal distributions. Continuous variables were expressed as means (SD) or median with (25th and 75th percentile) as appropriate. Statistical significance was based on a two-tailed P value of less than 0.05.

Univariable and multivariable logistic regression model was employed to evaluate the independent predictors of EHL (dependent variable). A repeated measures analysis was used to test the main effect of postoperative time (hours), HL group, and the time × group interaction to determine the change in lactate levels over the 10 time points by HL group (early versus late). In addition, the repeated measures analysis was used to determine the predictors of postoperative lactate levels where the response (dependent) variables are the lactate levels during the first 10 h after surgery and the between-subjects factor is diabetes mellitus while adjusting for glucose level and cardiopulmonary bypass time as covariates.

Details of univariable and multivariable logistic regression as well as repeated measures analysis are described in the Supplement (Sections 3 and 4).

Missing data analysis

A multiple imputation (5 imputations) to impute the 6.3% missing data points for all variables using Markov chain Monte Carlo multiple imputation method was employed. Details are provided in the Supplement (Section 5).

Results

Demographics and baseline clinical profile

Seventeen percent (n = 52) of the patients developed postoperative EHL while 83% (n = 253) did not. Of patients with no EHL, 70.8% (n = 179) had LHL. Only 24.3% (n = 74) of the entire population of this study did not develop postoperative hyperlactatemia (a lactate value < 3 mmol/L). Thus, even though EHL was not frequent after cardiac surgery, LHL was very common. The prevalence of diabetes mellitus was significantly lower in the EHL group compared to the LHL group (30% vs 51.4%, P = 0.006). There was a higher surgical complexity in the EHL group where the prevalence of combined CABG and valve(s) procedures was higher in the EHL group (21% vs. 9.5%, P = 0.038). There were no other significant differences between the two groups in other baseline characteristics. Details of patients' baseline characteristics are presented in Table 1.

Table 1 Demographics and baseline clinical profile

Variable	Early hyperlactatemia		
	No	Yes	*P* value
No. of patients	(253)	(52)	
Age (years)	54.3 ± 12.8	53.6 ± 14.9	0.79
BSA	1.84 ± 0.29	1.88 ± 0.22	0.45
BMI	29.3 ± 6.6	30.4 ± 7.4	0.32
Female	37.5% (95)	42.3% (22)	0.52
Euro Score ES II	3.5 ± (4.5)	3.6 ± (4.8)	0.94
Diabetes mellitus	51.4% (129)	30% (15)	0.006
Metformin use	24.5% (62)	15.4% (8)	0.15
Hypertension	53.6% (134)	54% (27)	0.96
Creatinine clearance	97.1 ± 38.5	99.8 ± 42.3	0.52
ESRD on dialysis	2.4% (6)	4% (2)	0.50
Operation category			0.038
Isolated CABG	35.2% (89)	23.1% (12)	
Isolated valve(s)[a]	49.2% (124)	50% (26)	
Combined CABG + valve(s)[a]	9.5% (24)	21.2% (11)	
Others[b]	6% (15)	5.8% (3)	
Cardioplegia type			0.96
Del Nido	75.8% (191)	75.5% (40)	
Cold blood	24.2% (61)	24.5% (13)	
Atrial Fibrillation	19.1% (48)	22% (11)	0.64
Ejection Fraction	50.1 ± (9.4)	49.4 (9.8)	0.64
Redo surgery (first and multiple)	11.1% (28)	7.7% (4)	0.47
Preoperative TIA or stroke	4% (10)	4% (2)	0.50
Systolic PAP (mmHg)	38.5 ± 17	36.8 ± 15.6	0.57
Hemoglobin (mg/dL)	12.3 ± 2.2	12 ± 1.9	0.40

BSA body surface area, *BMI* body mass index, *MI* myocardial infarction, *LVEF* left ventricular ejection fraction
[a]This includes single, double, or triple valve repair and/or replacements
[b]Others include aortic root replacement, ascending aorta, or aortic arch interventions such as type A dissection repair, post-myocardial VSD closure, and LV aneurysm repair, among others

Operative profile and postoperative outcomes

Cardiopulmonary bypass (181 (54) vs. 150 (56), P = 0.001) and aortic cross clamp (144 (49) vs. 120 (44), P = 0.001) times were significantly higher in the EHL group which is explained by the more prevalence of complex procedures in the EH group.

Early hyperlactatemia was associated with significant increase in mortality (3.7% vs. 0%, P = 0.009) and marked increase in the requirement for postoperative extracorporeal membrane oxygenation (ECMO) support (P < 0.001). Likewise, there was a sixfold increase in the rate of metabolic acidosis in the EHL group. Similarly, the prevalence of other postoperative complications such as stroke and surgical site infections was significantly higher in the EHL group. As a result, postoperative intensive care unit stay and hospital length of stay were both significantly longer in the EHL group. Operative and postoperative profiles are detailed in Table 2. Of note, there was almost 2.5-folds increase in the rate of postoperative IABP in the EHL group (7.7% vs. 3.2%). However, this difference did not reach a statistical significance (P = 0.1) with our current sample size.

Patterns of postoperative hyperlactatemia

Two distinguished patterns of HL were identified. Early hyperlactatemia (EHL) started early and these patients arrived to the intensive care unit with high lactate level, reached peak level at 3 h, and then started to decrease 5 h after ICU admission. In contrast, LHL developed few

Table 2 Operative profile and postoperative outcomes

Variable	Early hyperlactatemia		
	No	Yes	**P** value
Intraoperative variables			
Duration of CPB (min)	150 ± 56	181 ± 54	0.001
Clamp time (min)	120 ± 44	144 ± 49	0.001
Postoperative outcomes			
Operative mortality[a]	0 (0)	3.7% (2)	0.009
ECMO	0 (0)	5.7% (3)	< 0.001
IABP	3.2% (8)	7.7% (4)	0.10
Metabolic acidosis	2.8% (7)	17.3% (9)	< 0.001
Peak troponin T level (ng/mL)	0.9 (0.65–1.4)	1.1 (0.7–1.8)	0.03
Stroke	0.8% (2)	5.7% (3)	0.048
AKI requiring dialysis	2% (5)	1.9% (1)	0.98
Deep sternal infection	0(0)	5.7% (3)	< 0.001
ICU length of stay (days)	3 (2–5)	5 (3–6.5)	0.004
Hospital length of stay (days)	9 (7–14)	10 (7–17)	0.02

Metabolic acidosis was defined as a PH ≤ 7.3 with low HCO3 (< 22 mEq/L) on ABG during the first 10 h after surgery. Postoperative AKI was defined as any new postoperative renal failure that requires dialysis
AKI acute kidney injury, *CPB* cardiopulmonary bypass, *ECMO* extracorporeal membrane oxygenation, *ICU* intensive care unit.
[a]Operative mortality is defined as any in-hospital death

hours after arrival to the ICU, peaked at 7 h after ICU admission, and then started to decline after that. Details of patterns of HL are depicted in Fig. 1. Estimated marginal means for lactate levels with the 95% CI for each time point in both groups are detailed in the Supplement (Table S1).

Effect of blood glucose level on postoperative lactate levels

There was a positive relationship between glucose levels and lactate levels which is influenced by diabetes mellitus. Diabetes mellitus attenuated this relationship where a 1 mmol/L increase in glucose level was associated with 14 and 26% increase in the lactate level in patients with and without diabetes, respectively. This relationship is depicted in a scatter plot in Fig. 2.

Effect of diabetes mellitus on postoperative lactate levels

Importantly, diabetes mellitus was associated with a significant attenuation of lactate levels after cardiac surgery. As shown in Fig. 3, postoperative lactate levels were significantly lower in patients with diabetes mellitus ($P < 0.001$). Estimated marginal means for lactate levels with the 95% CI for each time point in both groups are detailed in the Supplement (Table S2). This negative association between DM and lactate levels is evident despite the fact that DM is associated with higher rate of hyperglycemia and higher glucose levels (mean glucose level is 10.1 (2.7) and 7.9 (2.6) mmol/L, $P < 0.001$) in patients with and without diabetes, respectively. The explanation for this important finding is detailed in the "Discussion" section.

Predictors of early hyperlactatemia

A logistic regression model was used to evaluate independent predictors of EHL. First, a univariable logistic regression model was employed to screen potential variables. All variables that had a P value of < 0.2 were included in a multivariable logistic regression model using the backward elimination method. On univariable analysis, glucose level, CPB time, cross-clamp time, and surgical complexity were all predictors of increased rate of EHL. In contrast, DM was a significant and strong predictor of lower rate of EHL (OR = 0.39; 95% CI, 0.20–0.75; $P = 0.005$).

On multivariable analysis, independent predictors of EH included glucose level (OR = 1.3; 95% CI, 1.1–1.3; $P = 0.003$), CPB time (OR = 1.02; 95% CI, 1.01–1.1; $P = 0.015$), and DM (OR = 0.26; 95% CI, 0.12–0.55; $P < 0.001$). Univariable and multivariable predictors are shown in Table 3, and the details of multivariable analysis methods including selection method, model calibration, model discrimination, and collinearity evaluation are described in Table 3 footnote and the Supplement (Section 3).

Discussion

In the present study, we examined the timing patterns of postoperative hyperlactatemia and their consequences in adult patients undergoing cardiac surgery. We found that early but not late hyperlactatemia was associated

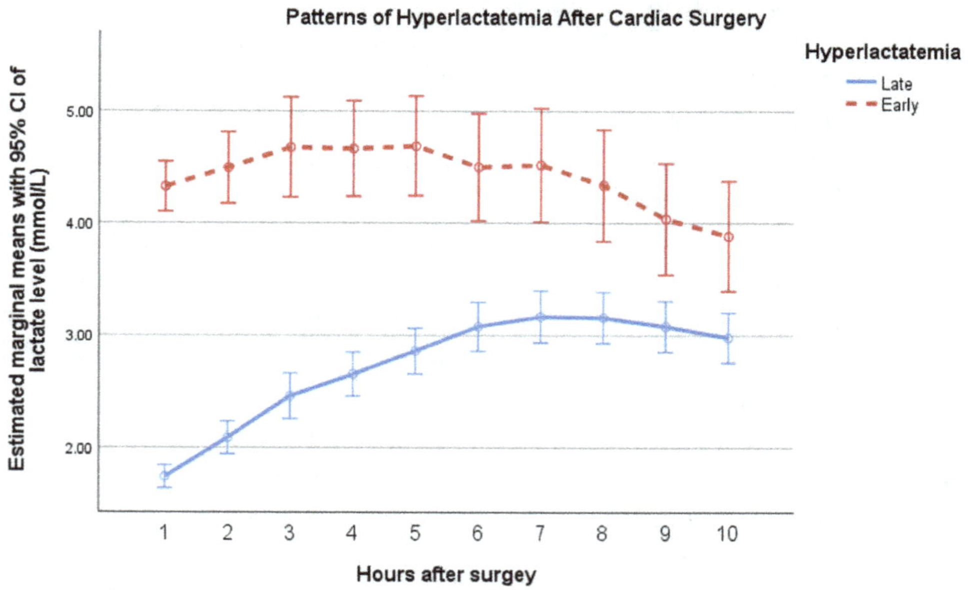

Fig. 1 Patterns of hyperlactatemia after cardiac surgery. Bars represent the 95% confidence intervals. The lactate levels change over time and it is significantly different in both groups (within-subjects P value < 0.001). Similarly, lactate levels are significantly different between the two groups at all time points (between-subjects P value < 0.001). Estimated marginal means for lactate levels with the 95% CI for each time point in both groups are detailed in the Supplement (Table S1)

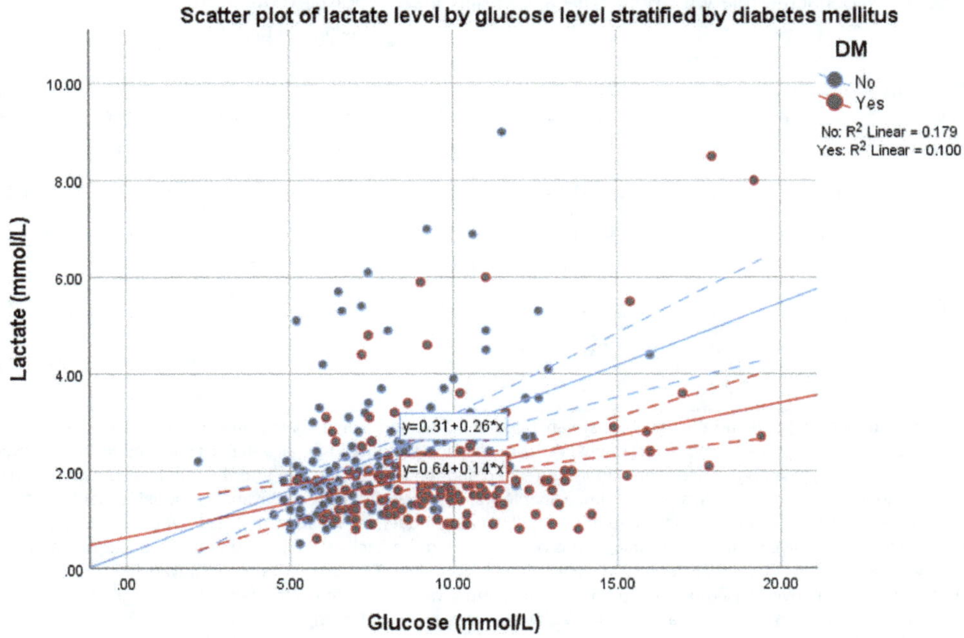

Fig. 2 Scatter plot for the relationship between glucose levels in mmol/L and the lactate levels in mmol/L stratified by diabetes mellitus. There is a positive relationship between the glucose level and the lactate level which is attenuated in patients with diabetes mellitus where a 1-mmol/L increase in glucose level is associated with 14 and 26% increase in the lactate level in patients with and without diabetes, respectively. The solid lines represent the fit lines for each category based on diabetes mellitus and the dotted lines represent the 95% confidence intervals.

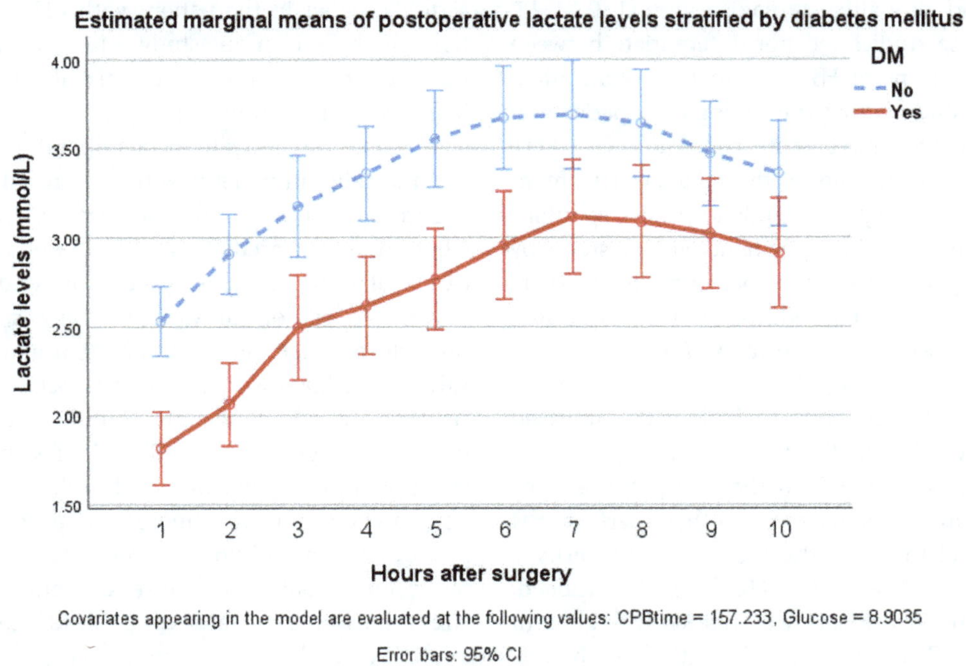

Fig. 3 The effect of diabetes mellitus on postoperative lactate levels while controlling for the effect of covariates (CPB time and glucose level). DM is associated with a significant attenuation of the postoperative lactate levels ($P < 0.001$). CPB indicates cardiopulmonary bypass. 95% CI indicates 95% confidence interval. DM indicates diabetes mellitus. Estimated marginal means for lactate levels with the 95% CI for each time point in both groups are detailed in the Supplement (Table S2)

Table 3 Predictors of early hyperlactatemia with univariate and multivariable logistic regression[a]

Univariable						Multivariable				
Variable	*β*	SE	OR	CI	*P*	*β*	SE	OR	CI	*P*
DM	− 0.94	0.33	0.39	0.20–0.75	0.005	− 1.3	0.4	0.26	0.12–0.55	< 0.001
Glucose	0.11	0.05	1.11	1.01–1.2	0.03	0.18	0.06	1.3	1.1–1.3	0.003
CPB time	0.09	0.03	1.1	1.03–1.14	0.001	0.07	0.03	1.02	1.01–1.1	0.015
Clamp time	0.10	0.03	1.1	1.04–1.17	0.001					
Procedure[a]					0.07					
Valve(s)	0.42	0.38	1.5	0.75–3.2	0.24					
Combined[b]	1.2	0.48	3.4	1.3–8.7	0.01					
Other	0.75	0.65	2.1	0.60–7.5	0.24					

CPB indicates cardiopulmonary bypass time (min) and the variables are analyzed at 10 min increment. Clamp time is also analyzed at 10 min increment. DM indicates diabetes mellitus. Glucose is analyzed at 1 mmol/L increment. Variance inflation factor (VIF) for all variables included in the multivariable model is < 4. Cross-clamp time and cardiopulmonary bypass (CPB) times were highly correlated and induced collinearity into the multivariable model (VIF = 5 for both variables when both are included in the model). Therefore, the cross-clamp time variable was removed from the multivariable model. Variables with *P* value > 0.2 on univariate analysis are not included in the table. Variables included in the multivariable model are variables that had a *P* value < 0.2 on univariate analysis and had no collinearity and these include (DM, glucose level, CPB time, and procedure) using the backward elimination method. Logistic regression multivariable model Hosmer and Lemeshow *P* value = 0.7. Area under the receiver operating characteristic (ROC) curve for the multivariable model is 0.71, *P* < 0.001. Bonferroni correction for *P* value adjustment was employed based on the number of explanatory variables tested with the univariate logistic regression model

[a]The reference group for surgical procedure variable is isolated coronary artery bypass grafting (CABG)

[b]Combined indicates combined CABG and valve(s) procedures

with increased mortality and morbidity. We also found that complexity of the procedure and cardiopulmonary bypass time and glucose level are important predictors of increased risk of EHL while diabetes mellitus attenuates this risk. Importantly, late hyperlactatemia (LHL) was very common after cardiac surgery and was benign and self-limiting.

Several studies have examined and confirmed the prognostic value of postoperative lactate levels in predicting mortality and morbidity after cardiac surgery [1, 2, 7, 15, 16]. However, these studies did not differentiate between different timing patterns of HL. The incremental finding from the present study is that the timing of hyperlactatemia is a critical determinant of its consequences where EHL is usually detrimental and needs aggressive treatment while LHL is usually benign and tends to resolve spontaneously. Our findings are in agreement with a study by Maillet and colleagues who found that immediate hyperlactatemia occurring on ICU admission was associated with fourfold increased risk of mortality (*P* < 0.001) compared to late hyperlactatemia [13].

The association of EHL but not LHL with increased morbidity and mortality in the present study may indicate different etiologies of HL in the two patterns. Anaerobic metabolism secondary to tissue hypoperfusion is the prevailing mechanism in the literature and perhaps represents the main etiology in EHL [7, 9, 17]. Indeed, the rate of metabolic acidosis was markedly higher in the patient with EHL in our study. Nonetheless, the etiology of hyperlactatemia after cardiac surgery is likely to be multifactorial. Large proportion of patients in the present study had no EHL but developed LHL several hours after arrival to the intensive care unit which did not increase the risk of morbidity or mortality. Increased lactate levels may occur under aerobic conditions secondary to increased catecholamine and inflammatory mediators after cardiac surgery without significant tissue hypoperfusion, and this latter mechanism may be the principle etiology of LHL [1].

The association of EHL with increased mortality and morbidity is perhaps linked to some extent to the acidifying effect of lactate. Indeed, metabolic acidosis was sixfolds higher in the patient with EHL compared to patients with LHL in our study. Metabolic acidosis leads to cellular dysfunction, myocardial depression, and hemodynamic compromise [16]. This may explain the significantly higher rate of postoperative ECMO support and mortality in patients with EHL in our study.

Cardiopulmonary bypass and aortic cross-clamp times were important predictors of EHL. Both are usually indicative of more complex or complicated cardiac procedures. Indeed, on univariable analysis, more complex procedures such as combined coronary and multiple valve procedures were strongly associated with increased risk of EHL. The longer the duration of CPB and clamp times, the higher the likelihood of sustaining systemic end-organ hypoperfusion which induces a state of anaerobic metabolism with increased glycolysis and lactate production. In addition, longer CPB time provokes systemic inflammatory response and induces cytokine and stress hormone release which leads to hyperglycemia and increased lactate production [18].

Glucose level was also an important predictor of lactate levels. Both lactate and glucose are involved in carbohydrate metabolism, and they serve as precursors for biosynthesis of one another [17]. Similarly, hyperlactatemia and hyperglycemia are common metabolic manifestations of response to stress induced by cardiac surgery and other major procedures [1, 2, 15]. Each 1-mmol increase in the glucose level was associated with 11% increase in the lactate level. Interestingly, diabetes mellitus strongly attenuated this relationship between glucose and lactate where each 1-mmol increase in the glucose level was associated with 14% increase in the lactate level in diabetic patients compared to 26% increase in the lactate level in non-diabetics. This may seem counter-intuitive as patients with diabetes are more likely to have hyperglycemia and therefore DM should presumably have a positive effect on lactate level. Nonetheless, DM had actually a suppressing effect on lactate level. Indeed, postoperative lactate levels (Fig. 3) are significantly attenuated by diabetes mellitus. Similar to our findings, Greco and associates evaluated the relationship between hyperlactatemia, glucose, and diabetes in 4098 patients after cardiac surgery and found that stress-induced increase in lactate levels is strongly attenuated in patients with DM [7]. Moreover, this suppressing effect of DM on stress hyperlactatemia has been also reported with stress hyperglycemia in several studies where the association between hyperglycemia and adverse outcomes is strongly suppressed in patients with DM [19–21].

These findings suggest that DM may grant a degree of protection against HL in patients undergoing cardiac surgery which is independent of the glucose level, surgical complexity, and CPB duration, among other confounders. Although mechanisms for this suppressing effect of DM on stress-induced hyperlactatemia are not fully understood, it can be to some extent explained by the state of relative insulin deficiency in patients with DM which leads to inhibition of glycolysis and lactate production since insulin is a positive regulator of glycolysis [7, 22]. Likewise, gluconeogenesis is inhibited by insulin, and therefore, with relative insulin deficiency in diabetic patients, gluconeogenesis pathway is stimulated and lactate utilization is increased through the lactic acid cycle resulting in increased lactate clearance [23]. Thus, the net result of relative insulin deficiency in diabetic patients is a reduction in synthesis and increase in utilization of plasma lactate by glycolysis inhibition and gluconeogenesis acceleration, respectively.

Our study has important clinical implications. First, the timing of HL, in our view, is the most important determinant of prognostic value of lactate levels after cardiac surgery. Early HL was strongly predictive of complications in the present study which may reflect end-organ hypoperfusion and tissue hypoxia as primary etiology in early HL. Therefore, EHL should be managed aggressively in order to reverse end-organ hypoperfusion and tissue hypoxia. In contrast, LHL occurred very commonly and was not associated with increased mortality or morbidity. Second, patients with DM may not exhibit significant HL despite significant tissue hypoperfusion as DM appears to mask and attenuates stress-induced hyperlactatemia. Thus, when the lactate level is used in evaluating end-organ perfusion in diabetic patients, this suppressing effect of DM on the lactate level should be considered.

Limitations

Our study has several limitations. This is an observational single-center retrospective study which makes it susceptible to inherent selection and information biases. However, the prospective nature of the data collection adds strength to the internal validity of the study. We attempted to use rigorous statistical regression analysis to control for confounders; however, we admit that regression analysis accounts only for known confounders that are included in the multivariable model and does not account for unknown or unmeasured confounders. Finally, we reported only short-term outcomes and weather EHL is associated with any long-term consequences is unknown from the present study.

Conclusions

After cardiac surgery, early but not late hyperlactatemia could be associated with increased morbidity and mortality. Increased surgical complexity, hyperglycemia, and cardiopulmonary bypass time were positive independent predictors of EHL. Diabetes mellitus significantly attenuated stress-induced hyperlactatemia after cardiac surgery, and this masking effect of DM on lactate level should be considered when lactate is used as a biomarker in evaluating end-organ perfusion in diabetic patients.

Supplementary information

Additional file 1: Supplement. **Table S1.** Estimated marginal means with 95% CI of lactate levels during the first 10 hours after cardiac surgery in patients with early and late patterns of hyperlactatemia. **Table S2.** Estimated marginal means with 95% CI of lactate levels during the first 10 hours after cardiac surgery in patients with and without diabetes mellitus. Adjusted for CPB time and Glucose level.

Abbreviations

CABG: Coronary artery bypass grafting; EHL: Early hyperlactatemia; HL: Hyperlactatemia; LHL: Late hyperlactatemia

Acknowledgements

Juan J Alfonso collected, maintained, and managed the adult cardiac surgery database from which the data for this study is generated.

Author's contributions

KDA designed the study, analyzed the data, and wrote and approved the final manuscript

References

1. Garcia-Alvarez M, Marik P, Bellomo R (2014) Stress hyperlactataemia: present understanding and controversy. Lancet Diabetes Endocrinol. 2:339–347
2. Kogan A, Preisman S, Bar A et al (2012) The impact of hyperlactatemia on postoperative outcome after adult cardiac surgery. J Anesth. 26:174–178
3. Svenmarker S, Häggmark S, Ostman M (2006) What is a normal lactate level during cardiopulmonary bypass? Scand Cardiovasc J. 40:305–311
4. Masyuk M, Wernly B, Lichtenauer M et al (2019) Prognostic relevance of serum lactate kinetics in critically ill patients. Intensive care medicine. 45:55–61
5. Alkozai EM, Mahmoodi BK, Decruyenaere J et al (2018) Systematic comparison of routine laboratory measurements with in-hospital mortality: ICU-Labome, a large cohort study of critically ill patients. Clinical chemistry and laboratory medicine. 56:1140–1151
6. Toraman F, Evrenkaya S, Yuce M et al (2004) Lactic acidosis after cardiac surgery is associated with adverse outcome. Heart Surg Forum. 7:E155–E159
7. Greco G, Kirkwood KA, Gelijns AC et al (2018) Diabetes is associated with reduced stress hyperlactatemia in cardiac surgery. Diabetes care. 41:469–477
8. Ranucci M, De Toffol B, Isgrò G et al (2006) Hyperlactatemia during cardiopulmonary bypass: determinants and impact on postoperative outcome. Crit Care. 10:R167
9. Naik R, George G, Karuppiah S, Philip MA (2016) Hyperlactatemia in patients undergoing adult cardiac surgery under cardiopulmonary bypass: causative factors and its effect on surgical outcome. Ann Card Anaesth. 19:668–675
10. Hajjar LA, Almeida JP, Fukushima JT et al (2013) High lactate levels are predictors of major complications after cardiac surgery. J Thorac Cardiovasc Surg. 146:455–460
11. Evans AS, Levin MA, Lin HM et al (2018) Prognostic value of hyperlactatemia and lactate clearance after mitral valve surgery. J Cardiothorac Vasc Anesth. 32:636–643
12. Lopez-Delgado JC, Esteve F, Javierre C et al (2015) Evaluation of serial arterial lactate levels as a predictor of hospital and long-term mortality in patients after cardiac surgery. Journal of cardiothoracic and vascular anesthesia. 29:1441–1453
13. Maillet JM, Le Besnerais P, Cantoni M et al (2003) Frequency, risk factors, and outcome of hyperlactatemia after cardiac surgery. Chest 123:1361–1366
14. Minton J, Sidebotham DA (2017) Hyperlactatemia and cardiac surgery. J Extra Corpor Technol. 49:7–15
15. Dungan KM, Braithwaite SS, Preiser JC (2009) Stress hyperglycaemia. Lancet. 373:1798–1807
16. Kraut JA, Madias NE (2014) Lactic acidosis. N Engl J Med. 371:2309–2319
17. Adeva-Andany M, López-Ojén M, Funcasta-Calderón R et al (2014) Comprehensive review on lactate metabolism in human health. Mitochondrion 17:76–100
18. Revelly JP, Tappy L, Martinez A et al (2005) Lactate and glucose metabolism in severe sepsis and cardiogenic shock. Crit Care Med. 33:2235–2240
19. Sechterberger MK, Bosman RJ, Oudemans-van Straaten HM et al (2013) The effect of diabetes mellitus on the association between measures of glycaemic control and ICU mortality: a retrospective cohort study. Crit Care. 17:R52
20. Greco G, Ferket BS, D'Alessandro DA et al (2016) Diabetes and the association of postoperative hyperglycemia with clinical and economic outcomes in cardiac surgery. Diabetes Care. 39:408–417
21. Krinsley JS, Egi M, Kiss A, et al. Diabetic status and the relation of the three domains of glycemic control to mortality in critically ill patients: an international multicenter cohort study. Crit Care. 2013;17:R37.
22. Wu C, Khan SA, Lange AJ (2005) Regulation of glycolysis—role of insulin. Exp Gerontol. 40:894–899
23. Consoli A, Nurjhan N, Reilly JJ Jr et al (1990) Mechanism of increased gluconeogenesis in noninsulin-dependent diabetes mellitus. Role of alterations in systemic, hepatic, and muscle lactate and alanine metabolism. J Clin Invest. 86:2038–2045

17

Surgery for autoimmune aortitis: unanswered questions

Amr A. Arafat

Abstract

Background: The aorta is rarely affected by autoimmune vasculitis, which can lead to aortic dilatation requiring surgery. Autoimmune aortitis may affect one aortic segment or the entire aorta, and in some cases, the aorta may be affected at different time intervals. Because of the rarity of the disease and the limited cases described in the literature, management of autoimmune aortitis is still controversial. We aimed to review the current literature evidence regarding these controversial aspects for the management of autoimmune aortitis and give recommendations based on this evidence.

Main text: Immunosuppressants are generally indicated in vasculitis to halt the progression of the disease; however, its role after the occurrence of aortic dilatation is debatable since further aortic dilatation would eventually occur because of the weakness of the arterial wall. In patients with a localized ascending aortic dilatation who required surgery, the optimal approach for the distal aorta is not known. If the probability of disease progression is high, it is not known whether the patients would benefit from postoperative immunosuppressants or further distal aortic intervention may be required. The risk of rupture of the weakened aortic wall was not established, and it is debatable at which diameter should these patients have surgery. In patients with previous ascending surgery for autoimmune aortitis, the endovascular management of the distal aortic disease has not been studied. The inflammatory process may extend to affect the aortic valve or the coronary vessels, which may require special attention during the procedure.

Conclusion: Patients with diagnosed autoimmune aortitis are prone to the development of the distal aortic disease, and endovascular intervention is feasible in those patients. Patients with concomitant aortic valve can be managed with the aortic valve-sparing procedure, and preoperative screening for coronary disease is recommended. Immunosuppressants should be used early before aortic dilatation, and its role postoperatively is controversial.

Keywords: Autoimmune aortitis, Giant cell aortitis, Takayasu aortitis, Non-infectious aortitis

Background

Autoimmune aortitis is a rare cause of aortic disease requiring surgery [1]. Several types of vasculitic disease can affect the aortic wall; however, the clinical features are non-specific, and the preoperative diagnosis is difficult, especially in patients with no extra-aortic disease [1, 2]. There are several unresolved issues related to autoimmune aortitis that can affect the surgical decision and patients' management. Autoimmune aortitis is classified based on the type of the vasculitis, and there are no anatomical or surgical classifications that can guide patient management. Patients with autoimmune aortitis may have distal disease progression after surgical correction of the proximal disease, and the role of immunosuppressants to halt this progression is debatable. Optimal management of the distal aortic disease is not settled, and it is not known if these patients may benefit from prophylactic interventions at the time of proximal aortic repair or staged endovascular repair could be warranted.

The European Society of Cardiology (ESC) guidelines for the management of aortic disease did not define a threshold at which surgery is recommended in patients with aneurysmal aortitis, and the risk of aortic rupture in these patients are not known compared to the

Correspondence: amr.arafat@med.tanta.edu.eg
Cardiothoracic Surgery Department, Faculty of Medicine, Tanta University, Al-Geish Street, Tanta, Gharbyia 31529, Egypt

atherosclerotic or connective tissue aneurysms [3]. The use of immunosuppressants modulates the course of the disease; however, its role after aortic dilatation and surgery is controversial. The probability of the involvement of the coronary arteries and the aortic valve with the inflammatory process is not established but may require special attention intraoperatively. We aimed to review the current literature evidence regarding these controversial aspects for the management of autoimmune aortitis and give recommendations based on this evidence.

Classification of autoimmune aortitis

Generally, vasculitis is classified according to the vessels and organs affected into large, medium, small, and variable vessels vasculitis, single organ vasculitis, vasculitis associated with systemic autoimmune disease [4], and vasculitis associated with probable etiology [5]. Despite being the largest artery, the aorta can be affected by all types of vasculitis. The aorta is mainly affected by large vessel vasculitis with its two variants giant cell and Takayasu arteritis [6]. Clinically, the American College of Rheumatology criteria are used to diagnose giant cell (GCA) and Takayasu arteritis [7, 8]. Takayasu tends to occur in patients younger than 40 years and has more predilection to the subclavian artery [5, 7]; on the other hand, GCA tends to affect patients above 50 years and affects more the carotid and vertebral arteries [5, 8]. Although giant cell and Takayasu arteritis are considered two distinct disorders based on the clinical presentation, some authors considered them as one disease entity, and their clinical picture represents a spectrum within a single disorder [9].

The prevalence of autoimmune aortitis in surgically resected aortas varies between 1.8 and 8.8% [1, 2, 10, 11]. Histologically, both GCA and Takayasu are granulomatous diseases affecting all layers of the aortic wall, which becomes infiltrated with lymphocytes, macrophages, and multinucleated giant cells [5]. The classic Takayasu's aortitis is a pan-aortitis, more commonly associated with intimal and adventitial thickening with intraluminal stenosis [10]. In GCA, the aorta is thickened mainly due to the involvement of the media with the destruction of the elastic lamina associated with medial necrosis and the development of an aneurysm [10], and it is characterized by focal arteritis and skip lesions [12].

The isolated aortitis—also known as single organ vasculitis—is an increasingly recognized form of aortitis mostly diagnosed after surgical treatment of an aortic aneurysm. Isolated aortitis is localized inflammation of the aortic wall, not associated with systemic disease and does not fit the diagnostic criteria of GCA or Takayasu arteritis [6, 13, 14].

Early diagnosed autoimmune aortitis requires immunosuppressant therapy. On the other hand, infectious aortitis requires antimicrobial therapy and surgical intervention. The diagnosis of autoimmune aortitis can be suspected from the associated clinical syndrome, and the American College of Rheumatology criteria [7, 8] can be used to diagnose GCA and Takayasu diseases. However, the preoperative diagnosis of the isolated variant presents a clinical challenge, especially in the absence of systemic symptoms. Several studies had attempted to identify the risk factors suspecting underlying inflammatory component of the aortic disease requiring surgery. Schmidt and associates found the incidence of aortitis was 6.1%, and the predictors of idiopathic aortitis were a history of connective tissue disorders, diabetes mellitus, age more than 67 years, and aortic valve disease [15]. Other studies found that patients undergoing surgery for aortitis complications had associated hypertension [16–18], peripheral vascular disease [18], coronary artery disease [18], shortness of breath, and aortic incompetence [16–18]. From Cleveland Clinic experience, they found that aortitis occurred more frequently in females and the majority of the patients are hypertensive and smokers and had associated aortic valve disease. All age groups can be affected by autoimmune aortitis ranging from 20 to 87 years old [1, 13]. Despite these trials to predict the inflammatory nature of the aneurysm, none of the risk factors are specific.

Imaging plays a vital role in diagnosing aortitis. Computed tomography and magnetic resonance imaging had replaced angiography as the modality of choice in aortitis [19]. Both of them show aortic wall thickening or thinning depending on the stage of the disease, vessel wall edema which could reflect disease activity, luminal narrowing, periaortic thickening, and wall ulceration, dissection or aneurysm formation [20]. MRI is superior to CT in demonstrating the vessel wall and the edema; however, CT can show wall calcification and disease progression. Despite the superiority of MRI in detecting vessel wall edema, the correlation of edema with disease activity is controversial. MRI showed a decrease in vessel wall edema in a patient with GCA after 2 weeks of steroid use [21]. However, in a previous study from Cleveland Clinic on 24 patients with Takayasu disease, there was no correlation between vessel wall edema shown on MRI and acute phase reactants [22]. Recently, FDG-PET CT was found to have a role in diagnosing aortitis, which shows an increase in FGD uptake in the aorta [23–25]. In our experience, the operative inspection may play an important role in the diagnosis of aortitis, and the glossy white intima with only some yellow streaks is considered the typical finding in GCA This glossy white look represents the change from the loss of elastic lamellae and smooth muscle cells and the formation of scar tissue rich in proteoglycans. All resected aortic tissue should be sent for histopathological examination to confirm the etiological diagnosis and identify the type of vasculitis [26].

Currently, there is no standard classification that can guide the decision of surgery. Svensson, Arafat, and their coworkers had classified the disease based on the possible etiological factor [1]. However, recognizing the disease preoperatively still presents an ongoing challenge and, in their series, more than half of their patients were diagnosed postoperatively. The diagnosis of autoimmune aortitis requires a high level of suspicious, female patients presented with ascending aortic dilatation with or without the distal disease, and elevated inflammatory markers should undergo further evaluation with MRI or PET scan.

The threshold for intervention

Autoimmune aortitis causes progressive thinning of the aortic wall, and the risk of rupture has not been evaluated before. In the series by Arafat and associates, 16% of the patients had a surgical intervention because of acute aortic syndrome or chronic dissection in the ascending aorta [13]. Development of aortic dissection in patients with aortitis was attributed to the delayed use of steroid from the time of onset of symptoms to the diagnosis, and it was found that dissection is an early complication of GCA compared with other causes of the aneurysm [27]. There is not enough evidence in the literature supporting the intervention at specific diameter in autoimmune aortitis [28], but considering the high incidence of acute events reported in the scarce series, intervention at lower aortic diameters than the atherosclerotic aneurysms could be warranted.

The distal aorta

The preoperative diagnosis of vasculitis is essential to guide the management of the distal aorta. Disease progression was not evaluated in large and several series; however, the largest series up to date by Clifford and Arafat and their colleagues found that 29% of the patients required distal aortic intervention during an 8-year follow-up and many patients developed other vascular lesions [13, 29]. Wang and associates found 7 of 15 patients with GCA who had ascending aortic surgery developed the distal aortic disease, and 5 required distal reinterventions in a mean time of 58 months. The risk of distal aortic disease was 11-fold in comparison to the control group [30]. The progressive aortic dilatation was noted in all levels from the arch to the infrarenal aorta after ascending aortic surgery [31].

Despite the limited studies on autoimmune aortitis, the current evidence supports distal disease progression in patients with GCA and isolated aortitis [32]. Those patients may benefit from additional prophylactic interventions during their primary surgery, such as the deliberate use of elephant trunk procedure to manage those patients. Further studies are required to adequately describe the optimal surgical procedure for the management of these patients.

Endovascular repair

Patients who had ascending aortic surgery for autoimmune aortitis are prone to frequent reinterventions, mostly involving the distal aortic segments. Disease progression in the distal aorta and progressive dilatation of the weakened inflamed distal aortic wall observed in those patients raise the question about the feasibility of endovascular aortic repair (TEVAR). Currently, there is not enough evidence for the feasibility of stent grafting in these patients. A study had evaluated the results of endovascular stenting in patients with aortopathy including Marfan, GCA, and Takayasu aortitis [33], technical success was 91.7%, endoleak occurred in 16.7%, and no aneurysm-related mortality was reported. Recent reports had a good outcome of TEVAR in patients with the genetic aortic disease [34]; however, reinterventions are common.

In a study by Arafat and coworkers, reinterventions after TEVAR occurred in the distal segments because of continuous disease progression, and aortic growth, three interventions for endoleak were reported, and all reinterventions were managed endovascularly [13]. In the same study, none of the Takayasu patients who had ascending aortic repair for aortitis required later TEVAR; this may reflect the progression of the aortic pathology in Takayasu patients, which tends to be obstructive [1]. On the other hand, patients who had isolated aortitis required more reinterventions after TEVAR than patients with GCA and aortitis associated with systemic autoimmune disease [1, 13].

Aortic diameters at the level of the mid arch and the maximum descending aortic diameters were decreased post-stenting. Although the decrease in diameters was not statistically significant, the stent graft succeeded to stop the progressive aortic expansion in patients with aortitis [1, 13, 29]. Patients with active inflammation of the aortic wall may benefit from endovascular interventions since open repair is associated with the formation of pseudoaneurysm at the suture line [35, 36]. The feasibility of endovascular interventions in inflammatory aortitis came from sporadic case reports [37, 38] and abdominal aortic aneurysm interventions [39]; however, the current evidence supports its feasibility. Additionally, several endovascular procedures are performed without a confirmatory aortic specimen to exclude vasculitis [40].

The aortic valve

Aortic valve pathology was a positive predictor of inflammatory origin of the aneurysm in several studies [16–18]. Concomitant aortic valve surgery was performed in 51%

and 80% of the patients [13, 31] who had ascending aortic surgery for autoimmune aortitis. The aortic valve can be affected as a part of the systemic disease as in Cogan's syndrome and Behcet disease [41] while aortic valve affection in Takayasu is rare. Long-term results of aortic valve repair and the durability of aortic bioprosthesis are not known in these patients. Mennandar and colleagues performed ascending aortic surgery in 100 patients with aortitis, 38 had an aortic valve-sparing procedure, 30 had aortic valve replacement, and 30 patients had competent valves. There was no difference in operative mortality and morbidity between groups. Postoperative echo was available in 59 patients with no significant difference between groups related to the valve and ventricular function. Two patients with prior aortic valve-sparing procedure had aortic valve replacement after 1 year, and one developed aortic regurge and treated conservatively. They concluded that the aortic valve-sparing procedure is technically feasible in patients with aortitis, but long-term results are unknown [42].

Aortic valve disease is associated with autoimmune ascending aortitis; however, the inflammatory nature of this association cannot be elicited, and reinterventions after aortic valve repair or aortic valve-sparing procedure is not common. This supports the feasibility of these procedures in patients with autoimmune aortitis.

Concomitant coronary artery disease

Autoimmune diseases causing aortitis are classified as large vessel vasculitis; however, they are not exclusive for large vessel disease. The blindness that can occur with GCA is attributed to small vessel affection of the ophthalmic vessels. Concomitant coronary artery bypass grafting (CABG) was reported in 25% of patients who had surgery for autoimmune aortitis [1, 13]. It is not clear whether the associated coronary lesions were atherosclerotic or vasculitis.

Several case reports described non-atherosclerotic coronary disease with or without associated aortitis [43, 44]. Many of these series reported the association of coronary artery disease with IgG4 disease [45] and used PET scan for screening [46]. The current guidelines do not address the management of coronary arteries in patients presenting for surgery for autoimmune aortitis. Many of those patients are young and asymptomatic, and screening for the coronary artery disease is not recommended. Based on the high association between aortitis and coronary artery disease in which the etiology of both lesions cannot be clearly separated, it is recommended to screen high-risk patients undergoing aortic surgery for the autoimmune cause for the presence of concomitant coronary artery disease. Patients with positive screening results can benefit from a PET scan to demonstrate the activity of the disease and assess the possibility of preoperative steroid therapy. There is no definitive recommendation on how to manage concomitant coronary lesions; however, a similar management plan to atherosclerotic coronary artery disease is recommended until we have enough evidence in literature towards alternate practice.

Follow-up and immunosuppressants

Current guidelines for the management of thoracic aortic disease recommend preoperative treatment with immunosuppressant drugs in patients with elevated inflammatory markers. However, there are no guidelines for postoperative management of these patients [11, 28]. Rojo-Leyva and associates recommended postoperative treatment with immunosuppressants if there is evidence of disease progression beyond the resected segment [11].

The effect of postoperative immunosuppressant on the incidence of reintervention is not known. In a large series from Cleveland Clinic, postoperative immunosuppressant did not affect the reintervention rate [1]. Blumstein and fellows found that GCA patients treated with steroids had complete resolution of the inflammation on histological analysis compared to non-treated patients indicating that the disease is steroid responsive [47]. Rojo-Leyva and colleagues treated 11 patients with steroids after aortic surgery and had a mean follow-up of 35.5 months without the development of an aneurysm; however, 6 of 25 that were not treated with steroid had a mean follow-up of 41.2 months and developed subsequent aneurysms [11]. Miller and coworkers found 10% of 21 patients with isolated aortitis developed aneurysms after surgical repair (2 treated with steroids) and 21% of 14 patients with GCA developed aneurysm even though 11 of them were on steroid (p value = 0.09) [10]. Wang and associates treated 3/15 patients with postoperative steroids, one of them developed distal aortic disease [30]. The ineffectiveness of postoperative immunosuppressants therapy on the incidence of distal reintervention in our experience could be attributed to the late presentation of these patients to surgery especially with lack of signs and symptoms suggestive of inflammatory nature of their aneurysms. Early discovery of these patients and treatment with immunosuppressants before developing surgical aortic disease could reverse the pathological process and slow disease progression before medial destruction occurs.

Conclusion and recommendations

Autoimmune aortitis is an under-recognized cause of aortic aneurysms. Preoperative diagnosis is challenging, especially with the isolated form. High level of suspicious is required to investigate the patients with MRI or PET scan further. Patients with diagnosed autoimmune aortitis are prone to the development of the distal aortic disease, and endovascular intervention is feasible in those patients. Patients with concomitant aortic valve can be managed with the aortic valve-sparing procedure, and preoperative screening for coronary disease is recommended. Immunosuppressants should be used early before aortic dilatation, and its role postoperatively is controversial.

Abbreviations

CABG: Coronary artery bypass grafting; CT: Computed tomography; ESC: European Society of Cardiology; GCA: Giant cell arteritis; IgG4: Immunoglobulin G4; MRI: Magnetic resonance imaging; PET: Positron emission tomography; TEVAR: Thoracic endovascular aortic repair

Acknowledgements

None.

Author's contributions

AA did the literature search, wrote the manuscript, and approved the final version.

References

1. Svensson LG, Arafat A, Roselli EE, Idrees J, Clifford A, Tan C et al (2015) Inflammatory disease of the aorta: patterns and classification of giant cell aortitis, Takayasu arteritis, and nonsyndromic aortitis. J Thorac Cardiovasc Surg 149(2 Suppl):S170–S175
2. De Martino A, Ballestracci P, Faggioni L, Pratali S, Morganti R, Pucci A et al (2018) Incidence of aortitis in surgical specimens of the ascending aorta clinical implications at follow-up. Semin Thorac Cardiovasc Surg https://www.ncbi.nlm.nih.gov/pubmed/30414447
3. Erbel R, Aboyans V, Boileau C, Bossone E, Bartolomeo RD, Eggebrecht H et al (2014) 2014 ESC Guidelines on the diagnosis and treatment of aortic diseases: document covering acute and chronic aortic diseases of the thoracic and abdominal aorta of the adult. The Task Force for the Diagnosis and Treatment of Aortic Diseases of the European Society of Cardiology (ESC). Eur Heart J 35(41):2873–2926
4. Arafat AA, Torky MA, Elhamshary M, Aboelnasr M (2019) Immunoglobulin G4 thymic tumor. Ann Thorac Surg 108(4):e229-e23. https://www.ncbi.nlm.nih.gov/pubmed/30914283
5. Jennette JC, Falk RJ, Bacon PA, Basu N, Cid MC, Ferrario F et al (2013) 2012 revised International Chapel Hill Consensus Conference Nomenclature of vasculitides. Arthritis Rheum 65(1):1–11
6. Jennette JC (2013) Overview of the 2012 revised International Chapel Hill Consensus Conference nomenclature of vasculitides. Clin Exp Nephrol 17(5): 603–606
7. Arend WP, Michel BA, Bloch DA, Hunder GG, Calabrese LH, Edworthy SM et al (1990) The American College of Rheumatology 1990 criteria for the classification of Takayasu arteritis. Arthritis Rheum 33(8):1129–1134
8. Hunder GG, Bloch DA, Michel BA, Stevens MB, Arend WP, Calabrese LH et al (1990) The American College of Rheumatology 1990 criteria for the classification of giant cell arteritis. Arthritis Rheum 33(8):1122–1128
9. Grayson PC, Maksimowicz-McKinnon K, Clark TM, Tomasson G, Cuthbertson D, Carette S et al (2012) Distribution of arterial lesions in Takayasu's arteritis and giant cell arteritis. Ann Rheum Dis 71(8):1329–1334
10. Miller DV, Isotalo PA, Weyand CM, Edwards WD, Aubry MC, Tazelaar HD (2006) Surgical pathology of noninfectious ascending aortitis: a study of 45 cases with emphasis on an isolated variant. Am J Surg Pathol 30(9):1150–1158
11. Rojo-Leyva F, Ratliff NB, Cosgrove DM 3rd, Hoffman GS (2000) Study of 52 patients with idiopathic aortitis from a cohort of 1,204 surgical cases. Arthritis Rheum 43(4):901–907
12. Gravanis MB (2000) Giant cell arteritis and Takayasu aortitis: morphologic, pathogenetic and etiologic factors. Int J Cardiol 75(Suppl 1):S21–S33 discussion S5–6
13. Arafat A, Roselli E, Clifford A, Idrees J, Tan C, Svensson L et al (2013) Abstract 16022: is proximal aortic repair sufficient for autoimmune aortitis? Circulation 128(suppl_22):A16022-A
14. Pipitone N, Salvarani C (2011) Idiopathic aortitis: an underrecognized vasculitis. Arthritis Res Ther 13(4):119
15. Schmidt J, Sunesen K, Kornum JB, Duhaut P, Thomsen RW (2011) Predictors for pathologically confirmed aortitis after resection of the ascending aorta: a 12-year Danish nationwide population-based cross-sectional study. Arthritis Res Ther 13(3):R87
16. Kerr LD, Chang YJ, Spiera H, Fallon JT (2000) Occult active giant cell aortitis necessitating surgical repair. J Thorac Cardiovasc Surg 120(4):813–815
17. Lee A, Luk A, Phillips KR, Lim KD, David TE, Butany J (2011) Giant cell aortitis: a difficult diagnosis assessing risk for the development of aneurysms and dissections. Cardiovasc Pathol 20(4):247–253
18. Zehr KJ, Mathur A, Orszulak TA, Mullany CJ, Schaff HV (2005) Surgical treatment of ascending aortic aneurysms in patients with giant cell aortitis. Ann Thorac Surg 79(5):1512–1517
19. Gornik HL, Creager MA (2008) Aortitis. Circulation 117(23):3039–3051
20. Restrepo CS, Ocazionez D, Suri R, Vargas D (2011) Aortitis: imaging spectrum of the infectious and inflammatory conditions of the aorta. Radiographics 31(2):435–451
21. Bley TA, Ness T, Warnatz K, Frydrychowicz A, Uhl M, Hennig J et al (2007) Influence of corticosteroid treatment on MRI findings in giant cell arteritis. Clin Rheumatol 26(9):1541–1543
22. Tso E, Flamm SD, White RD, Schvartzman PR, Mascha E, Hoffman GS (2002) Takayasu arteritis: utility and limitations of magnetic resonance imaging in diagnosis and treatment. Arthritis Rheum 46(6):1634–1642
23. Blockmans D, Stroobants S, Maes A, Mortelmans L (2000) Positron emission tomography in giant cell arteritis and polymyalgia rheumatica: evidence for inflammation of the aortic arch. Am J Med 108(3):246–249
24. Rahman MS, Storrar N, Anderson LJ (2013) FDG-PET/CT in the diagnosis of aortitis in fever of unknown origin with severe aortic incompetence. Heart 99(6):435–436
25. Trad S, Bensimhon L, El Hajjam M, Chinet T, Wechsler B, Saadoun D (2013) 18F-fluorodeoxyglucose-positron emission tomography scanning is a useful tool for therapy evaluation of arterial aneurysm in Behcet's disease. Joint Bone Spine 80(4):420–423
26. Cozijnsen L, Ter Borg EJ, Braam RL, Seldenrijk CA, Heijmen RH, Bouma BJ et al (2019) Ascending aortic aneurysm secondary to isolated noninfectious ascending aortitis. J Clin Rheumatol 25(4):186–194
27. Nuenninghoff DM, Hunder GG, Christianson TJ, McClelland RL, Matteson EL (2003) Mortality of large-artery complication (aortic aneurysm, aortic dissection, and/or large-artery stenosis) in patients with giant cell arteritis: a population-based study over 50 years. Arthritis Rheum 48(12):3532–3537
28. Hiratzka LF, Bakris GL, Beckman JA, Bersin RM, Carr VF, Casey DE Jr et al (2010) 2010 ACCF/AHA/AATS/ACR/ASA/SCA/SCAI/SIR/STS/SVM guidelines for the diagnosis and management of patients with thoracic aortic disease: executive summary. A report of the American College of Cardiology Foundation/American Heart Association Task Force on Practice Guidelines, American Association for Thoracic Surgery, American College of Radiology, American Stroke Association, Society of Cardiovascular Anesthesiologists, Society for Cardiovascular Angiography and Interventions, Society of Interventional Radiology, Society of Thoracic Surgeons, and Society for Vascular Medicine. Catheter Cardiovasc Interv 76(2):E43–E86
29. Clifford AH, Arafat A, Idrees JJ, Roselli EE, Tan CD, Rene Rodriguez E, Svensson LG, Blackstone E, Johnston D, Pettersson G, Soltesz E, Hoffman GS (2019) Outcomes among 196 patients with non-infectious proximal aortitis. Arthritis Rheumatol (Hoboken, NJ) https://doi.org/10.1002/art.40855. https://www.ncbi.nlm.nih.gov/pubmed/30730604
30. Wang H, Smith RN, Spooner AE, Isselbacher EM, Cambria RP, MacGillivray TE et al (2012) Giant cell aortitis of the ascending aorta without signs or symptoms of systemic vasculitis is associated with elevated risk of distal aortic events. Arthritis Rheum 64(1):317–319
31. Gagne-Loranger M, Dumont E, Voisine P, Mohammadi S, Garceau C, Dion B et al (2016) Giant cell aortitis: clinical presentation and outcomes in 40 patients consecutively operated on. Eur J Cardio-thoracic Surg 50(3):555–559
32. Cinar I, Wang H, Stone JR (2017) Clinically isolated aortitis: pitfalls, progress, and possibilities. Cardiovasc Pathol 29:23–32
33. Baril DT, Carroccio A, Palchik E, Ellozy SH, Jacobs TS, Teodorescu V et al (2006) Endovascular treatment of complicated aortic aneurysms in patients with underlying arteriopathies. Ann Vasc Surg 20(4):464–471
34. Preventza O, Mohammed S, Cheong BY, Gonzalez L, Ouzounian M, Livesay JJ et al (2014) Endovascular therapy in patients with genetically triggered thoracic aortic disease: applications and short- and mid-term outcomes. Eur JCardio-thorac Surg 46(2):248–253 discussion 53

35. Ogino H (2019) Surgical strategy for refractory aortitis. Gen Thorac Cardiovasc Surg 67(1):25–31
36. Gaudric J, Dennery M, Jouhannet C, Kagan N, Saadoun D, Chiche L et al (2016) Aortitis and surgery. La Revue de Medecine Interne 37(4):284–291
37. Arworn S, Orrapin S, Chakrabandhu B, Reanpang T, Settakorn J, Laohapensang K (2018) Aorto-enteric fistula after endovascular abdominal aortic aneurysm repair for Behcet's disease patient: a case report. EJVES Short Rep 39:54–57
38. Imai S, Tahara N, Hiromatsu S, Fukumoto Y, Tanaka H (2018) Endovascular repair for inflammatory abdominal aortic aneurysm. Eur Heart J Cardiovasc Imaging 19(10):1191–1192
39. Duque Santos A, Reyes Valdivia A, Romero Lozano MA, Aracil Sanus E, Ocana Guaita J, Gandarias C (2018) Outcomes of open and endovascular repair of inflammatory abdominal aortic aneurysms. Vascular 26(2):203–208
40. Arafat A, Roselli EE, Idrees JJ, Feng K, Banaszak L, Eagleton M et al (2016) Stent grafting acute aortic dissection: comparison of DeBakey extent IIIA versus IIIB. Ann Thorac Surg 102(5):1473–1481
41. Jansen M, Saleh S, Bolster M, O'Donnell A, Ahern T, Spence L et al (2010) Thoracic vasculitis presenting as surgical problems. Virchows Archiv 456(1):91–96
42. Mennander AA, Miller DV, Liang KP, Warrington KJ, Connolly HM, Schaff HV et al (2008) Surgical management of ascending aortic aneurysm due to non-infectious aortitis. Scand Cardiovasc J 42(6):417–424
43. Nishimura S, Amano M, Izumi C, Kuroda M, Yoshikawa Y, Takahashi Y et al (2016) Multiple coronary artery aneurysms and thoracic aortitis associated with IgG4-related disease. Internal medicine (Tokyo, Japan) 55(12):1605–1609
44. Zambetti BR, Garrett E Jr (2016) Plasmacytic aortitis with occlusion of the right coronary artery. Am J Case Rep 17:549–552
45. Tran MN, Langguth D, Hart G, Heiner M, Rafter A, Fleming SJ et al (2015) IgG4-related systemic disease with coronary arteritis and aortitis, causing recurring critical coronary ischemia. Int J Cardiol 201:33–34
46. Oyama-Manabe N, Yabusaki S, Manabe O, Kato F, Kanno-Okada H, Kudo K (2018) IgG4-related cardiovascular disease from the aorta to the coronary arteries: multidetector CT and PET/CT. Radiographics 38(7):1934–1948
47. Blumstein H, Kerr LD, Fallon JT (2006) Giant cell aortitis with histopathologic and clinical response to steroid therapy: a case report. J Thorac Cardiovasc Surg 132(6):1467–1468

18

Evaluation of the predictive value of thorax trauma severity score (TTSS) in thoracic-traumatized patients

Mohamed Reda Zahran[1*], Amr Abd El Monem Abd Elwahab[2], Mohamed Mahmoud Abo El Nasr[3] and Mohamed Ahmed El Heniedy[4]

Abstract

Background: Thorax trauma severity score (TTSS) combines patient-related parameters with the anatomical and physiological parameters, and it can be easily calculated in the emergency room. The validity of this score in the Egyptian population has not been tested; therefore, the objective of this study was to evaluate the prognostic role of TTSS to predict the outcome of thoracic trauma in the Egyptian patients in two centers.

Results: The study included 284 male patients (94.7%) with a mean age of 41 years. Fifty-six patients (18.7%) had conservative management, 216 had morbidity (72%), and 28 patients died (9.3%). One hundred forty-eight patients (49.3%) had a thoracostomy tube, and thoracotomy was required in 4 patients (1.3%). Respiratory rate above 20 cycles/min at admission was associated with mortality (n = 28 (9.3%); $p < 0.001$). One hundred thirty-six patients had TTSS between 0 and 5 points; 56 of them were discharged and 80 of them were admitted to the inpatient ward with a good prognosis. Twenty-four patients had TTSS between 21 and 25 points; all the 24 patients had a fatal prognosis. A cut-off value of 7 points or more of TTSS was 100% sensitive and 97.73% specific to poor and fatal prognosis, and it was significantly associated with acute respiratory distress syndrome and the need for mechanical ventilation (n = 64; $p < 0.001$; AUC = 0.998).

Conclusion: The outcome of thoracic trauma patients could be predicted based on the thorax trauma severity score. A score of 7 points or above was associated with increased morbidity, and a score of 20 points or above predicted a fatal prognosis and prolonged mechanical ventilation.

Keywords: Thorax trauma severity score, Thoracic trauma, Outcome prediction

Background

The outcome of thoracic trauma is variable and is affected by the interaction between several demographics and anatomical factors [1, 2]. Although most of the life-threatening injuries can be managed with minor surgical interventions [3, 4], the reported mortality in thorax trauma ranged from 15 to 25% [5]. Additionally, predictors of morbidity and mortality after thoracic trauma vary widely in the literature, and the associated extra-thoracic injuries have a significant role in determining the outcome s[4].

Several scores were developed to predict the outcomes of thoracic injuries such as the trauma and injury severity score, which is used in poly-traumatized patients, and Wagner score for the pulmonary contusion [6]. Trauma and injury severity score may underestimate thoracic injuries, in addition to its difficulty in the calculation [7]. In 2000, Pape and coworkers developed a new score, thorax trauma severity score (TTSS), that combined the patient-related parameters with the anatomical and physiological parameters [8]. TTSS is composed of five parameters; age, PaO2/FiO2, pleural injuries, lung contusion, and rib fractures, and the score ranges from 0 to 25 points.

The validity of this score in the Egyptian population has not been evaluated; therefore, the objective of this

* Correspondence: medozamzam1@gmail.com
[1]Emergency Medicine, Faculty of Medicine, Tanta University, Mansoura, Egypt
Full list of author information is available at the end of the article

study was to assess the prognostic role of TTSS to predict the outcome of thoracic trauma in the Egyptian patients in two centers.

Methods

Patients and design

We conducted a prospective cohort study on 300 chest trauma patients in two emergency departments during the period from May 2018 through April 2019. We included adult patients aged 18 years or above. Patients with a burn, chronic respiratory diseases, pregnancy, malignancy, end-organ failure, and patients with associated mediastinal, severe abdominal, pelvic injuries, or brain injuries with Glasgow Coma Score (GCS) below 13 were excluded.

Ethical considerations

The study was approved by the local Ethical Committee of the participating centers, and the need to obtain informed consent was waived.

Trauma management

We managed the patients according to the Advanced Trauma Life Support (ATLS) guidelines. All patients had routine laboratory investigations including random blood glucose, complete blood count, and arterial blood gases (ABG). We performed a chest X-ray, computed tomography scan, electrocardiogram for all patients, and echocardiography if a cardiac injury was suspected.

Scoring system

TTSS (thorax trauma severity score) was used to evaluate the severity of the trauma, and its components are shown in Table 1. The outcome was recorded along with the patient's data and the scoring system. The prognosis of the patients was classified into the following categories: normal; which included discharged patients, good; which included patients who were admitted to inpatient ward up to 7 days, or patients with pneumothorax, or hemothorax who were managed with simple thoracostomy, fair; which included patients who were admitted to inpatient ward more than 7 days, patients with pneumothorax with persistent air leak, patients with hemothorax who needed open thoracotomy, or patients who were admitted to ICU but did not require mechanical ventilation, poor; which included patients who were admitted to ICU and needed mechanical ventilation, fatal; which included patients who died. Morbidity was presented with a good, fair, and poor prognosis, and mortality with the fatal prognosis.

Statistical analysis

Quantitative data were presented as mean and standard deviation (SD) and qualitative data as frequencies and percentages. The chi-square or Fisher exact tests were used to compare qualitative data. A probability value of less than 0.05 was considered statistically significant. Regression analysis was used to explore the relation between TTSS, and the duration of mechanical ventilation and ICU stay. The receiver operator curve (ROC) was used to evaluate the statistical significance of sensitivity and specificity and to choose suitable cut-off points to make decisions. SPSS (Statistical Package for Social Science; SPSS for IBM, USA) version 23 for Microsoft Windows was used to perform the analysis.

Results

Patients' data

The study included 284 male patients (94.7%), and 68 of the patients (22.7%) were below 30 years, 108 patients (36.0%) were between 30 and 41 years, 60 patients (20.0%) were between 42 and 54 years, 44 patients (14.7%) were between 55 and 70 years, 20 patients (6.7%) were above 70 years, the mean age was 41 years and the standard of deviation was ± 14. Ninety-six patients (32.0%) had penetrating trauma, and 204 patients had blunt trauma (68.0%) including, fall from height in 40 patients (13.33%), road traffic accident (RTA) in 52 patients (17.33%), and crush injury in 4 patients (1.33%).

Respiratory rate was associated with patients' outcomes; all fatalities had a respiratory rate above 20 cycle/min ($p < 0.001$). All patients with heart rate (HR) below 100 beats per minute were discharged, and HR above 100 beats per minute was associated with an increase in morbidity and mortality ($p < 0.001$) (Table 2).

Table 1 Items of the thorax trauma severity score (TTSS) [8]

Grade	PaO2/FiO2	Rib fractures	Lung contusion	Pleura	Age	Points
0	> 400	0	No	No	< 30	0
I	300–400	1–3	Unilobar unilateral	Pneumothorax	30–41	1
II	200–300	3–6 (will use 4 to 6) unilateral	Unilobar bilateral or bilobar unilateral	Hemothorax or hemo/pneumothorax unilateral	42–54	2
III	150–200	> 3 bilateral	Bilateral < 2 lobes	Hemothorax or hemo/pneumothorax bilateral	55–70	3
IV	< 150	Flail chest	Bilateral ≥ 2 lobes	Tension pneumothorax	> 70	5

Notes: (a) For calculation of the total score, all categories are summed. (b) A minimum value is of 0 points and a maximum value is of 25 points

Table 2 The effect of vital signs on patients' outcomes

Vital signs		Discharge N = 56	Morbidity N = 216	Mortality N = 28	*p* value
SBP					<0.001
	<90	0 (0.00%)	48 (16.00%)	20 (6.70%)	
	90–109	4 (1.3%)	44 (14.70%)	0 (0.00%)	
	>110	52 (17.3%)	124 (41.30%)	8 (2.70%)	
RR					<0.001
	1219	52 (17.30%)	44 (14.70%)	0 (0.00%)	
	20–29	4 (1.30%)	148 (49.30%)	0 (0.00%)	
	>30	0 (0.00%)	24 (8.00%)	28 (9.30%)	
HR					<0.001
	<100	56 (18.70%)	60 (20.00%)	0 (0.00%)	
	100–120	0 (0.00%)	128 (42.70%)	12 (4.00%)	
	120–140	0 (0.00%)	28 (9.30%)	12 (4.00%)	
	>140	0 (0.00%)	0 (0.00%)	4 (1.30%)	

(Categorical variables are presented as number and percentage)
HR: Heart rate, *RR*: respiratory rate, *SBP*: systolic blood pressure

Fifty-six patients (18.7%) were discharged with conservative management, 216 patients had morbidity (72%), and 28 patients died (9.3%); all of them had life-threatening thoracic injuries (Table 3). One hundred forty-eight patients (49.3%) had closed thoracostomy or observation in the inpatient ward, 24 patients (8%) needed observation ICU, and 44 patients (14.7%) needed mechanical ventilation. Thoracotomy was required in 4 patients (1.3%).

TTSS and patients' outcome

One hundred thirty-six patients had TTSS between 0 and 5 points; 56 of them were discharged and 80 of them were admitted to the inpatient ward with a good prognosis.

Ninety-two patients had TTSS between 6 and 10 points; 60 of them were admitted to inpatient ward (40 patients had a good prognosis 20 patients had a fair prognosis), and 32 patients were admitted to ICU (16 patients had a fair prognosis and16 patients had a poor prognosis).

Twenty-four patients had TTSS between 11 and 15 points; eight of them were admitted to the inpatient ward and had a fair prognosis, and 16 patients were admitted to ICU (8 patients had a fair prognosis and eight patients had a poor prognosis).

Twenty-four patients had TTSS between 16 and 20 points; 20 of them were admitted to ICU and had a poor prognosis and four patients died after 34–38 days of ICU stay.

Twenty-four patients had TTSS between 21 and 25 points; 12 of them died in the emergency room (ER) and 12 died after 30–40 days in the ICU. All the 24 patients had a fatal prognosis.

TTSS of 7 points or more was associated with developing acute respiratory distress syndrome (ARDS) and the need for mechanical ventilation (n = 64). Increased TTSS was associated with increased duration of mechanical ventilation and prolonged ICU stay (p < 0.001) (Figs. 1 and 2). A cut-off point of 7 or above of TTSS had a 100% sensitivity to fair, poor, and fatal prognosis, and 97.73 % specificity to good and normal prognosis, with 96.88% positive predictive value and 100.00 % negative predictive value. The area under the curve was 0.998 (Fig. 3).

Discussion

Our study showed that the TTSS value of 7 points or above points had 100% sensitivity and 97.73 % specificity to morbidity and mortality of patients of isolated thoracic trauma after exclusion of associated severe extra-thoracic injuries. This result agrees with Elbaih and coworkers, who found that the TTSS value of 7 or above was 100% sensitive and 100% specific to poor prognosis [9]. Similarly, Elnaby and associates found that the TTSS value of 8 or above had a sensitivity of 92.3% and a specificity of 100% in the prediction of poor outcome and mortality [10]. In another study, TTSS of 8 points had a sensitivity of 80% and a specificity of 94% to predict complications and death [11].

In our study, the area under the curve was 0.998 showing that TTSS has a strong predictive value for morbidity and mortality. In a study by Hildebrand and associates, they found that TTSS had the best predictive value in comparison to CT-dependent Wagner score for pulmonary contusion and CT-independent scoring system [12]. On the other hand, Moon and associates found that thorax and trauma injury severity score (TRISS) was superior to TTSS in predicting the mortality of severe thoracic trauma [13]. However, the study was retrospective with possible selection biases.

Mortality occurred in 28 patients (9.3%) and had TTSS ranging from 20 to 23. Subhani and coworkers had 9.8% mortality, and high TTSS was associated with increased mortality. (14) We noticed that bilateral lung contusion more than two lobes had a significant effect on mortality, which is consistent with other studies [14].

Flail chest was associated with a mortality rate of 66% in our study. In another study, the flail chest had a mortality of 36% [14].

We found that 76 patients (25.3%) had lung contusion injuries in the absence of thoracic bony fractures. Shorr and colleagues declared that severe parenchymal lung injuries could be present even if thoracic bony injuries are absent [15]. The majority of rib fracture injuries were managed with conservative treatment. Mechanical ventilation was not indicated except when signs of respiratory failure were developed [16, 17].

Table 3 Patients' outcome distributed according to thorax trauma severity score (TTSS)

TTSS parameters		Prognosis of patients			*p* value
		Discharge	Morbidity	Mortality	
		N = 56	*N* = 216	*N* = 28	
Pleural involvement	No	56(18.70%)	20(6.70%)	0(0.00%)	< 0.001
	Pneumothorax	0(0.00%)	76(25.30%)	0(0.00%)	
	Hemothorax or hemo/pneumothorax unilateral	0(0.00%)	84(28.00%)	0(0.00%)	
	Hemothorax or hemo/pneumothorax bilateral	0(0.00%)	32(10.70%)	8(2.70%)	
	Tension pneumothorax	0(0.00%)	4(0.00%)	20(6.70%)	
Lung contusion	No	56(18.70%)	100(33.30%)	0(0.00%)	< 0.001
	Unilobar unilateral	0(0.00%)	32(10.70%)	0(0.00%)	
	Unilobar bilateral or bilobar unilateral	0(0.00%)	28(9.30%)	0(0.00%)	
	Bilateral < 2 lobes	0(0.00%)	20(6.70%)	0(0.00%)	
	Bilateral > 2 lobes	0(0.00%)	36(12.00%)	28(9.30%)	
Rib fractures	No	56(18.70%)	144(48.00%)	0(0.00%)	< 0.001
	1–3 Fracture ribs	0(0.00%)	28(9.30%)	4(1.30%)	
	3–6 Fracture ribs	0(0.00%)	28(9.30%)	0(0.00%)	
	> 3 Bilateral fracture ribs	0(0.00%)	8(2.70%)	8(2.70%)	
	Flail chest	0(0.00%)	8(2.70%)	16(5.30%)	
PaO2/FiO2	> 400	56(18.70%)	24(8.00%)	0(0.00%)	< 0.001
	300–400	0(0.00%)	80(26.70%)	0(0.00%)	
	200–300	0(0.00%)	60(20.00%)	0(0.00%)	
	150–200	0(0.00%)	28(9.30%)	0(0.00%)	
	< 150	0(0.00%)	24(8.00%)	28(9.30%)	

(Categorical variables are presented as number and percentage)

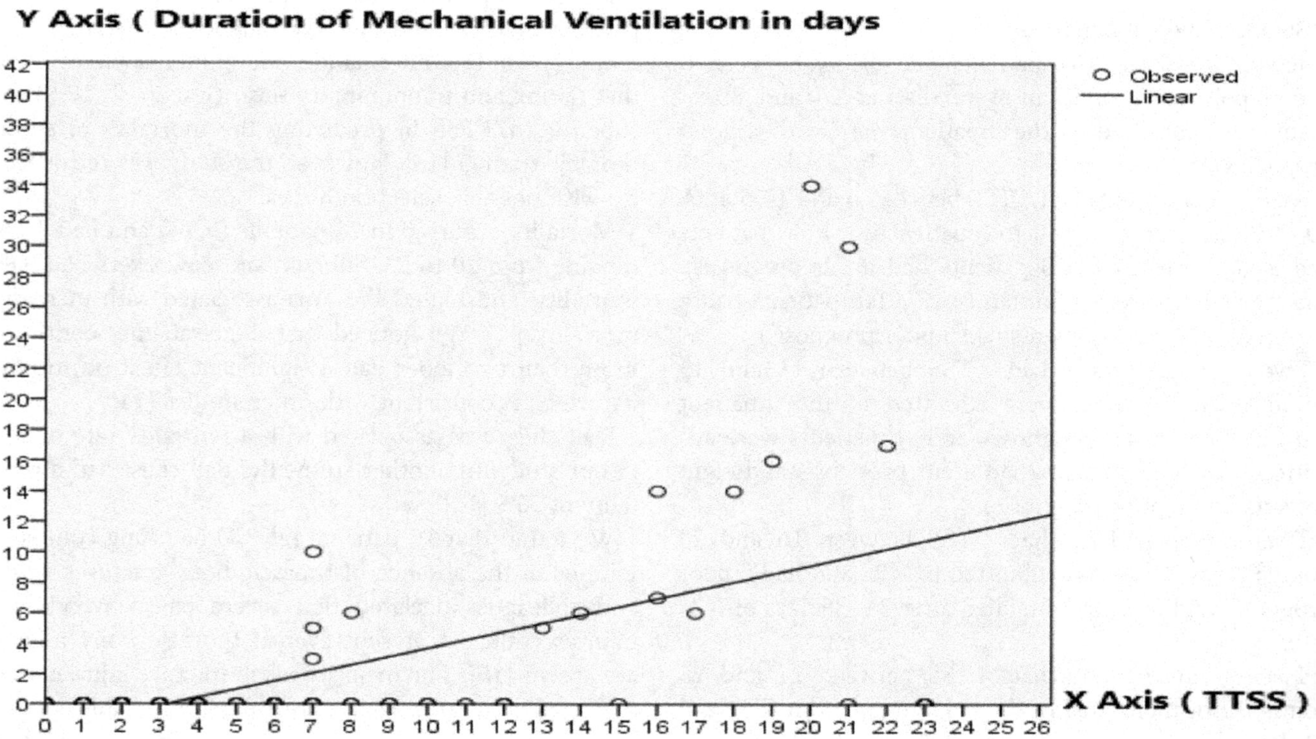

Fig. 1 Regression curve showing the effect of increasing TTSS (X-axis) on the duration of mechanical ventilation (Y-axis). ($p < 0.001$)

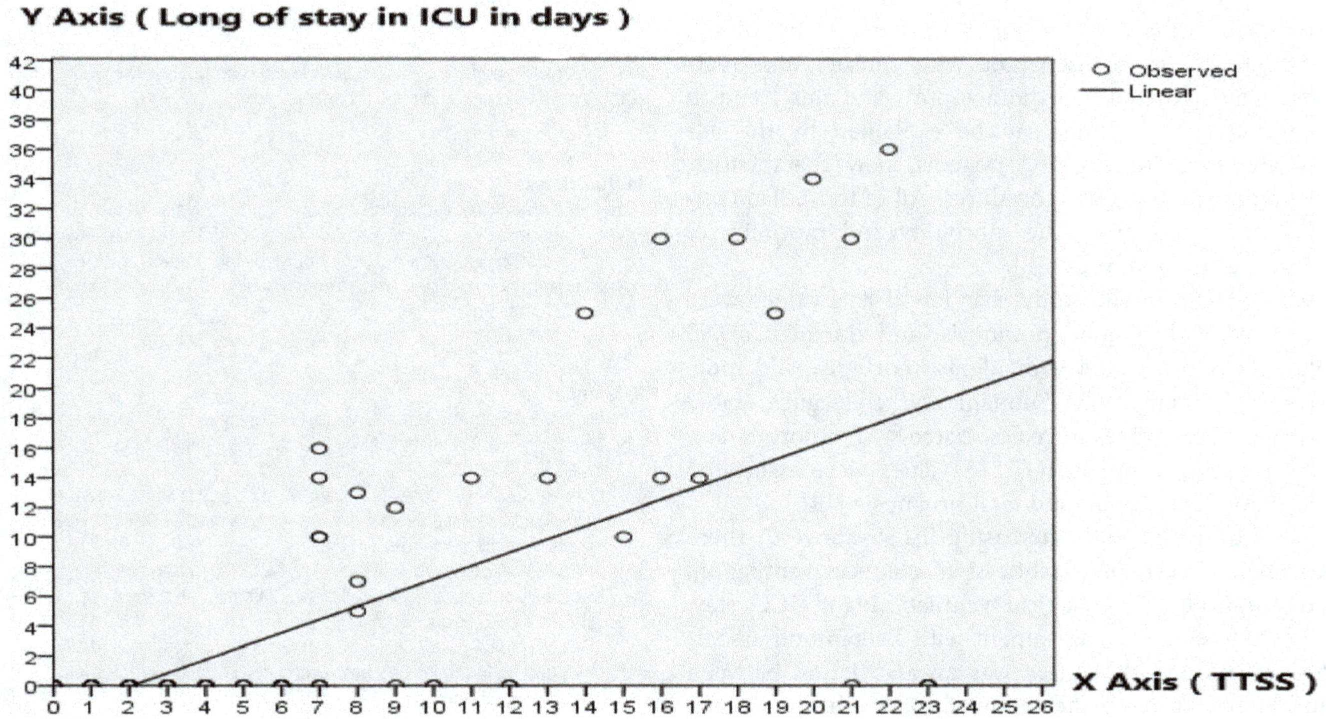

Fig. 2 Regression curve showing the effect of increasing TTSS (X-axis) on the duration of ICU stay (Y-axis). ($p < 0.001$)

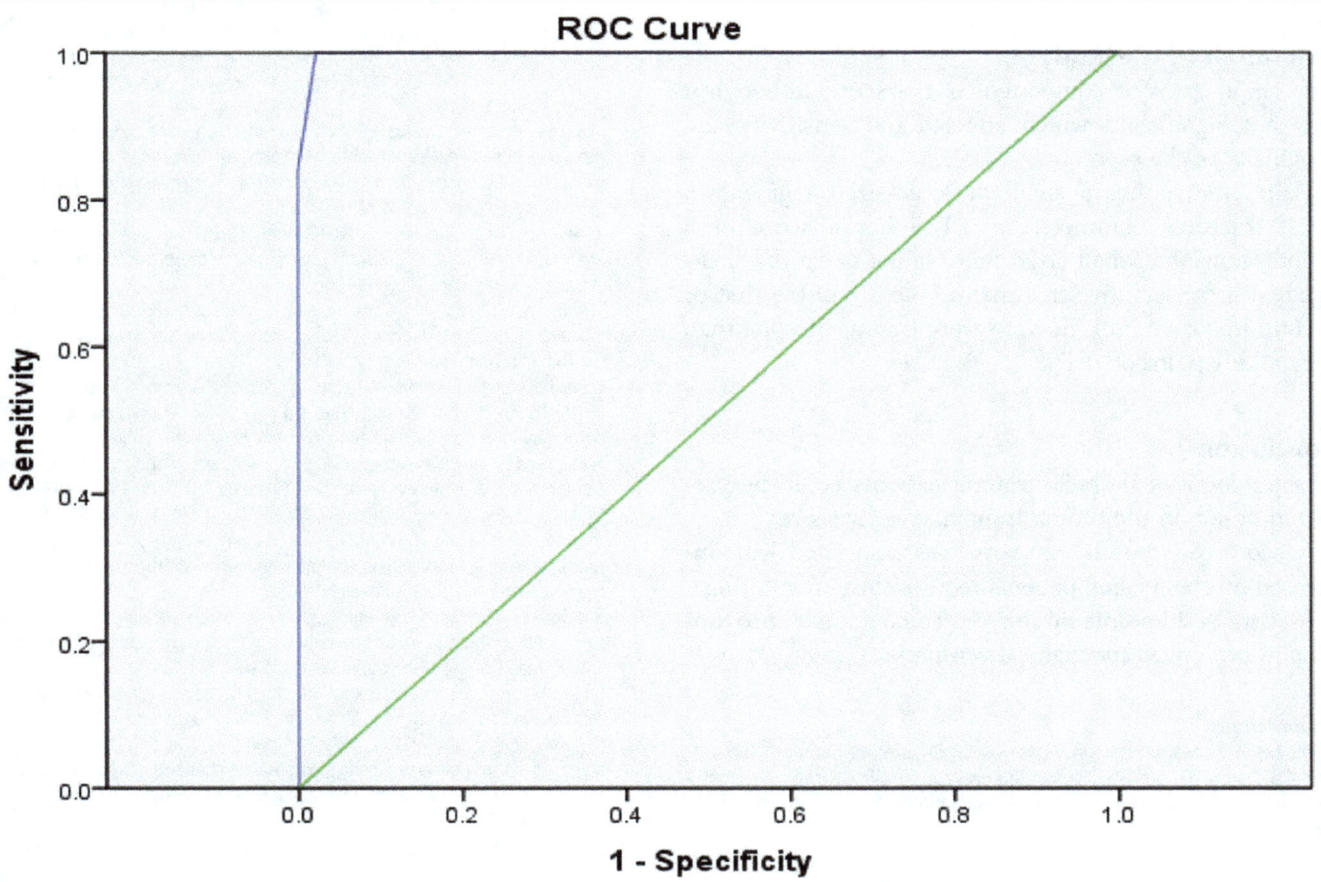

Fig. 3 The receiver operator curve (ROC) of the predictability of thorax trauma severity score (TTSS) with area under the curve equals 0.998

In our study, most patients were managed with simple procedures without any major complications, and 56 patients (18.7%) were discharged with conservative treatment. Four patients had thoracotomy, and this trend in managing chest trauma can be explained by the advancement of the imaging systems, new therapeutics, and minimally invasive procedures. All of those had contributed in decreasing the morbidity and mortality of thoracic trauma injuries [18].

We noticed in our study that low TTSS values were associated with a good prognosis, and the high TTSS values were associated with higher morbidity and mortality. Correspondingly, Subhani and colleagues stated that low TTSS values were associated with a normal and good prognosis, and high TTSS values were associated with a good, fair, poor, and fatal prognosis [14].

We found that with increasing TTSS above 7, there was an increased probability of mechanical ventilation, and duration of mechanical ventilation and ICU stay. This study comes in agreement with Balkan and associates, who found that there was an association between morbidity, mortality, and the need for mechanical ventilation [19].

TTSS, with a cut-off value of 7 points or above, was associated with ARDS, which is consistent with other studies [20, 21].

Limitation of the study

The age is a major component of the score, although it was not significant, which affected the sensitivity and specificity of the score.

Flail chest, either a small or large-sized segment in chest fractures parameter in TTSS has a score of 5 points; however, small-sized flail segments can be managed with conservative treatment. Fracture of the first or second ribs is an indicator of severe trauma; despite that, they take 1 point on TTSS.

Conclusion

The outcome of thoracic trauma patients could be predicted based on the thorax trauma severity score.

A score of 7 points or above was associated with increased morbidity, and patients require close monitoring.

A score of 20 points or above predicted a fatal prognosis and prolonged mechanical ventilation.

Abbreviations

ARDS: Acute respiratory distress syndrome; ER: Emergency Room; HR: Heart rate; ICU: Intensive Care Unit; RR: Respiratory rate; RTA: Road traffic accident; SBP: Systolic blood pressure; TRISS: Trauma and Injury Score; TTSS: Thorax trauma severity score

Acknowledgements

Very thankful and grateful to all who helped me to complete this work.

Authors' contributions

MZ participitated in collection of data and writing the thesis. AA was the supervisor participated in statistical analysis, writing the thesis and pioneering the ideas. MMA and MAE participated in writing and guiding the work . All authors have read and approved the manuscript.

Author details

Emergency Medicine, Faculty of Medicine, Tanta University, Mansoura, Egypt. [2]Cardiothoracic Surgery, Faculty of Medicine, Tanta University, Tanta, Egypt. [3]Cardiothoracic Surgery, Faculty of Medicine, Tanta University, Tanta, Egypt. [4]Emergency Medicine Department, Faculty of Medicine, Tanta University, Tanta, Egypt.

References

1. Bozorgi F, Mirabi A, Chabra A, Mirabi R, Hosseininejad SM, Zaheri H (2018) Mechanisms of Traumatic Injuries in Multiple Trauma Patients. Int J Med Invest 7(2):7–15
2. Dongel I, Coskun A, Ozbay S, Bayram M, Atli B (2013) Management of thoracic trauma in emergency service: Analysis of 1139 cases. Pakistan journal of medical sciences 29(1):58
3. Walls, R., Hockberger, R., & Gausche-Hill, M. (2017). Rosen's Emergency Medicine-Concepts and Clinical Practice E-Book (9th ed., Vol 1 , pp. 382-391) . Elsevier Health Sciences.
4. Mirka H, Ferda J, Baxa J (2012) Multidetector computed tomography of chest trauma: indications, technique and interpretation. Insights into imaging 3(5):433–449
5. Peters S, Nicolas V, Heyer CM (2010) Multidetector computed tomography-spectrum of blunt chest wall and lung injuries in polytraumatized patients. Clinical radiology 65(4):333–338
6. Mommsen P, Zeckey C, Andruszkow H, Weidemann J, Frömke C, Puljic P et al (2012) Comparison of different thoracic trauma scoring systems in regards to prediction of post-traumatic complications and outcome in blunt chest trauma. *Journal of surgical research 176*(1):239–247
7. Domingues, C. D. A., Nogueira, L. D. S., Settervall, C. H. C., & Sousa, R. M. C. D. (2015). Performance of Trauma and Injury Severity Score (TRISS) adjustments: an integrative review. Revista da Escola de Enfermagem da USP, 49(SPE), 138-146.
8. Pape HC, Remmers D, Rice J, Ebisch M, Krettek C, Tscherne H (2000) Appraisal of early evaluation of blunt chest trauma: development of a standardized scoring system for initial clinical decision making. J Trauma Acute Care Surgery 49(3):496–504
9. Elbaih AH, Elshapowry IM, Kalil NG, El-Aouty H (2016) Evaluation of thoracic trauma severity score in predicting the outcome of isolated blunt chest trauma patients. IJSM 2(3):100–106
10. Elnaby, M.A., Saffan, M.M., Wahdan, A.M., & Saad, D. (2018). Assesement Of Isolated Blunt Chest Trauma Patients In Benha University Hospital According To Thoracic Trauma Severity Score .
11. Casas IM, Marchante MAA, Paduraru M, Olea AIF, Nolasco A, Medina JC (2016) Thorax trauma severity score: is it reliable for patient's evaluation in a secondary level hospital? Bulletin Emergency Trauma 4(3):150
12. Hildebrand F, van Griensven M, Garapati R, Krettek C, Pape HC (2002) Diagnostics and scoring in blunt chest trauma. Eur J Trauma 28(3):157–167
13. Moon SH, Kim JW, Byun JH, Kim SH, Choi JY, Jang IS et al (2017) The thorax trauma severity score and the trauma and injury severity score: Do they predict in-hospital mortality in patients with severe thoracic trauma?: A retrospective cohort study. Medicine 96(42)
14. Subhani SS, Muzaffar MS, Khan MI (2014) Comparison of outcome between low and high thoracic trauma severity score in blunt trauma chest patients. J Ayub Med College Abbottabad 26(4):474–477
15. Shorr RM, Crittenden M, Indeck M, Hartunian SL, Rodriguez A (1987) Blunt thoracic trauma. Analysis of 515 patients. Annals Surgery 206(2):200
16. Simon B, Ebert J, Bokhari F, Capella J, Emhoff T, Hayward T III et al (2012) Management of pulmonary contusion and flail chest: an Eastern Association for the Surgery of Trauma practice management guideline. J Trauma Acute Care Surgery 73(5):S351–S361
17. Menditto VG, Gabrielli B, Marcosignori M, Screpante F, Pupita G, Polonara S et al (2012) A management of blunt thoracic trauma in an emergency department observation unit: pre-post observational study. J Trauma Acute Care Surgery 72(1):221–226

18. Trinkle JK, Richardson JD, Franz JL, Grover FL, Arom KV, Holmstrom FM (1975) Management of flail chest without mechanical ventilation. Annals Thoracic Surgery 19(4):355–363
19. Balkan EM, Oktar LG, Kayt-Cangtr A (2002) Emergency thoracotomy for blunt thoracic trauma. Annals Thoracic Cardiovasc Surgery 8(2):78–82
20. Aukema TS, Beenen LF, Hietbrink F, Leenen LP (2011) Validation of the Thorax Trauma Severity Score for mortality and its value for the development of acute respiratory distress syndrome. Open Access Emergency Med 3:49
21. Daurat A, Millet I, Roustan JP, Maury C, Taourel P, Jaber S et al (2016) Thoracic Trauma Severity score on admission allows to determine the risk of delayed ARDS in trauma patients with pulmonary contusion. Injury 47(1): 147–153

Modified selective aortic root reconstruction with valve repair for treatment of Stanford A aortic dissection

Mohammed Abd Al Jawad

Abstract

Background: Acute aortic dissection is a serious emergency with a significant impact on mortality and morbidity. Many patients present with hemodynamic instability that may prevent them from being transported to more experienced centers. We aim to present our experience with a modified limited root approach in terms of the operative details and early results.

Results: This retrospective study included 27 patients who presented with Stanford A aortic dissection and underwent modified selective root replacement. All patients were followed up using transthoracic echocardiography at 6 months postoperatively and at yearly intervals thereafter. Computed tomography (CT) angiography was performed 12 months after the initial surgery.

A total of 92.6% of patients required concomitant aortic valve repair. There was no operative mortality related to the operation itself; however, four patients died during the follow-up period. One patient developed new severe aortic regurgitation in the 6th month of follow-up. One patient developed a pseudoaneurysm related to the suture line that was diagnosed by CT angiography in the 16th month of follow-up.

Conclusions: The early results of modified selective root reconstruction with aortic valve repair are promising. This procedure is a quick, reliable, easily reproducible, and technically undemanding valve-sparing treatment for acute aortic root dissection.

Keywords: Aortic dissection, Aortic root, Stanford type A, Root reconstruction, Valve sparing

Background

Acute Stanford type A aortic dissection is one of the most challenging scenarios encountered in the emergency room (ER), a true emergency that is associated with very high risks of morbidity and mortality [1]. The surgical management of aortic dissection has evolved along a circuitous path and is constantly being challenged by many authors. The main concerns are the extent and length of the operation in this fragile group of patients [2].

The trend toward aggressive root replacement with the addition of valve-sparing procedures demands a new level of expertise and has a slow learning curve for many surgeons, necessitating the concept of an "aortic center" [2, 3].

Unfortunately, the concept of an "aortic center" may not be feasible for developing countries, and even if such a center exists, unnecessary transport delays hinder properly timed definitive management. If a simpler intervention was developed many rural areas with cardiac surgery capabilities and acceptable levels of training could save many high-risk or hemodynamically unstable patients without the risks involved in transporting them.

In this study, we aim to present our experience by evaluating the clinical and echocardiographic results of modified limited root reconstruction in the context of aortic dissection.

Correspondence: mohammed_abdaljawad@med.asu.edu.eg
Department of Cardiothoracic Surgery, Faculty of Medicine, Ain Shams University, Abbaseya Square, Cairo, Egypt

Methods

This retrospective observational study included 27 patients who had Stanford type A aortic dissection involving the root and underwent modified selective root reconstruction with or without aortic valve repair. The study took place in the Ain Shams University Hospitals, spanning from July 2014 until October 2019. The study protocol was revised and approved by the Ethical Committee at our institute, by which patient consent was waived due to the retrospective nature of the study.

All patients were followed up using transthoracic echocardiography at 6 months postoperatively and on a yearly basis afterward or whenever clinical symptoms are indicated. Computed tomography (CT) angiography was performed 12 months after the initial operation to evaluate false lumen thrombosis and remodeling in the native residual aortic segments. Positive aortic remodeling was defined by obliteration of the proximal entry point with subsequent reduction of the false lumen along with a corresponding increase in the size of the true lumen and, ultimately, obliteration of the false lumen. Negative remodeling was defined as a failure of reduction of the false lumen, pseudoaneurysm formation, or persistence of the side branch arising from the false lumen [4].

The primary endpoint of the study was operative mortality. The secondary endpoints were all-cause mortality during follow-up; the occurrence of new aortic regurgitation (AR) above grade 2+ on transthoracic echocardiogram or of residual dissection or pseudoaneurysm on CT angiography by the 12-month follow-up; reoperation for AR; residual dissection or pseudoaneurysm; and significant postoperative complications.

Surgical technique

Cardiopulmonary bypass (CPB) was performed through femoral artery cannulation in 24 patients and innominate artery cannulation in 3 patients. Venous cannulation was determined according to associated procedures, e.g., mitral replacement. The target temperature range was 20.1-28 °C (moderate hypothermia) as measured by a nasopharyngeal probe.

Once the heart entered cardioplegic arrest, the aorta was incised, and the root was carefully examined. If dissection involved the root at the noncoronary sinus and/

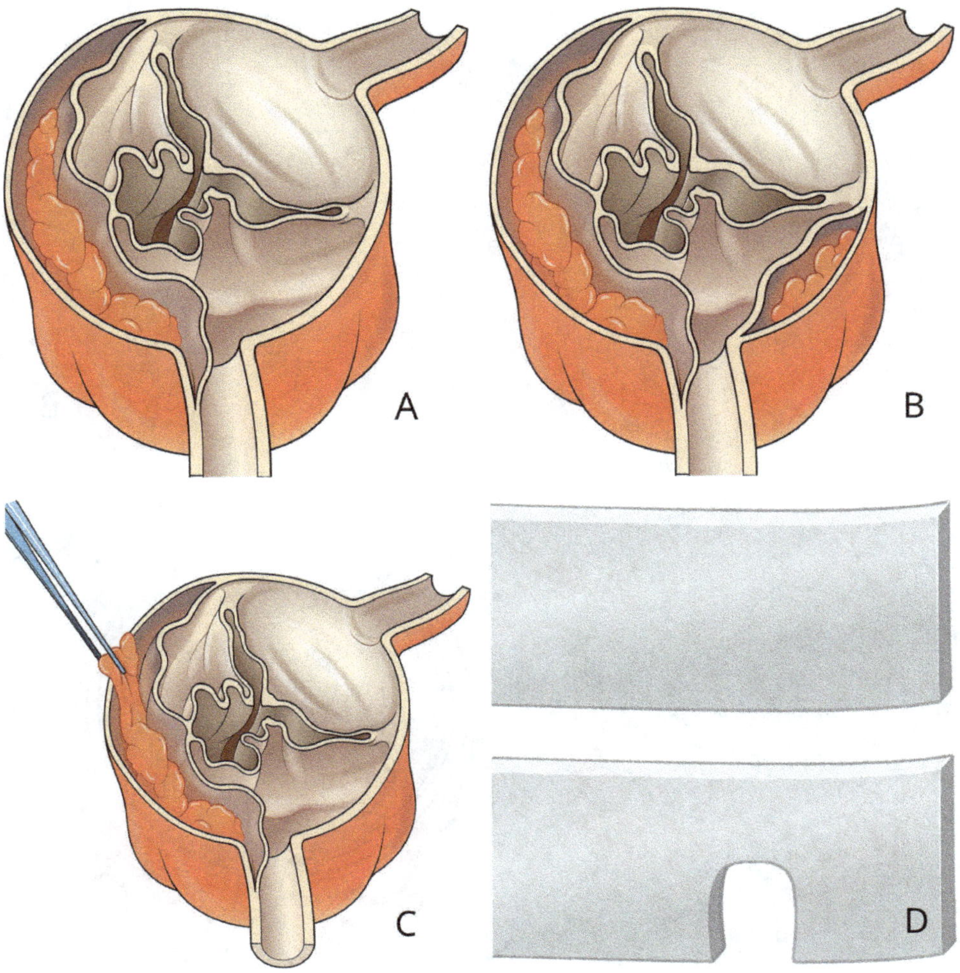

Fig. 1 Operative sighting of the aortic root and preparation for the procedure

or the right coronary sinus, i.e., sparing the left coronary sinus and ostium, the repair was carried out even if there was an extension of the flap to the right coronary ostia (Fig. 1a, b). The valve leaflets were thoroughly examined to determine whether they were bicuspid or tricuspid and to assess their leaflet pliability, calcification, and raphe fibrosis in bicuspids. Additionally, the geometric height of the leaflets (gH) was roughly estimated. If this value was less than 17 mm in the tricuspid valve or less than 20 mm in the bicuspid valve, repair was not carried out.

The root was debrided from any thrombi or blood clots and then irrigated with normal saline solution to remove any nonvisible particles; this debridement must reach as far down into the root as possible (Fig. 1c).

A polytetrafluoroethylene (PTFE) patch was cut and fashioned as a strip (for the noncoronary sinus) and/or a strip with an arched opening (to fit in the shape of a saddle above the right coronary ostia) (Fig. 1d).

The patch(es) were then squeezed in the dissected sinuses, reaching as down as possible in the root. The patches were held in place using interrupted 5/0 polypropylene sutures from the inside (Fig. 2a).

Just before the sutures were tightened, a very thin film of BioGlue was applied on both sides of the patch. The film was both thin and homogenous to prevent any bumps on the endothelial side (Fig. 2b).

A sharp scissor was used to trim the upper edges of the patch to achieve an orderly, circular, uniform new aortic wall (Fig. 2c). This step was followed by valve resuspension, subcommissural annuloplasty, and/or leaflet plication as an adjunct repair to nullify residual AR (Fig. 2d).

Aortic valve repairs included resuspension and subcommissural annuloplasty as a basic step in all patients. Any leaflet calcification or raphe fibrosis was gently shaved away with a sharp scalpel to increase the pliability of the leaflet. A 6/0 Prolene suture was passed through the central free margin of each leaflet, stretching every pair of leaflets together to identify any excess tissue that might cause leaflet to prolapse. The prolapsed leaflet was then plicated with a 6/0 Prolene suture to

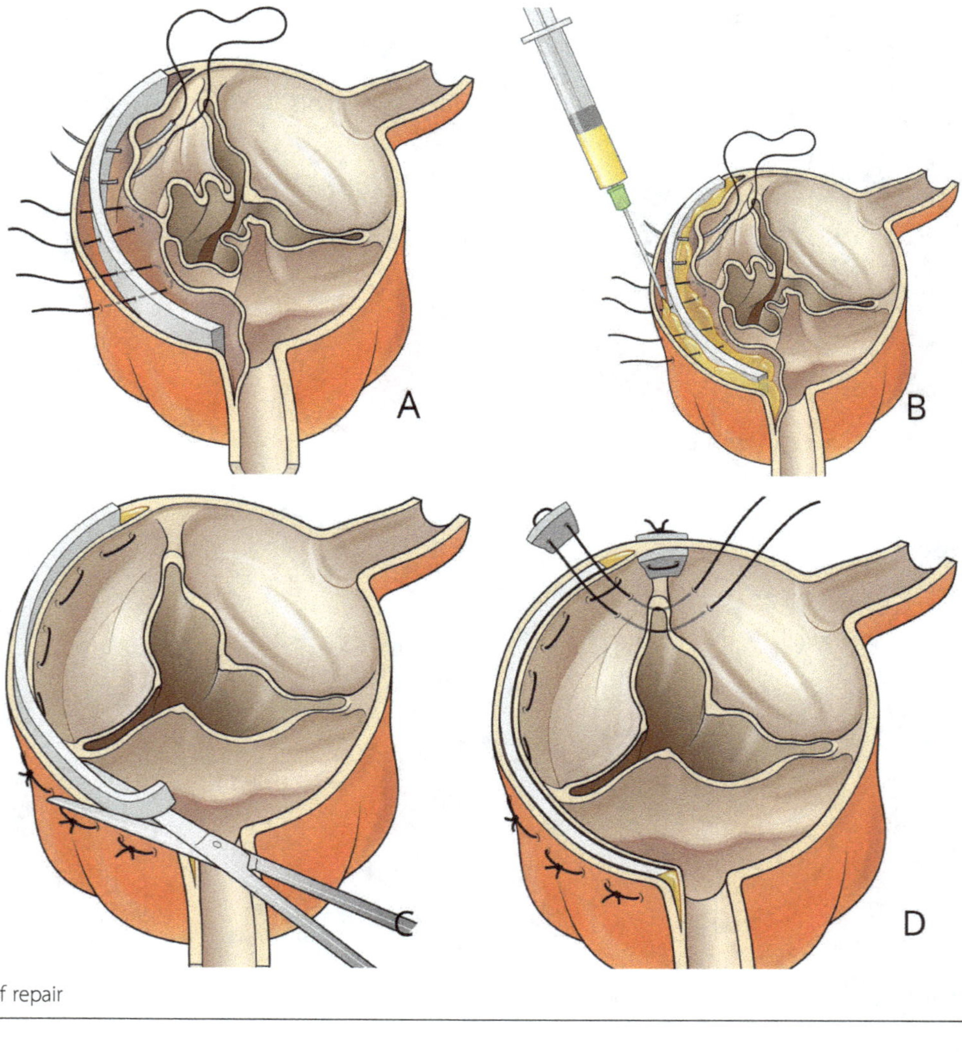

Fig. 2 Basic steps of repair

achieve equal length. The central plication was used to increase the effective height of the leaflet (eH).

The key element of leaflet repair is to achieve good coaptation between all leaflets at two levels: above the annulus and at the annulus. Due to the lack of a special caliper in our institute, more difficult repairs were discouraged.

These steps were followed by an interposition graft to replace the ascending aorta. The dissected distal end of the aorta was obliterated by another patch of PTFE with an additional external PTFE support from the outside. Total circulatory arrest was needed in 3 patients to achieve good distal anastomosis, and all three patients were given unilateral antegrade cerebral perfusion via innominate artery cannulation.

Statistical analysis

The results were expressed as numbers (mean values and standard deviation, median, and range) and percentages as appropriate. Kaplan-Meier survival analysis was performed using MedCalc® v.14.8.1.

Results

The mean age of the patients included in the study was 48.15 ± 10.92 years, denoting a relatively young cohort; 85.1% of patients were male with systemic hypertension as a comorbidity; 77.8% of patients presented with acute Stanford type A dissection (Table 1).

Table 1 Patients' demographics and characteristics

	Selective root + repair *n* = 27	
Age (years)	48.15 ± 10.92	
Sex (male)	23	85.1%
NYHA I-II	11	40.7%
NYHA III-IV	16	59.3%
Comorbidities		
• HTN	19	70.4%
• DM	2	7.4%
• CAD	1	3.7%
• COPD	4	14.8%
• CT disease	0	0%
• Cerebral malperfusion	0	0%
• Renal impairment (Cr > 1.7 mg/dl)	1	3.7%
• Malperfusion of another organ	2	7.4%
Aortic dissection		
• Acute	21	77.8%
• Chronic	6	22.2%

Values are shown as numbers, percentages, mean ± SD. *NYHA* New York Heart Association class, *HTN* hypertension, *DM* diabetes mellitus, *CAD* coronary artery disease, *COPD* chronic obstructive pulmonary disease, *CT* connective tissue, *Cr* creatinine, *mg/dl* milligram(s) per deciliter

A total of 85.2% of patients had more than grade 2 AR as an echocardiographic finding, and 74% of patients had a tricuspid aortic valve configuration (Table 2).

A total of 92.6% of patients required additional aortic valve repair rather than valve resuspension and/or subcommissural annuloplasty. Additional procedures included 2 patients who required an additional saphenous vein graft (SVG) to the right system, one patient who required SVG to the left anterior descending artery (LAD), and one patient who required a concomitant mitral valve replacement. Operative details are shown in Table 3.

There was no operative-related mortality; however, during the follow-up period, four patients were deceased. The first patient sustained a significant neurological disability causing severe bulbar affection and died during the first month of follow-up. The second death was due to a newly developed severe AR, causing heart failure diagnosed in the 6th month of follow-up; the patient was operated on for aortic valve replacement (AVR) and died 1 month after the second operation. The third patient developed a pseudoaneurysm related to the suture line that was diagnosed by CT angiography in the 16th month of follow-up, he was operated on, and the sac was found to be infected. He later died of septicemia. The fourth death was mostly due to sudden fatal arrhythmia in the 23rd month (Tables 4 and 5).

Kaplan-Meier survival analysis showed a 5-year survival rate of 83% for the study cohort (Fig. 3).

During a follow-up period of 30.96 ± 17.82 (median 29 months), 96.3% of patients had ≤ 2 AR by echocardiography. Of the 27 patients included in the study, 22 patients reached the one-year milestone at which follow-up CT angiography showed thrombosis of the false lumen and positive remodeling with no residual dissection in 21 patients (Table 5).

Discussion

The Bentall procedure was one of the earliest approaches of acute aortic dissection involving the root by replacing the ascending aorta and valve with a prefabricated valved conduit [1, 2].

Table 2 Preoperative echocardiographic findings

	Selective root + repair *n* = 27	
EF	52.53 ± 9.17	
Aortic insufficiency		
• ≤ 2	4	14.8%
• > 2	23	85.2%
Aortic valve morphology		
• Bicuspid	7	26%
• Tricuspid	20	74%

Values are shown as numbers, percentages, mean ± SD. *EF* ejection fraction

Table 3 Operative details

	Selective root + repair n = 27	
ACX time (min)	124.4 ± 22.2	
Bypass time (min)	194 ± 53	
Arterial cannulation		
• Innominate artery	3	11.1%
• Femoral artery	24	88.9%
Lowest temperature, °C	23.74 ± 3.87	
Circulatory arrest	3	11.1%
Circulatory arrest time (min)	26 ± 12.16	
Cerebral perfusion during circulatory arrest		
• Antegrade	3	100%
• Retrograde	0	0%
Concomitant procedures	4	
• CABG (SVG to RCA)	2	
• CABG (SVG to LAD)	1	
• MVR	1	
Aortic valve repair (leaflet other than SCA and resuspension)	25	92.6%

Values are shown as numbers, percentages, mean ± SD. *ACX* aortic cross-clamp, *min* minutes, *CABG* coronary artery bypass grafting, *SVG* saphenous vein graft, *RCA* right coronary artery, *LAD* left anterior descending coronary artery, *MVR* mitral valve replacement, *SCA* subcommissural annuloplasty

For a long time, it has been considered the gold standard for root replacement [5]. Since its first adoption, it underwent several modifications that decreased rates of reoperation following the primary procedure [6]. Most of the Bentall procedures performed today utilize mechanical valves owing to their longer duration, yet this carries its own risk of thromboembolic complications and life-long commitment to anticoagulation [7].

However, this was challenged later by the trend of sparing the native valve in younger patients without apparent leaflet disease [8]. The adoption of valve-sparing techniques revolutionized the concept of managing such pathology [9].

Table 4 Postoperative in-hospital outcomes

	Selective root + repair n = 27	
Operative mortality	0	0%
Other mortality (ICU, ward)	0	0%
Permanent neurological impairment	1	3.7%
Transient neurological impairment	3	11.1%
New onset of dialysis	0	0%
GIT complications	0	0%
Re-exploration	2	7.4%

Values are shown as numbers, percentages, mean ± SD. *ICU* intensive care unit, *GIT* gastrointestinal tract

Whether first introduced by Yacoub as "remodeling" [10] or later by David as "reimplantation" [11], both share the same principle of replacing the ascending aorta and root with a prosthetic conduit while preserving the native aortic valve, differing only in the treatment of the aortic sinuses [11, 12]

This revolutionary concept came with the high technical cost of replacing the whole ascending aorta, valve repair, and reimplanting the coronary buttons. Additionally, extensive experience is required both to perform the operation and to select the suitable patient who will benefit from such complicated procedures with the least unfavorable results, with many experienced centers not recommending the procedure for high-risk and elderly patients [2].

Since then, surgeons have realized that restoration of normal root geometry can indeed restore aortic valve competence [9]. Additionally, David and colleagues showed that a reduction of the sinotubular junction (STJ) diameter can achieve even better coaptation of the aortic valve with normal leaflets, leading to a newer concept of "isolated aortic valve repair" [13].

One of the most basic and efficient valve repair techniques is "central plication" of the free margin of the leaflet; shortening the free margin causes the effective height (eH) to increase, thus ensuring better coaptation. A surgeon must ensure that residual leaflet tissue is available before proceeding with the repair; as a rule of thumb, the geometric height (gH) should be at least 17 mm in the tricuspid valve and at least 20 mm in the bicuspid valve for all leaflets together [14].

It is difficult to calculate the long-term outcome of many valve-sparing procedures since most published data include the repair of both tricuspid and bicuspid valves. However, for isolated valve repair, the 5-year freedom from intervention was 95% if the AR was due to prolapse and no leaflet restriction [15].

The mere adhesion of a dissected aortic wall by means of biocompatible glue is a simple and efficient way to

Table 5 Postoperative follow-up data

	Selective root +repair n = 27	
Follow-up death	4	14.8%
Follow-up period	30.96 ± 17.82	Median 29
Aortic insufficiency		
• ≤ 2	26	96.3%
• > 2	1	3.7%
Reoperation for aortic valve	1	3.7%
Reoperation for residual dissection	0	0%
Reoperation for pseudoaneurysm	1	3.7%
1-year remodeling (n = 22)	21 (positive)	95.4%

Values are shown as numbers, percentages, mean ± SD

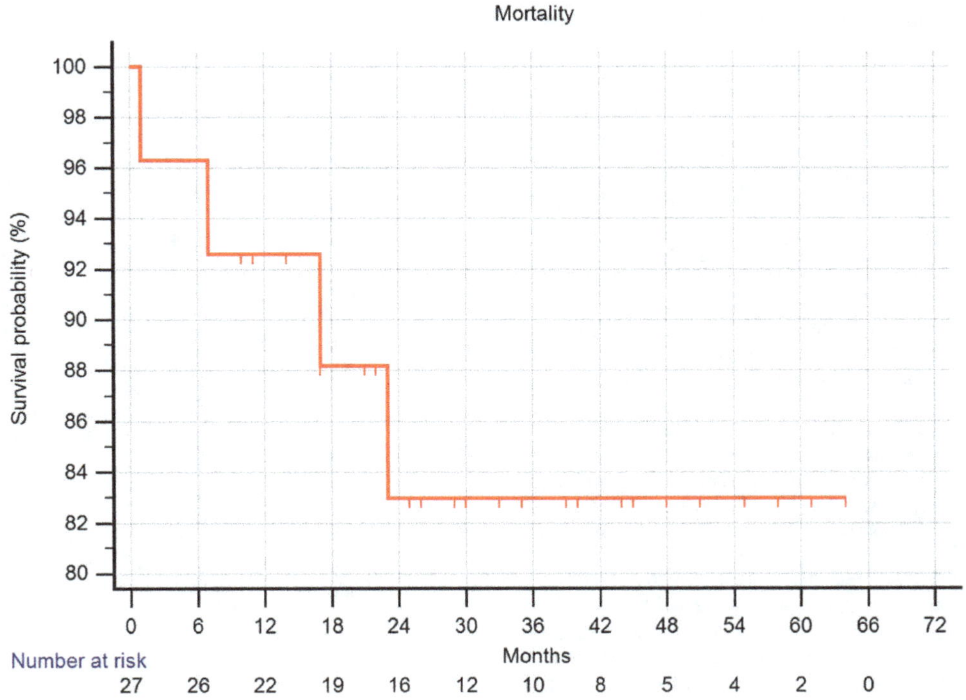

Fig. 3 Kaplan-Meier survival analysis

restore the aortic root configuration. This technique is beneficial in reconstructing dissected sinuses in fragile, severely ill patients who might benefit from short, simple interventions [1]. The critical drawback of this technique is that it is noncurative, potentially resulting in the need for reoperation [2].

The principle of our technique is based on combining three approaches. The first approach is the Stanford and Cleveland Clinic approach, which has always been conservative in dealing with a dissected root using a supracoronary graft, valve resuspension, and/or sinus repair [2]. To achieve a reduction in the sinotubular junction (STJ), we tend to use a graft size of 30 for males and 28 for females. The second approach is that of the Leipzig group, who found that "limited root remodeling" to replace one or two sinuses, i.e., the Uni/Bi Yacoub procedure, has results comparable to those of David's reimplantation procedure [1, 16]; hence, we used sandwiched PTFE patches in selected sinuses. The third approach is the concept of utilizing BioGlue to reconstruct aortic wall sinuses.

Limitations of the study

Our study has some limitations that should be acknowledged. In particular, the design is retrospective, and the number of patients is small. Furthermore, this study is limited to short-term data, and a longer follow-up is needed. Due to the extremely low rate of adverse events, it is not possible to determine small differences in favor of this technique or its alternatives.

In our belief, this technique should be reserved for high-risk patients in whom the risk of open surgery risk outweighs the benefit and medical treatment alone is not effective; patients who will not tolerate complex procedures; patients who would usually be recommended for endovascular interventions rather than open procedures; and critically ill patients who present to cardiac centers offering only basic services and cannot be transferred to a center with advanced aortic services, e.g., a hybrid room and proper cerebral monitoring systems, without a high risk of immediate mortality.

Conclusion

The early results of modified selective root reconstruction with aortic valve repair are excellent. This method provides a quick, reliable, easily reproducible, and technically undemanding valve-sparing technique for acute aortic root dissection.

Abbreviations

CT: Computed tomography; ER: Emergency room; AR: Aortic regurgitation; PTFE: Polytetrafluoroethylene; CPB: Cardiopulmonary bypass; SVG: Saphenous vein graft; LAD: Left anterior descending artery; AVR: Aortic valve replacement; gH: Geometric height; eH: Effective height; STJ: Sinotubular junction

Acknowledgements

Not applicable

Availability of data and material

Data are available with the corresponding author upon request. All data were retrieved from the patient archives of the Cardiothoracic Academy of Ain Shams University.

Author's contributions

The author has contributed to the content of the article. The author read and approved the final manuscript.

References

1. Pape L, Awais M, Woznicki E (2016) Presentation, diagnosis, and outcomes of acute aortic dissection: seventeen-year trends from the international registry of acute aortic dissection. J Vasc Surg *63*(2):552–553. https://doi.org/10.1016/j.jvs.2015.12.012
2. Chiu P, Miller DC (2016) Evolution of surgical therapy for Stanford acute type A aortic dissection. Ann Cardiothorac Surg 5(4):275–295. https://doi.org/10.21037/acs.2016.05.05
3. Urbanski PP, Hijazi H, Dinstak W, Diegeler A (2013) Valve-sparing aortic root repair in acute type A dissection: how many sinuses have to be repaired for curative surgery?†. Eur J Cardio Thorac Surg 44(3):439–444. https://doi.org/10.1093/ejcts/ezt042
4. Patterson BO, Cobb RJ, Karthikesalingam A, Holt PJ, Hinchliffe RJ, Loftus IM, Thompson MM (2014) A systematic review of aortic remodeling after endovascular repair of type B aortic dissection: methods and outcomes. Ann Thorac Surg *97*(2):588–595. https://doi.org/10.1016/j.athoracsur.2013.07.128
5. Mookhoek A, Korteland NM, Arabkhani B, Centa ID, Lansac E, Bekkers JA et al (2016) Bentall procedure: a systematic review and meta-analysis. Ann Thorac Surg 101(5):1684–1689. https://doi.org/10.1016/j.athoracsur.2015.10.090
6. Aomi S, Nakajima M, Nonoyama M, Tomioka H, Bonkohara Y, Satou W et al (2002) Aortic root replacement using composite valve graft in patients with aortic valve disease and aneurysm of the ascending aorta: twenty years experience of late results. Artificial Organs 26(5):467–473. https://doi.org/10.1046/j.1525-1594.2002.06957.x
7. Girardi LN (2008) Composite root replacement with a mechanical conduit. Oper Tech Thorac Cardiovasc Surg 13(3):148–160. https://doi.org/10.1053/j.optechstcvs.2008.06.004
8. Gaudino M, Franco AD, Weltert L, Benedetto U, Lau C, Gambardella I et al (2017) The role of neo-sinus reconstruction in aortic valve-sparing surgery. J Cardiac Surg *32*(6):328–333. https://doi.org/10.1111/jocs.13143
9. Vojáček J, Žáček P, Dominik J (2017) Aortic valve repair and valve sparing procedures. Cor Et Vasa 59(1). https://doi.org/10.1016/j.crvasa.2017.01.025
10. Fagan, A., Pillai, R., Radleysmith, R., & Yacoub, M. H. (1983, January). Results of new valve conserving operation for treatment of aneurysms or acute dissection of aortic root. In British Heart Journal (Vol. 49, No. 3, pp. 302-302). BRITISH MED ASSOC HOUSE, TAVISTOCK SQUARE, LONDON, ENGLAND WC1H 9JR: BRITISH MED JOURNAL PUBL GROUP.
11. David TE, Feindel CM (1992) An aortic valve-sparing operation for patients with aortic incompetence and aneurysm of the ascending aorta. J Thoracic Cardiovasc Surg 103(4):617–622. https://doi.org/10.1016/s0022-5223(19)34942-6
12. Sarsam MA, Yacoub M (1993) Remodeling of the aortic valve anulus. J Thoracic Cardiovasc Surg 105(3):435–438. https://doi.org/10.1016/s0022-5223(19)34225-4
13. David TE, Feindel CM, Armstrong S, Maganti M (2007) Replacement of the ascending aorta with reduction of the diameter of the sinotubular junction to treat aortic insufficiency in patients with ascending aortic aneurysm. J Thoracic Cardiovasc Surg 133(2):414–418. https://doi.org/10.1016/j.jtcvs.2006.09.049
14. Schäfers H-J, Schmied W, Marom G, Aicher D (2013) Cusp height in aortic valves. J Thoracic Cardiovasc Surg 146(2):269–274. https://doi.org/10.1016/j.jtcvs.2012.06.053
15. Kerchove LD, Boodhwani M, Glineur D, Poncelet A, Rubay J, Watremez C et al (2009) Cusp prolapse repair in trileaflet aortic valves: free margin plication and free margin resuspension techniques. Ann Thorac Surg 88(2):455–461. https://doi.org/10.1016/j.athoracsur.2009.04.064
16. Subramanian S, Leontyev S, Borger MA, Trommer C, Misfeld M, Mohr FW (2012) Valve-sparing root reconstruction does not compromise survival in acute type A aortic dissection. Ann Thorac Surg *94*(4):1230–1234. https://doi.org/10.1016/j.athoracsur.2012.04.094

20

Tricuspid three-dimensional ring versus fashioned flexible band annuloplasty in management of functional tricuspid valve regurge: comparative long term study

Abdallah Nosair[1*], Mohamed Elkahely[2], Sherif Nasr[3] and Hesham Alkady[1]

Abstract

Background: Functional tricuspid valve regurgitation due to left sided valve lesions remains a common finding. Nowadays, different types of three-dimensional rings and flexible bands are considered to be the gold standard techniques for repair of such functional regurgitation. Our study aimed for long-term comparison of the durability and effectiveness of those techniques.

Results: The data of 170 adult patients with moderate or more functional tricuspid regurgitation secondary to mitral stenosis or regurgitation receiving tricuspid valve repair using either rigid 3D rings (contour 3D or MC3 ring) or prosthetic fashioned bands (Dacron or PTFE) and mitral valve surgery between March 2013 and September 2018 were collected and analysed. Patients were classified in two matched groups: ring group (group A) consisting of 90 cases and band group (group B) consisting of 80 cases. follow-up period ranged from 55.2 to 78 months (mean 67.2 ± 10.8), during this period New York heart association for dyspnea functional class evaluation and full echocardiographic assessment were done and was scheduled as following: before hospital discharge, after 6 months of surgery and finally, every 2 years. In-hospital mortality was 1(1.1%) and 2 (2.5%) with *p* value 0.49 after ring or band annuloplasty, respectively. No significant differences in both groups regarding hospital mortality and morbidities. There was statistically significant decrease in NYHA class, degree of TR, and PASP within the 2 groups postoperatively with *p* value of 0.03, 0.04, and 0.033, respectively, with no statistically significant difference between both groups (p value > 0.05). There was statistically significant difference in the freedom from recurrent TR and need for reoperation during the follow-up period between both groups with lower recurrence and reoperation rates in group A, (*p* value 0.03 and 0.001, respectively).

Conclusion: Tricuspid valve repair with different annuloplasty rigid three dimensional rings or fashioned flexible bands for functional tricuspid regurgitation offers good long-term outcome. Yet, the rigid rings maintain their benefits on the rate of recurrent TR and the need for reoperation.

Keywords: Functional tricuspid regurgitation, Band annuloplasty, Tricuspid 3D ring

* Correspondence: abdallah_nosair@live.com
[1]Department of Cardiothoracic Surgery, Faculty of Medicine, Cairo University, Cairo, Egypt
Full list of author information is available at the end of the article

Backgrounds

Functional tricuspid regurgitation (FTR) remains a common finding in patients with left-sided valvular heart diseases especially mitral valve regurgitation or stenosis. It is mainly caused by dilatation and flattening of the tricuspid valve (TV) annulus as a result of right ventricular (RV) enlargement and is inevitably affected by the RV function [1]. Multiple studies support the better outcome of using rigid ring annuloplasty over suture repair for treating FTR in concern with the durability and freedom from residual regurgitation. These studies refer the superiority of rigid ring annloplasty to the three-dimensional configuration achieved by such rings which matches the normal tricuspid annulus and, at the same time, to the rigid support of the annulus [2–6]. On the other hand, other studies support the use of flexible prosthetic bands like Dacron or polytetrafluroethilin (PTFE), especially over suture techniques, due to their easy applicability and availability with good postoperative results [7, 8]. Therefore, suture annyloplasty became nowadays less convenient for FTR repair since both flexible bands and rigid rings appeared to offer good mid-term outcomes in recent meta-analysis studies [9, 10]. However, the ideal annuloplasty method for repairing FTR is still debatable between the three-dimensional (3D) rigid rings versus flexible prosthetic bands regarding the long-term outcome. In this retrospective comparative study, we share our experience with long-term outcome of using 3D rigid rings and flexible fashioned bands in FTR.

Methods

Study method

Between March 2013 and September 2018, a total of 367 patients with moderate or more FTR secondary to mitral stenosis or regurgitation underwent tricuspid valve repair and mitral valve surgery at Cairo University hospitals. Of these, 90 cases received tricuspid valve repair with rigid 3D rings (contour 3D or MC3 ring) while the rest (277 cases) received tricuspid valve repair with prosthetic fashioned bands (Dacron or PTFE). The data of the patients receiving tricuspid valve repair with rigid rings were collected and reviewed (group A). Another group of 80 cases receiving tricuspid valve repair with bands were matched to group A using propensity scores according to preoperative patient characteristics (group B). Cases with organic tricuspid regurgitations, recurrent tricuspid valve disease (TVD), endocarditis affecting the TV, associated tricuspid stenosis, congenital TR, associated aortic or pulmonary valve affection, and concomitant ischemic heart disease were not included in our study. This study was approved by our ethical committee. An informed consent was obtained from all patients for the planned operations and due to its retrospective nature the consent for enrolment of patient data in the study was waived. The indication for surgery for the tricuspid valve in our study was based on the American Heart Association (AHA) guidelines; when TR was severe or if moderate but with tricuspid annular dilatation (˃ 40 mm) or pulmonary artery systolic pressure (PASP) above 50 [11]. The TR severity was assessed by the M mode, two dimension and Doppler echocardiography. Moderate TR (grade 2+) was defined by a width of vena contracta of 4–7 mm and a jet area of 5–10 cm^2. Severe TR (grade 3+ and 4+) was defined by a width of vena contracta of 7 ˃ mm and a jet area of 10 ˃ cm^2 with systolic flow reversal in hepatic veins. Data were categorized into; preoperative, operative, postoperative, and follow-up which ranged from 4.6 to 6.5 years (mean 5.6 ± 0.9). In-hospital mortality was defined by deaths within 30 days of the operation. Recurrent TR was defined by postoperative moderate or more TR (grade 2+ or more).

Data collection:

Full data was recorded and analyzed as following:

Preoperative data: age, sex, New York Heart Association (NYHA) class for dyspnea, transthoracic echo (TTE) findings including: ejection fraction (EF), left ventricle end diastolic dimensions (LVEDD), left ventricle end systolic dimensions (LVESD), systolic pulmonary pressure (SPAP) in mmHg. We will consider it as mild, moderate, and severe pulmonary hypertension, respectively, with the values of 30–45 mmHg, 45–70 mmHg, and > 70 mmHg.TR Jet area (cm2), vena contracta width which measures the narrowest distance of the tricuspid jet in mm, tricuspid annular plane systolic excursion (TAPSE), which measures the longitudinal systolic motion of the free edge of the tricuspid valve annulus, tricuspid annulus (TA) diameter, and mid RV diameter in short axis

Operative data

Full records of cardiopulmonary bypass time, cross clamp time, intra-operative findings, type of ring or band in each group, and type of mitral valve intervention.

Postoperative data

Duration of mechanical ventilation, need for pacemaker, intensive care unit (ICU) stay, hospital stay, morbidities, mortality, and follow-up echo data as scheduled by TTE preoperatively as a baseline, then, intra-operative trans-oesophageal echocardiography (TEE) for correlation with the preoperative echo, postoperative TTE before hospital discharge, then, in outpatient clinic after 6 months of surgery and finally, every 2-year of follow-up for all patients in both groups with comparison with the preoperative NYHA,TR grade, PASP, and EF. Follow-up period ranged from 55.2 to 78 months (mean 67.2 ± 10.8).

Operative procedure

Surgery was done in all cases through full median sternotomy and cardiopulmonary bypass (CPB) was achieved with routine bicaval cannulation. Myocardial protection was carried out with multi-dose cold blood cardioplegia every 30–40 min delivered in an ante-grade mode with systemic cooling to 32 °C. After aortic cross-clamping the concomitant mitral valve surgery, whether repair or replacement, was done first through left atriotomy. Tricuspid valve repair was then performed through right atriotomy during the rewarming period on flaccid heart with either band (Dacron or Gortex) or using rigid 3D tricuspid rings (Contour 3D (Medtronic, Minneapolis, MN) ring or MC3) which were fixed to the annulus with interrupted non-pledgetted 2/0 non-absorbable (Ethibond) sutures avoiding the area of the AV node. The choice of the type of tricuspid repair was carried out according to the surgeon´s preference. Sizing for rigid rings by different sizers took place according to the base of the septal leaflet (or one size smaller than the anterior tricuspid leaflet surface area). For band annuloplasty, bands of Dacron or Gortex were fashioned in a width of 3–4 mm and a length of 5 to 7 cm depending on the operative assessment of the surgeon. Finally, testing of the repair was done by saline injection into the tricuspid valve while closing the pulmonary valve before the right atrium closure (Fig. 1).

Statistical analysis

A propensity score matching (PSM) analysis to create comparable risk groups for comparing the outcome of using the two different techniques on degree of postoperative tricuspid regurge and freedom from reoperation with respect to covariates as demographics and preoperative characteristics. In PSM standardized difference were calculated to compare features before and after matching with imbalance being defined as an absolute value greater than 0.10 (small effect size). Matching was performed using the nearest neighbor algorithm with a calliper distance of 0.0001. All preoperative variables > 90% missing data were excluded from analysis. Data were reviewed and coded to facilitate data manipulation and double entered into Microsoft Access and data analysis was performed using Statistical Package of Social Science (SPSS) software version 25 in Windows 7. Quantitative data were summarized using mean ± standard deviation while categorical data were presented as frequency (count) and relative frequency (percentage). For two independent groups of quantitative parametric data non-paired Student's t test was used while for qualitative data chi-squared test was used. Two-way ANOVA test was implied for repeated measures. A p value < 0.05 was considered the cut-off value for significance.

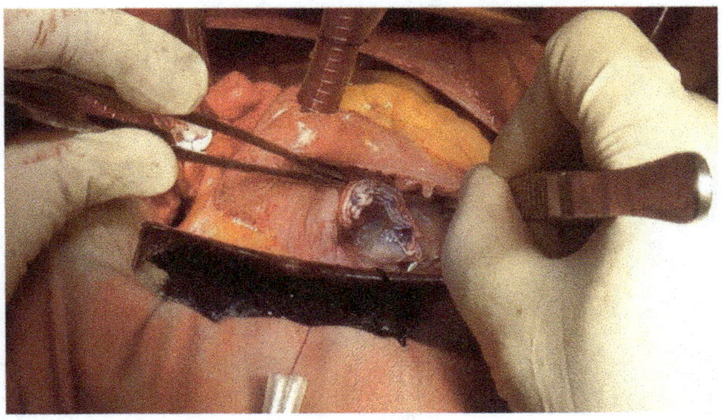

Fig. 1 tricuspid fashioned Dacron band after saline test

Results

Early results

Preoperative patient characteristics are summarized in Table 1 including epidemiological, clinical, and echocardiological data. There was no statistical significant difference between both groups, which indicates proper

Table 1 Preoperative data in both study groups

Variables		Ring group (n = 90)	Band group (n = 80)	p value
Sex				
Male		33(36.7%)	28(35%)	0.8
Female		57(63.3%)	52 (65%)	
Age (years)		39.7 ± 6.5	37.9 ± 7.5	0.08
TR grads	II	36(40%)	24(30%)	0.15
	III	18(20%)	12(15%)	
	IV	36(40%)	44(55%)	
Mitral valve lesions		74 (82%)	65 (81%)	0.75
Stenosis		4 (5%)	2 (2.5%)	
Regurgitation		12 (13%)	13 (16.5%)	
Stenosis and regurgitation				
NYHA class		2.9 ± 0.85	3.1 ± 0.92	0.14
LVEF %		53.3 ± 16.8	55.2 ± 18.9	0.49
LVSD (cm)		3.7 ± 0.0.98	3.92 ± 0.53	0.07
LVEDD (cm)		6.04 ± 0.98	5.87 ± 0.56	0.16
TAPSI (cm)		1.8 ± 0.43	1.9 ± 0.3	0.08
RV short axis (cm)		2.93 ± 0.37	2.99 ± 0.4	0.13
TA diameter (cm)		4.8 ± 0.4	4.7 ± 0.5	0.15
PASP (mmHg)		63.52 ± 9.95	61.23 ± 10.25	0.14

TR tricuspid regurgitation, *NYHA* New York Heart Association, *LVEF* left ventricular ejection fraction, *LVEDD* left ventricle end diastolic dimensions, *LVESD* left ventricle end systolic diameter, *TAPSE* tricuspid annular plane systolic excursion, *RV* right ventricular, *TA* tricuspid annulus, *SPAP* systolic pulmonary artery pressure matching between the two study groups. The pathology of the mitral valve affection was rheumatic in origin in all cases of the study. The sizes of the rigid rings (MC3 in 20 cases and Contour 3D in 70 cases) used in group A ranged from 28 to 34 cm with a mean value of 30.5 cm. On the other hand, fixed lengths of 5 to 7 cm of flexible fashioned bands (Dacron in 70 cases and Gortex in 10 cases) were used in group B. There was statistical significant difference of bypass time and cross clamp time being shorter in group B. Other operative and post-operative parameters are shown in Table 2 with no statistically significant differences between both groups. One case (1.1%) died in group A due to multi-organ failure while two cases (2.5%) died in group B from refractory low cardiac output in one patient and respiratory failure due to pneumonia and prolonged ventilation in the other case with no significant difference. On comparison between the preoperative and postoperative values for NYHA class, degree of TR, and PASP, there was statistically significant decrease in the immediate postoperative period within the 2 groups with a p value of 0.03, 0.04, and 0.033, respectively. However, there was no statistically significant difference between both groups (p value = 0.065).

Late results and follow-up

Our complete long-term follow-up was achieved in 134 (78.82%) cases due to mortalities and patients non-compliance (8.8%). Follow-up period ranged from 55.2 to 78 months (mean 67.2 ± 10.8). Late deaths occurred in 18 (10.58%) of cases. Ten cases in group A as well as in 8 case in group B due to infective endocarditis in 4 cases, stuck mitral valves in 3 cases, cerebrovascular events in 3 cases, renal failure in 2 cases, malignancy in 2 cases, and 4 unknown causes with no statistically significant difference (Fig. 2).

There was no statistically significant difference in the mean NYHA class during the follow-up period between both groups (0.91 in group A and 0.92 in group B) with a p value of 0.09 (Fig. 3). Also, PASP and EF% showed no statistical difference in the same follow-up periods between both groups. However, there was a statistically significant difference in the mean degree of TR improvement at the same follow-up period in favor of group A (1 in group A and 1.5 in group B) with a p value of 0.03. The degree of improvement and severity of TR in the follow-up period is shown in Fig. 4.

In addition, 7 cases (8.75%) out of the 80 patients in group B and 4 (4.4%) out of the 90 patients in group A had recurrent TR during follow-up period. Four patients from the 7 cases with recurrent TR in the band group needed reoperation with replacement of the tricuspid valve due to recurrent right sided heart failure despite maximal medical treatment. On the other side, the four patient with recurrent TR in ring group continued their follow-up period without reoperation. There was statistically significant difference in the freedom from recurrent TR and need for reoperation during the follow up period

Table 2 Operative and outcome data in both study groups

Variables	Ring group (n = 90)	Band group (n = 80)	p value
Bypass time (min)	116 ± 25.41	105.6 ± 20.33	**< 0.001***
Cross clamp time (min)	91 ± 28.6	76.7 ± 30.2	**< 0.001***
Concomitant mitral valve surgery Repair	6(6.7%)	4(5%)	0.64
Replacement	84(93.3%)	76(95%)	
Types of ring or band	MC3 20: (22.2%) Contour 3D: 70 (77.8%)	Dacron: 70(87.5%) Gortex: 10(12.5%)	
Postoperative mechanical ventilation (h)	8.1 ± 1.9	7.7 ± 1	0.08
ICU stay (days)	2.9 ± 0.76	2.6 ± 1.3	0.07
Hospital stay (days)	7.4 ± 1.2	7.8 ± 1.5	0.06
Postoperative complications Reoperation for bleeding	5(5.6%)	3(3.8%)	0.9
Renal failure	2(2.2%)	2(2.5%)	
Cerebrovascular stroke	1(1.1%)	1(1.3%)	
New pacemaker insertion	1(1.1%)	0(0%)	
Tracheostomy	0(0%)	1(1.25%)	
Pneumonia	0(0%)	2(2.5%)	
In-hospital mortality	1(1.1%)	2(2.5%)	0.49
Reoperation for recurrence	0(0%)	4(5%)	**0.001***

ICU intensive care unit

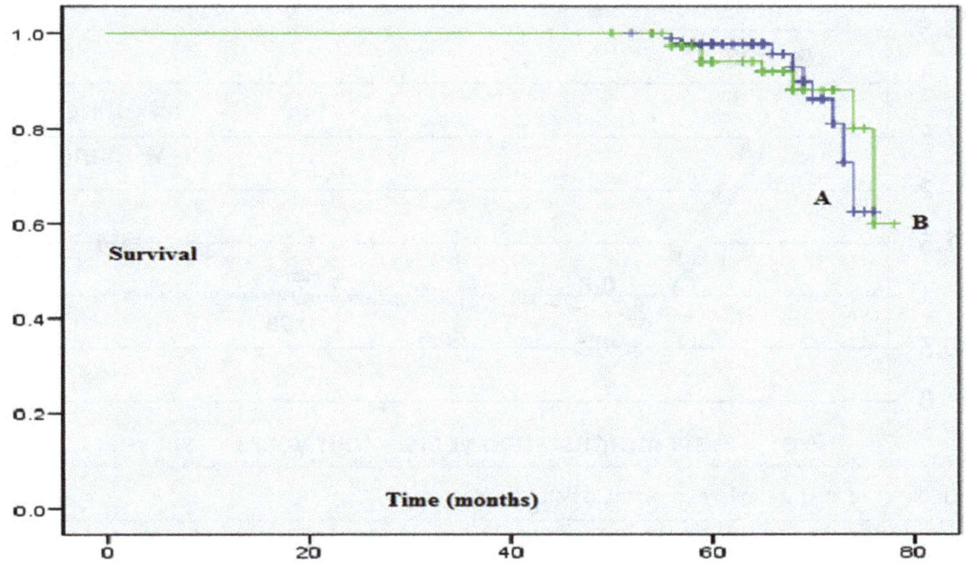

Fig. 2 Kaplan-Meier curve for survival

between both groups with lower recurrence and reoperation rates in group A with a p value of 0.03 and 0.001 respectively (Fig. 5).

Discussion

Secondary FTR is very common at the time of left sided valve surgery due to progressive annular dilatation mainly leading to lack of proper tricuspid leaflets coaptation and regurge. Furthermore, the changes that occurs in valve geometry and the more planer the tricuspid annulus that become with prolonged dilatation.

Current data suggest that the dilatation that occurs in cases of FTR especially with left-sided valve lesions is an on-going process that continues to progress unless surgical annuloplasty is done at the time of left-sided valve surgery to prevent future progression of the disease [12]. Without intervention, persistent TR is currently associated with poor outcome even if not sever and therefore, the recommendations for repairing the FTR nowadays changed to lesser threshold for regurgitation [13].

The main difference between both rigid 3D rings and flexible fashioned bands is that rigid rings restore the saddle, non-planner, and tricuspid annulus which have been proven by the studies using 3D echocardiography to improve annular symmetrical contractions during the cardiac cycle. In addition, rigid rings seem to give more long-term stability of the tricuspid annulus [14]. On the other hand, flexible bands maintain the physiological motion of the tricuspid annulus during cardiac contractions which is now well-recognized by many researches but its clinical importance and role are not yet fully investigated [15].

In our study, the mean size of used rigid rings was 30.5 (range 28–34). We simply used one size smaller of the 3D ring (contour 3D or MC3) since some studies showed that the exact annular size is relatively smaller when the heart is beating than when arrested. Also,

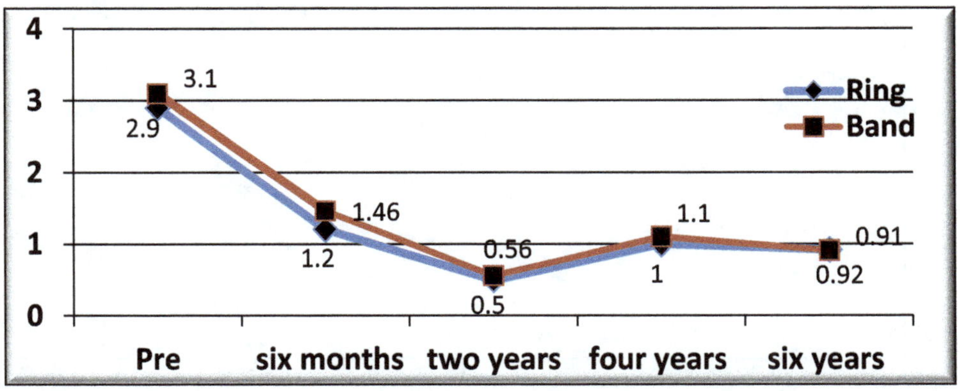

Fig. 3 Postoperative NYHA class follows-up in study groups

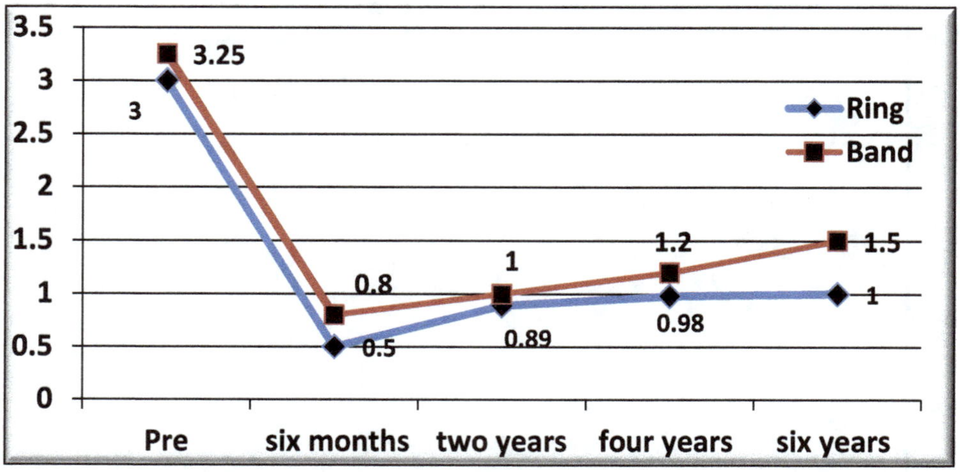

Fig. 4 Postoperative TR pattern during the follow-up period in both study groups

other studies recommended routine downsizing in all cases whether performing the tricuspid repair on beating or arrested heart with comparable results [3, 16]. However, multiple studies failed to identify a concrete relation between the ring size, as a risk factor, and recurrent TR with no much benefits of aggressive downsizing [17, 18].

On the other hand, we fashioned the bands to a width of 3 mm and a length of 5 to 7 cm to plicate the anterior and posterior annulus depending upon the intra-operative measurement of the tricuspid annulus and the degree of TR. Although the fact that there are no solid guidelines for this measurement, but this length has been obtained in previous studies from the average circumferences of most used ring sizers. In addition, it has been shown in previous studies that the tricuspid annulus measured by preoperative echocardiography from the mid-anterior to the mid-septal leaflet in the end-diastole using the apical four chamber view differs from the transvers annulus measured surgically from the antero-septal commissure to the antero-posterior commissure. For example, an annulus estimated by pre-operative echocardiography to be 4 cm would be measured surgically 7 cm [19].

In the band group, we used Dacron or Gortex assuming that both has nearly equal flexibility with fashioning the band 3 mm width and from 5 to 7 cm length depending upon the intraoperative measurement of the tricuspid annulus and to what degree the TR present and the needs for the proper downsizing with no solid guidelines for measurement but, we took this measurement previously from average circumferences of most used ring sizers.

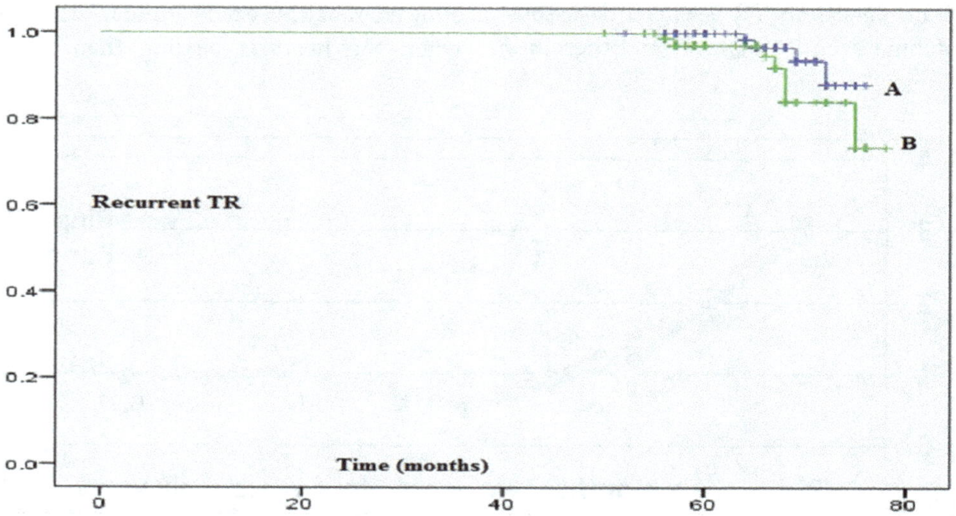

Fig. 5 Freedom from recurrent TR at different follows up periods in the study groups

In our series, we have succeeded effectively to reduce the tricuspid annulus size by either the rigid rings or fashioned flexible bands with no statistically significant difference in both modalities in the aspect of improving the TR degree, PASP and NYHA class in the early post-operative period. However, rigid 3D rings significantly maintained long-term effects on the repair with less re-intervention and recurrent TR during our follow-up. This finding agrees with previous multiple studies and meta-analysis comparing rigid rings with flexible band devices, not fashioned (custom made) bands, as we tried. We use these intra-operatively fashioned bands for easy accessibility and applicability with similar concepts [9, 10, 20–22]. Moreover, some studies used native pericardium fashioned into similar bands as it is widely available for all patients with encouraging results [8, 23].

Nevertheless, most of the studies addressing the risk factors for recurrent TR after surgical repair of FTR reported LV dysfunction, high preoperative PASP and the presence of tricuspid valve tethering [24, 25] these studies could not identify the type of annuloplasty as a risk factor for recurrent TR which implies the importance of multi-centric prospective studies with long term results. We could not include TV tethering in our preoperative echo parameters, and we did not study the risk factors for recurrence as PASP, also, mean LVEF was in normal rang in our preoperative data and maintained in the long-term follow-up with no significant changes to be a risk factor.

Study limitations

Our study has several limitations. The retrospective nature of the study and the sample size was relatively small. There is procedural difference between fashioned bands which cover the anterior and posterior annulus only and rigid rings which cover in addition part of septal annulus. There were no standard guidelines for sizing the fashioned tricuspid bands. The risk factors for recurrence have not been studied. Finally, the study did not compare different annuloplasty material used in bands or different manufactured rigid rings.

Conclusion

Tricuspid valve repair with different annuloplasty rigid three-dimensional rings or fashioned flexible bands for functional tricuspid regurgitation offers good long-term outcome. Yet, the rigid rings on the long run maintain their benefits on decreasing the rate of recurrent TR and the need for reoperation.

Abbreviations

AHA: American heart association; CPB: Cardiopulmonary bypass; EF: Ejection fraction; FTR: Functional tricuspid regurgitation; ICU: Intensive care unit; LVEDD: Left ventricle end diastolic dimensions; LVESD: Left ventricle end systolic dimensions; NYHA: New York Heart Association; PTFE: Polytetrafluroethilin; RV: Right ventricular; SPAP: Systolic pulmonary pressure; SPSS: Statistical Package of Social Science; TR: Tricuspid regurgitation; TVD: Tricuspid valve disease; TTE: Transthoracic echo; TAPSE: Tricuspid annular plane systolic excursion; TA: Tricuspid annulus; TEE: Trans-oesophageal echocardiography; 3D: Three dimensions

Acknowledgements

Thanks to our statistical member in this study Dr. Asma Elsary who did great effort in organizing and illustrating the data to be clear in our results.

Authors' contributions

All authors participated in getting the conception, data collection, analysis, and manuscripts writing. ME was a major contributor in analysis and interpreted the patient data regarding the comparative parameters. AN was a major contributor in writing the manuscript. SN was major contributor in revising and editing the manuscript. HE was major contributor in revising and editing the manuscript. All authors read and approved the final manuscript.

Author details

[1]Department of Cardiothoracic Surgery, Faculty of Medicine, Cairo University, Cairo, Egypt. [2]Department of Cardiothoracic Surgery, Faculty of Medicine for Girls, Al-Azhar University, Cairo, Egypt. [3]Department of Cardiothoracic Surgery, Faculty of Medicine, Fayoum University, Fayoum, Egypt.

References

1. Rashwan O, Nosair A et al (2017) Mid-term results of three dimentional annuloplasty ring repair in treating functional tricuspid valve regurgitation. Journal of the Egyptian Society of Cardiothorac Surg. 25:316–322
2. Naqshband MS, Abid AR, Akhtar RP, Waheed A, Khan JS (2010) Functional tricuspid regurgitation in rheumatic heart disease: surgical options. Ann Thorac Cardiovasc Surg 16:417–425
3. Ghoreishi M, Brown JM, Stauffer CE, Young CA, Byron MJ, Griffith BP et al (2011) Undersized tricuspid annuloplasty rings optimally treat functional tricuspid regurgitation. Ann Thorac Surg 92:89–96
4. Basel H, Aydin U, Kutlu H, Dostbil A, Karadag M, Odabasi D et al (2010) Outcomes of De Vega versus biodegradable ring annuloplasty in the surgical treatment of tricuspid regurgitation (mid-term results). Heart Surg Forum 13:233–237
5. Navia JL, Brozzi NA, Klein AL et al (2012) Moderate tricuspid regurgitation with left-sided degenerative heart valve disease: to repair or not to repair? Ann Thorac Surg 93:59–67 discussion 68–9
6. Ren WJ, Zhang BG et al (2015) Outcomes of tricuspid annuloplasty with and without prosthetic rings: a retrospective follow-up study. Journal of Cardiothorac Surg. 10:81
7. Abdelfattah I, Omar A (2014) Early outcome of tricuspid repair for functional tricuspid regurgitation associated with rheumatic mitral valve disease modified flexible band annuloplasty vs. suture annuloplasty. Journal of the Egyptian Society of Cardio-Thoracic Surgery 22:13–18
8. Chang BC, Song SW, Lee S, Yoo KJ, Kang MS, Chung N (2008) Eight-year outcomes of tricuspid annuloplasty using autologous pericardial strip for functional tricuspid regurgitation. Ann Thorac Surg 86:1495–1493
9. Zhu TY, Wang JG, Meng X (2013) Is a rigid tricuspid annuloplasty ring superior to a flexible band when correcting secondary tricuspid regurgitation? Interactive CardioVascular and Thoracic Surgery. 17:1009–1014
10. Wang N, Phan S, Tian DH et al (2017) Flexible band versus rigid ring annuloplasty for tricuspid regurgitation: a systematic review and meta-analysis. Ann Cardiothorac Surg 6:194–203
11. Nishimura Rick A, Otto Catherine M, Bonow Robert O et al (2014) AHA/ACC guideline for the management of patients with valvular heart disease: a report of the American college of cardiology/American heart association task force on practice guidelines. Circulation 129
12. Dreyfus GD, Corbi PJ, Chan KM, Bahrami T (2005) Secondary tricuspid regurgitation or dilatation: which should be the criteria for surgical repair? Ann Thorac Surg 79:127–132

13. Seo HS, Ha JW, Moon JY et al (2008) Right ventricular remodeling and dysfunction with subsequent annular dilatation and tethering as a mechanism of isolated tricuspid regurgitation. Circ J 72:1645–1649
14. Jouan J, Pagel MR, Hiro ME et al (2007) Further information from a sonometric study of the normal tricuspid valve annulus in sheep: geometric changes during the cardiac cycle. J Heart Valve Dis 16:511–518
15. Ton-Nu TT, Levine RA, Handschumacher MD et al (2006) Geometric determinants of functional tricuspid regurgitation: insights from 3-dimensional echocardiography. Circulation. 114:143–149
16. Filsoufi F, Salzerg SP, Coutu M, Adams DH (2006) A three-dimensional ring annuloplasty for the treatment of tricuspid regurgitation. Ann Thorac Surg 81:2273–2278
17. McCarthy PM, Bhudia SK, Rajeswaran J et al (2004) Tricuspid valve repair: Durability and risk factors for failure. J Thorac Cardiovasc Surg 127:674–685
18. Izutani H, Nakamura T, Kawachi K (2010) Flexible band versus rigid ring annuloplasty for functional tricuspid Regurgitation. Heart International 5:13
19. Gatti G, Dell'Angela L, Morosin M et al (2016) Flexible band versus rigid ring annuloplasty for functional tricuspid regurgitation: two different patterns of right heart reverse remodeling. Interactive Cardiovascular and Thoracic Surgery 23:79–89
20. Guenther T, Mazzitelli D, Noebauer C et al (2013) Tricuspid valve repair: is ring annuloplasty superior? Eur J Cardiothorac Surg 43:58–65
21. Gatti G, Dell'Angela L, Morosin M et al (2016) Flexible band versus rigid ring annuloplasty for functional tricuspid regurgitation: two different patterns of right heart reverse remodeling. Interactive Cardiovascular and Thoracic Surgery. 23:79–89
22. Adas A, Elnaggar A, Balbaa Y, Elashkar A, Alkady HM (2019) Ring, band or suture in tricuspid annuloplasty for functional tricuspid regurgitation; which is better and more durable? Heart Surg Forum. 22:411–415
23. Abdou Ettish AA, Etmanb WG, Ramadan AM, Ramadan BA (2019) Flexible band made of autologous pericardium for functional tricuspid regurgitation repair. Alexandria journal of medicine 55:44–48
24. Fukuda S, Gillinov AM, McCarthy PM et al (2006) Determinants of recurrent or residual functional tricuspid regurgitation after tricuspid annuloplasty. Circulation 114:I582–I587
25. Fukuda S, Song JM, Gillinov AM et al (2005) Tricuspid valve tethering predicts residual tricuspid regurgitation after tricuspid annuloplasty. Circulation 111:975–979

21

Spontaneous pneumothorax associated with primary lung cancer: a retrospective study

Walid Abu Arab* and Abdel-maguid Ramadan

Abstract

Background: The occurrence of spontaneous pneumothorax in primary lung cancer patients is infrequent. No exact theory could explain its mechanism of association. It could be either a primary manifestation or a late complication of primary lung cancer. The aim of this study is to analyze the association of the spontaneous pneumothorax with the primary lung cancer.

Results: A retrospective revision of patients' files that presented with spontaneous pneumothorax and admitted at the Cardiothoracic Surgery Department during the period between January 2000 and January 2018 was done. Twenty-three patients were included in this study. Seventy-four percent of them were males (n = 17). Age ranged between 48 and 77 years (62.3 ± 7.3 years). Twelve patients (52%) were known to have advanced primary lung cancer, while seven patients (30%) had SPnx as a primary presentation for the primary lung cancer that was discovered during radiological assessment for SPnx. The remaining four patients had SPnx and were treated via surgery. In three of them, bullectomy and pleurodesis was performed; the postoperative histo-pathological examination of excised bullae revealed a primary non-small cell lung cancer (NSCLC). While in one patient, who had bullectomy, the primary lung cancer was discovered accidently during surgery.

Conclusion: Pneumothorax as a first manifestation for lung cancer is infrequent. Its relation to the prognosis has not been yet clear. Recurrent spontaneous pneumothorax in old, heavy smoker patient, or emphysema patient should raise the suspicion for the possibility of association of lung carcinoma.

Keywords: Pulmonary carcinoma, Spontaneous, Pneumothorax, Spontaneous pneumothorax

Background

Spontaneous pneumothorax (SPnx) in young adults is not infrequent [1, 2]. The overall incidence is estimated to be around 5–10/100,000 per year. It is higher in young adult males (1/500 young males) [3]. SPnx is generally caused by rupture of sub-pleural blebs or emphysematous bullae [4–8]. Meanwhile, it can complicate primary or secondary lung tumors [4, 9–16]. Authors reported that sarcomas are the most common malignant neoplasm that causes pneumothorax [5, 9]. On contrary, SPnx is rarely related to primary pulmonary carcinomas [4, 12, 14]. The estimated incidence of its occurrence is about 0.03–0.05% for the primary pulmonary carcinoma [4, 5]. The aim of this retrospective study is to analyze the association of pneumothorax with the primary lung cancer.

Methods

Retrospective revision of the files of the patients who presented with SPnx and admitted to the Cardiothoracic Surgery Department during the period from January 2000 to January 2018 was performed following approval

* Correspondence: walidabuarab@yahoo.com

Meeting Presentation: The preliminary work was presented as an oral presentation at the annual meeting of the World Society of Cardiovascular and Thoracic Surgery (WSCTS2015) that was held at Edinburgh- Scotland during 19-22 September 2015. The abstract of the preliminary work is published on line by the Journal of Cardiovascular Surgery.

Cardiothoracic Surgery Department, Faculty of Medicine, University of Alexandria, Middan Al-Khartoum, Alexandria, Egypt from the Ethical Research Committee. The files were searched for association of SPnx with primary pulmonary carcinoma. Patients who had SPnx in association with pulmonary metastases were eliminated. Data analysis was performed with the SPSS 22.0 statistical software (SPSS, USA). Quantitative data with normal distribution were expressed as mean ± SD and compared by student *t* test. Categorical data were expressed as frequency and percentage, and assessed by the X^2 and Wilcoxon rank sum tests for nominal and ordinal variables, respectively $p < 0.05$ was considered statistically significant.

Results

Revision of 2536 files related to patients with SPnx was taken place. Those who have been proven to have primary lung cancer constituted twenty-three patients (0.9%) and were included in this study. Seventeen patients (74%) were males while female patients constituted only 36%. Age ranged between 48 and 77 years (62.3 ± 7.3 years). All patients included had CT-Chest as part of evaluation of the recurrent SPnx (Figs. 1 and 2). Twelve patients (52%) were known to have advanced primary lung cancer and were on therapy, while seven patients (30%) had the SPnx as a primary presentation for the primary lung cancer, which was discovered during radiological assessment for the SPnx. The remaining four patients had surgery for SPnx. In three of them, bullectomy and pleurodesis were performed; the postoperative histo-pathological examination of the excised bullae revealed a primary non-small cell lung cancer (NSCLC). They received formal lobectomy later. While

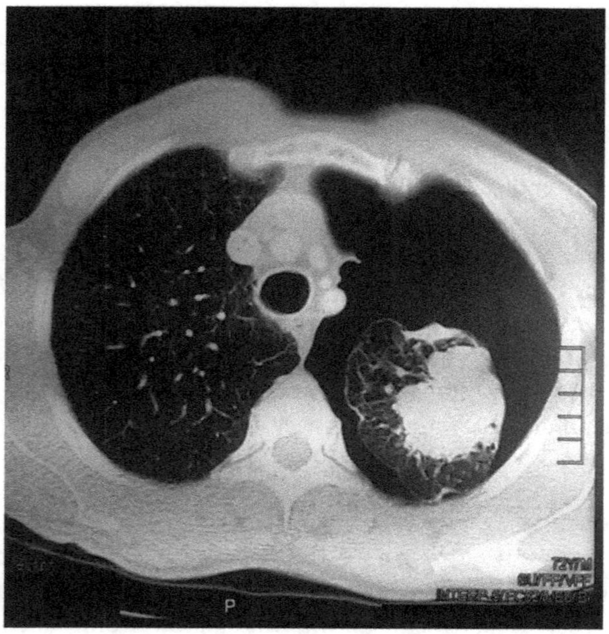

Fig. 1 CT-Chest (pulmonary window) showing mass lesion in the middle left lung zone with partial pneumothorax

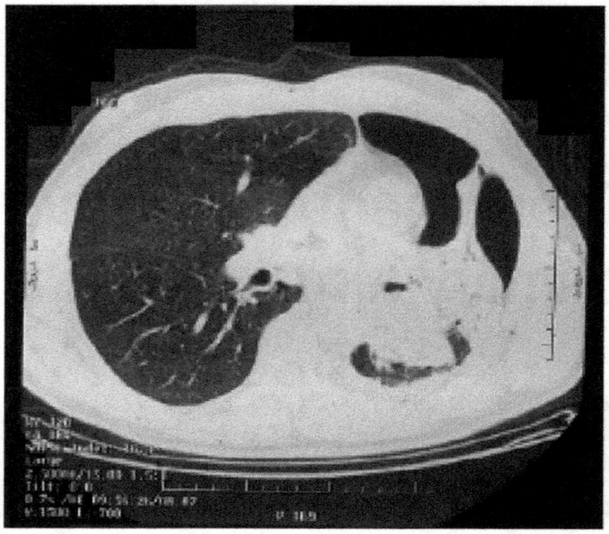

Fig. 2 CT-Chest (pulmonary window) showing a large left lung mass, measuring about 7 × 5.5 × 4.5 cm showing cavitations with thick irregular walls and foci of air

one patient, out of the four had bullectomy for large lung bulla; the surgeon felt a small nodule at the junction of the lung bulla and the normal remaining lung tissue during the surgical procedure. This nodule was resected with the lung bulla, and frozen section examination revealed a primary lung cancer. Hence, surgeon decided to proceed into formal lobectomy. Eighteen patients out of the twenty-three (78%) were smokers. For the nineteen patients who were preoperatively diagnosed with primary lung cancer, seven patients of them (36.8%) had an adenocarcinoma while twelve patients of them (63.2%) had squamous cell NSCLC. The preoperative staging revealed that 5.3% had stage IIA, 21.1% had stage IIB, 26.3% had stage IIIA, and 47.4% had stage IIIB NSCLC. Six patients out of the nineteen (31.6%) had surgical pulmonary resection following primary intervention for the pneumothorax for treatment of NSCLC. Surgery performed was in the form of lobectomy ($n = 5$) and pneumonectomy ($n = 1$). No perioperative mortality was encountered. Complications were found in three patients; one patient had post-operative cardiac arrhythmia, and two patients had superficial wound infection. Table 1 showed the demographic data of the studied group.

For facilitating discussion of the results, authors have divided the patients into four groups. This classification was not intended during planning for the methodology of the research protocol. Group I included patients who were diagnosed with primary lung cancer and were receiving chemotherapy, radiotherapy, or both, and they had SPnx during the course of their treatment. Group II included patients who had SPnx first, and primary lung cancer was discovered during investigations performed.

Table 1 Demographic data

No.	Sex	Age	Initial Dx.	Stage	Smoking	On therapy	Pnx during course of treatment	Pnx as primary presentation	Surgery	Type of surgery
Group I										
1	M	65	LSCC	IIIB	Y	Y	Y	N	N	
2	M	60	LSCC	IIIB	Y	Y	Y	N	N	
3	F	59	LAC	IIIB	N	Y	Y	N	N	
4	M	70	LSCC	IIIB	Y	Y	Y	N	N	
5	M	66	LSCC	IIIA	Y	Y	Y	N	N	
6	M	77	LAC	IIIA	Y	Y	Y	N	N	Pneumonectomy
7	M	54	LSCC	IIIB	Y	Y	Y	N	Y	
8	F	67	LAC	IIIB	N	Y	Y	N	N	
9	M	66	LSCC	IIIB	Y	Y	Y	N	N	
10	F	59	LSCC	IIIA	Y	Y	Y	N	N	
11	M	60	LSCC	IIIB	Y	Y	Y	N	N	
12	M	71	LSCC	IIIB	Y	Y	Y	N	N	
Group II										
13	M	62	LSCC	IIB	Y	N	N	Y	Y	Lobectomy
14	M	63	LAC	IIB	Y	N	N	Y	Y	Lobectomy
15	M	59	LAC	IIB	Y	N	N	Y	Y	Lobectomy
16	M	65	LSCC	IIIA	Y	N	N	Y	N	
17	M	59	LAC	IIB	N	N	N	Y	Y	Lobectomy
18	F	73	LAC	IIIA	N	N	N	Y	N	
19	M	69	LSCC	IIA	N	N	N	Y	Y	Lobectomy
Group III										
20	F	56	Rec.SPnx	N/A	Y	N	N	Y	Y	Bullectomy and lobectomy
21	M	49	Rec. SPnx	N/A	Y	N	N	Y	Y	Bullectomy and lobectomy
22	M	48	Rec.SPnx	N/A	Y	N	N	Y	Y	Bullectomy and lobectomy
Group IV										
23	F	56	Rec. SPnx	N/A	Y	N	N	Y	Y	Bullectomy and lobectomy

M male, *F* female, *Initial Dx.* initial diagnosis, *LSCC* lung squamous cell carcinoma, *LAC* lung adenocarcinoma, *Rec. SPnx* recurrent spontaneous pneumothorax, *Y* yes, *N* no

Group III included patients who were presented with SPnx, and an evident lung bullae at chest X-ray or chest-CT and post-operative histo-pathological examination of the resected lung bullae revealed an early primary lung cancer. While group IV included patients, who were presented with SPnx and lung bullae, and the primary lung cancer was discovered accidently at the operating room during resection of the bullae.

Group I

This group included twelve patients, three females and nine males. Age ranged between 54 and 77 years old

(64.5 ± 6.4 years). Patients with stage IIIB constituted 75% of patients in this group, while 25% of them had stage IIIA. The majority of patients (75%) had squamous cell lung cancer while 25% had adenocarcinoma. All patients except one had a smoking history. All of the patients had primary intervention for SPnx (pigtail and underwater seal; n = 3; intercostal drain and underwater seal; n = 9). Four patients (33.3%) had prolonged air leak, and they received blood patch. One of the three patients with stage IIIA had formal pneumonectomy later following down staging via preoperative chemo-radiotherapy.

Group II

Seven patients were included in this group; six patients (85.7%) were males. Age ranged between 59 and 73 years old (64.3 ± 5.2 years). All patients presented with SPnx, and the diagnosis of associated primary lung cancer was established during the management of SPnx. Four patients (57.1%) had a history of smoking. Stage IIB was the most frequently encountered stage in this group (57.1%) while stage IIA was found in one patient and stage IIIA in two patients. Pathological subtypes of NSCLC were either squamous cell lung cancer (42.9%) or adenocarcinoma of the lung (57.1%). All patients were managed for pneumothorax (insertion of pigtail and underwater seal (n = 1) and insertion of intercostal drain and underwater seal (n = 6)). One patient had prolonged air leak, and blood patch was performed. Most of patients (71.4%) included in this group had further management for lung cancer in the form of lobectomy.

Group III

This group included three patients. Two patients (66.7%) were males. Age ranged between 48 and 56 years (51 ± 4.4 years). These patients were presented with SPnx, and investigations revealed bullous lung disease. Following bullectomy, histo-pathological examination revealed primary lung cancer at the specimen of the resected lung bullae. All patients had an intercostal drain primarily inserted and underwater seal followed by video-assisted bullectomy. Following the pathology reports, all patients (100%) had surgical management of NSCLC in the form of lobectomy.

Group IV

This group includes one patient (female; smoker, 56 years old), who presented initially with SPnx and bullous lung disease. Intercostal drain and underwater seal was inserted. Bullectomy was scheduled and during the procedure, the surgeon felt a small nodule at the base of the large lung bulla. The nodule was included in the resected bullae. The specimen was sent for frozen section and pathological examination. Pathology revealed primary NSCLC. Lobectomy was performed at the same setting, and final pathological examination revealed brocho-alveolar carcinoma.

Discussion

SPnx could be either primary or secondary. Primary SPnx mostly affects healthy young adults while the secondary SPnx can develops as a result of bronchial obstruction, infarction, infection, neoplasm, or diffuse lung diseases [7]. SPnx as a complication of pulmonary carcinoma is rare [7, 12, 17]. Only 2% of all SPnx coexist with malignant lung diseases either primary or secondary. This tumor complication must be suspected in older patients [18]. In our series, the incidence of the primary lung cancer associated with SPnx was found to be 0.9%.

Only few small series and some case reports were published about SPnx occurring in association with primary pulmonary carcinoma. The largest four series [4, 5, 18, 19] in the literature are listed in Table 2. The largest one was that published by Cicénas et al. on 2011 that included 27 patients [18]. Our retrospective study included 23 patients during 18 years.

Several theories have been published in the literature regarding the mechanisms of the occurrence of the SPnx in patients with primary lung cancer. The first theory explained that pneumothorax could be due to necrosis of the cancer that directly ruptured into the pleural space [13]. This may be what is actually happened to some patients in group I and II who presented with a mass lesion that showed necrosis and air cavities. The second theory stated that endobronchial neoplasm could act as a check-valve that leads to dilatation and eventual rupture of the distal alveolar spaces [20]. This theory could explain the occurrence of the pneumothorax in some of patients who had partial obstruction of the lobar bronchus with the tumor that was evident at the radiological investigations. Majority of these patients were included in group II. The third theory stated that pneumothorax may arise from rupture of small subpleural blebs, and this may explain the occurrence of pneumothorax in the three patients included in group III. Fourth theory proposed that most patients with lung cancer have chronic obstructing pulmonary disease (COPD) or emphysematous bullae that may rupture following the disturbance of the pulmonary architecture due to bronchial carcinoma [7, 20]. This theory may explain the SPnx in the patient who had SPnx, and pathological examination revealed a pulmonary carcinoma at the base of excised large lung bulla.

In the majority of our patients, it was noted that the stage of lung cancer is advanced, stage IIIB (n = 9) and stage IIIA (n = 5). Laurens et al. [21] documented that the association of SPnx with lung cancer is an ominous

Table 2 Largest publications documented pneumothorax in association with primary lung cancer

Serial	Author	Publication year	Duration of the study	Number of patients
1	Yilmaz et al. [4]	2005	N/A*	5
2	Stienhauslin et al. [5]	1985	1959–1983	6
3	Cicénas et al. [18]	2011	1970–2009	27
4	Citron et al. [19]	1959	N/A*	6

*N/A = Non-applicable

sign. He explained this bad prognostic association by vascular invasion mechanism during the process of the tumor necrosis. However, this could not be confirmed at our study. Moreover, in four patients included in our series, the SPnx and surgery for emphysematous bulla helped to early discover the pulmonary carcinoma, and this is infrequent. Finally, there are some limitations in this study including that it is a retrospective study, small number of patients is included, and wide period that extended to 18 years. Moreover, some missing clinical data could not be obtained from the patient files especially old ones.

Conclusion

In conclusion, SPnx is a rare association with primary lung cancer. It could complicate advanced stages of pulmonary carcinoma. SPx occurring in heavy smokers, elderly patients with emphysema can be an alert for thoracic surgeons to exclude pulmonary carcinoma. However, SPnx in patients with lung cancer could not be proved an ominous sign, and its relation to final diagnosis should be furtherly investigated.

Abbreviations

SPnx: Spontanous pneumothorax; NSCLC: Non-small cell lung cancer; COPD: Chronic obstructive pulmonary disease

Acknowledgements

N/A

Authors' contributions

WA has made substantial contributions to the design of the work and the acquisition, analysis, and interpretation of the data and has drafted the work and revised it. AR has made substantial contributions to the design of the work and interpretation of the data and revised the draft. Authors have approved the submitted manuscript for publication and have agreed both to be personally accountable for the author's own contributions and to ensure that questions related to the accuracy or integrity of any part of the work, even ones in which the author was not personally involved, are appropriately investigated, resolved, and the resolution documented in the literature.

References

1. Solak O, Sayar A, Metin M, Turna A, Pekçolakar A, Gurses A (2006) Bronchial carcinoma presenting with pneumothorax. Eur J Med 3(2):78–79
2. Choi YK, Kim KC (2015) Spontaneous pneumothorax as the first manifestation of lung cancer: two case report. Journal of thoracic disease 7(8):E252
3. De Barrin J (1937) Haemopneumothorax spontane dans une metastase pulmonaire de sarcoma osseux. Bull Mem Soc Radiol Fr 25:73
4. Yilmaz A, Akkaya E, Guneylioğlu D, Duzgun S (2005) Spontaneous pneumothorax complicating primary lung cancer: analysis of five cases. Turkish Respiratory Journal 6(1):56–58
5. Steinhauslin CA, Cuttat JF (1985) Spontaneous pneumothorax: a complication of lung cancer? Chest 88:709–713
6. Ohata M, Suzuki H (1980) Pathogenesis of spontaneous pneumothorax with special reference to the ultrastructure of emphysematous bullae. Chest 77: 771–776
7. Vencevičius V, Cicénas S (2009) Spontaneous pneumothorax as a first sign of pulmonary carcinoma. World Journal of Surgical Oncology 7:57–59
8. Bauman MH, Noppen M (2004) Pneumothorax. Respiratory 9:157–164
9. Dines DE, Cortese DA, Brennan MD, Hahn RG, Payne WS (1973) Malignant pulmonary neoplasms predisposing to spontaneous pneumothorax. Mayo Clin Proc 48:541–544
10. Hoag JB, Sherman M, Fasihuddin Q, Lund ME (2010) A comprehensive review of spontaneous pneumothorax complicating sarcoma. Chest. 138(3): 510–518
11. Fayda M, Kebudi R, Dizdar Y, Gorgun O, Gun F, Aksu G, Ayan I (2012) Spontaneous pneumothorax in children with osteosarcoma: report of three cases and review of the literature. Acta Chir Belg 112(5):378–381
12. Galbis CJM, Mafe MJJ, Baschwitz GB, Perez CA, Rodriguez PJM (2001) Spontaneous pneumothorax as the first sign of pulmonary carcinoma. Arch Bronconeumol 37:397–400
13. Minami H, Sakai S, Watanabe A, Shimokata K (1991) Check-valve mechanism as a cause of bilateral spontaneous pneumothorax complicating bronchioloalveolar cell carcinoma. Chest 100:853–855
14. Mahajan V, Kupferer CF, Van Ordstrand HS (1975) Pneumothorax: a rare manifestation of primary lung cancer. Chest 68:730–732
15. Arab WS, Abdel-Aziz AM, Ramadan AM (2015) Spontaneous pneumothorax associated with primary lung cancer. In Journal of cardiothoracic surgery 10(1):A242
16. Kurokawa T, Morikawa T, Ohtake S, Kaji M, Sugiura H, Okushiba S, Kondo S, Katoh H (2002) Spontaneous pneumothorax secondary to radiographically occult lung metastasis from parapharyngeal synovial sarcoma: report of a case. Surg Today 32:267–269
17. O'Connor BM, Ziegler P, Spaulding MB (1992) Spontaneous pneumothorax in small cell lung cancer. Chest 102(2):628–629
18. Cicénas S, Vencevičius V (2011) Malignant pulmonary neoplasms predisposing to pneumothorax. Acta Medica Lituanica 18(2):53–55
19. Citron KM (1959) Spontaneous pneumothorax complicating bronchial carcinomas. Tubercle 40:384
20. Okada D, Koizumi K, Haraguchi S, Kawamoto M, Mikami I, Tanaka S (2002) Pneumothorax manifesting primary lung cancer. J Thorac Cardiovasc Surg 50(3):133–136
21. Laurens RG Jr, Pine JR, Honig EG (1983) Spontaneous pneumothorax in primary cavitating lung carcinoma. Radiology 146:295–297

22

Chemical pleurodesis for malignant pleural effusion: which agent is perfect?

Mohamed Elshabrawy Saleh, Gehad Awad and Mohammed Sanad*

Abstract

Background: Pleurodesis is defined as symphysis between two layers of pleura to prevent recurrence of effusion, and it is the best available treatment for recurrent effusions of incurable malignancies. An ideal agent must be highly effective, safe, inexpensive, and readily available which is yet to be identified.

The aim of this study was to assess our results of medical pleurodesis, using 3 different chemical agents: bleomycin ampoules, doxycycline capsules, povidone–iodine solution, through two different routes, chest tube and small bore indwelling catheter.

Over a period of 5 years, 104 patients with malignant recurrent pleural effusion underwent pleurodesis at our university hospital, using 3 different agents and two routes of delivery.

Results: Fifty patients were male, patients' age ranged from 22 to 74 years (57.55 ± 9.02). Fifty-nine patients (56.7%) had right-sided effusion, 61 patients (58.7%) had massive effusion. All patients were dyspneic. The rout of effusion drainage and sclerosing agent instillation was chest tube in 64 patients (61.5%) and small indwelling catheter in 40 patients. Forty-three patients received bleomycin, 36 patients received doxycycline, and 25 patients received povidone–iodine. The total success rate was 78.8%.

Conclusion: Pleurodesis is a safe acceptable palliative procedure for malignant pleural effusion with not yet definite ideal agent or rout. Hence, the availability and the expense of agent are important.

Keywords: *Pleurodesis, Malignant effusion, Pleural, Chemical pleurodesis, Pleurex*

Background

The mainstream of malignant pleural effusion (MPE) is produced by metastatic disease: typically, bronchogenic carcinoma in men and breast cancer in females. These two cancers combined account for 50–65% of all MPE [1]. Mesothelioma is the most common type of primary pleural tumor and is associated with MPE in more than 90% of cases. Even with the advancement in cancer treatment, the management of MPE is palliative, with median survival ranging from 3 to 12 months [1]. Patients' prognosis is extremely variable and rests on several influences (primary cancer, stage, performance status, and pleural fluid proteins). The LENT (pleural fluid lactate dehydrogenase, Eastern Cooperative Oncology Group performance score (ECOG), neutrophil-to-lymphocyte ratio and tumor type) prognostic score was recently proposed as a tool for the accurate prediction of survival [2].

The foremost target of management of MPE is prompt and effective relief of symptoms with minimal discomfort, negligible affection of everyday activity, and cost-effectiveness. Treatment options comprise repeated thoracentesis, chest tube, or catheter drainage with pleurodesis, pleuroperitoneal shunt, pleurectomy, and thoracoscopy.

Pleurodesis is defined as the induction of symphysis between the two layers of pleura to prevent recurrence of effusion. Chemical pleurodesis is the best palliative

* Correspondence: mams@mans.edu.eg; mohamedsanad2008@yahoo.com
Department of Cardiothoracic Surgery, Faculty of Medicine, Mansoura University, Mansoura, Egypt

treatment for recurrent effusions of end stage malignancies [3].

The ideal agent has to be highly effective, easy to administer, safe with minimal side effects, cheap, and readily available. Such agent is still a target to be identified [4].

Most of the agents used for pleurodesis cause pleural injury and inflammatory reaction with subsequent activation of the coagulation system and production of fibrogenic cytokines. All of these lead to the production of collagen that can result in a pleurodesis [5]..

The aim of this study is to assess our results of medical pleurodesis for MPE, using three different chemical agents; bleomycin ampoules, doxycycline capsules, povidone–iodine solution, through two different routes, chest tube and small bore indwelling catheter.

Methods

This retrospective cohort study started in January 2011 till January 2016. We retrospectively reviewed all cases of malignant pleural effusion who were managed palliatively in our cardiothoracic surgery department at our university hospitals by pleurodesis. We compared our techniques with various agents. We did not extend the study beyond this date because pleurodesis was then performed by chest medicine department.

Approval of the institutional research board of our university was obtained. We followed the Declaration of Helsinki as regards trials on humans [6].

Our cohort study included 104 consecutive patients, 50 males and 54 females. Their ages ranged from 22–74 years (57.55 ± 9.02).

Three sclerosing agents were used: 43 patients received bleomycin, 36 patients received doxycycline, and 25 patients received povidone–iodine.

Two routes of delivery applied were either chest tube (64 patients (61.5%)), or indwelling small catheter (40 patients (38.5%)).

For all patients with symptomatic malignant pleural effusion, initial pleurocentesis was applied first. Many patients did not develop recurrence or died before being in need for further pleurocentesis. Other benefited from recurrent pleurocentesis as the rate of accumulation was very gradual. So, symptomatic patients with recurrent malignant pleural effusion whose general condition was reasonable and whose lungs showed no entrapment were our targets for pleurodesis. All our patients had either grade 3 or grade 4 dyspnea.

For all patients, chest X-ray (CXR) was done. Computed tomography (CT) chest was not mandatory except in cases of wide mediastinum and cases of total opacity without mediastinal shift to exclude hilar mass.

The grading of pleural effusion was conducted according to the standard grading system of free-flowing effusion proposed by Smargiassi A. et al. [7] and published in the European respiratory journal as mentioned in Table 1.

We used either chest tube 28–32 French gauge, or a 12 Fr. Pig tail catheter inserted under complete aseptic conditions using local anesthesia. We followed up the patient for evacuation of all fluid with fully inflated lung proved by CXR. The sclerosing agent of choice (500 mg of vibramycin capsules, bleomycin 60 mg ampoules, or 20 mL of 10% povidone–iodine) was then added to a solution of 50cm^3 of sterile saline 0.9% and 10 ml of 2% xylocaine. The chest tube or the catheter was then clamped for 4 h, with rotation of the patient in all possible positions for 1 h to ensure uniform distribution of the agent. The drain was then opened. The patient was followed up over the next few days for the success of the maneuver in achieving drainage less than 100 cc per day and an expanded lung on CXR which enabled us to remove the tube or pig-tail catheter. For all cases with pig-tail and all stable cases of chest tube, the maneuver was performed at outpatient bases.

Table 1. Radiological description of free-flowing pleural effusions as proposed by Smargiassi A. et al. [7]

Grading	Description	Landmarks	Intercostal spaces
Grade 1 *Minimum*	Limited to the costophrenic sinus	Diaphragmatic dome partially evident	Limited to costophrenic sinus
Grade 2 *Small*	Lower lung lobe partially involved	Diaphragmatic dome completely evident	1 intercostal space
Grade 3 *Small to medium*	Lower lung lobe partially collapsed	Lower lung lobe partially atelectatic, pulmonary hilum not visible	2–3 intercostal spaces
Grade 4 *Medium*	Lower lung lobe completely collapsed	Atelectasis of the lower lung lobe, pulmonary hilum visible.	3–4 intercostal spaces
Grade 5 *Large*	Upper lung lobe partially collapsed	Atelectasis of the lower lobe, upper lung lobe partially atelectatic	4 intercostal spaces or more
Grade 6 *Massive*	Lung fully collapsed	Atelectasis of the whole lung, Hilum completely visible	

The choice of the agent was dependent upon operator preference and the availability of the agent. Patients transferred from Oncology Department were usually prescribed bleomycin. Patients with known thyroid malfunction were not subjected to betadine. Most operators preferred chest tube thoracostomy for rapid evacuation of the effusion and better delivery of the sclerosing agent. Some preferred catheter for less pain. In case of wide mediastinum on radiographs, central bronchogenic carcinoma, trapped lung, low pressure of the effusion at time of pleurocentesis, or absent mediastinal shift despite total or near total opacity, we used catheter as from our previous experience in many of these mentioned conditions, we were unable to remove the tube and many patients developed air-fluid level and subsequent empyema.

We considered success either the ability to prevent further re-accumulation of more fluid (< 100 cc/day) and elimination of effusion related extra dyspnea with absence of fluid reaccumulating on chest radiographs until death or loss of follow-up. The partial response entailed diminution of dyspnea related to the effusion and asymptomatic fluid re-accumulation (less than 50% of the initial radiographic evidence of fluid) that needs no further therapy. Failure is considered when patient recurred with pleural effusion in need for intervention with the lack of success as defined above [8, 9].

We followed up all patients for at least 1 month; extended follow up for all these patients was problematic. Usually cases of malignant pleural effusion are end stage with expected survival for few months, and patients have other morbidities. Patients with failed pleurodesis or recurrent effusion were obliged to follow up for further management. So, lack of further follow-up signified either successful pleurodesis or patient's death.

Results

Our study included 104 patients with recurrent malignant pleural effusion, all of them were dyspneic. Fifty patients were male (48.1%) and the remainder 54 patients were female (51.9%). Patients' age ranged from 22 to 74 years (mean 57.55 ± 9.02).

Fifty-nine patients had a New-York heat association (NYHA) IV class of dyspnea (56.7%), 36 patients had NYHA III class of dyspnea (34.6%), and 9 patients (8.6%) had only NYHA II class of dyspnea. As regards other symptoms, 32 patients had chest pain, 39 patients had cough, and 24 patients had both. The rate of pleural effusion re-accumulation was rapid in 55 patients and gradual in 49 patients.

Chest X-ray showed right side effusion in 59 patients (56.7%) and 45 had left-sided pleural effusion. Sixty-one patients (58.7%) had massive effusion and 72 patients (69.2%) had mediastinal shift to the opposite side. The

Table 2. Baseline demographic data, presentation of 104 patients with malignant pleural effusion

Characteristic	Mean ± SD *n*	Range %
Age (mean ± SD, range), years	57.55 ± 9.02	22–74
Male, *n* (%)	50	48.1
Diabetes mellitus	24	23.7
Hypertension	57	54.8
Congestive heart failure	13	12.5
Hepatic dysfunction	8	7.7
Smoker	28	26.9
Side of intervention, right, *n* (%)	59	56.7
ECOG score, *n* (%)		
0–2	80	76.9
3–4	21	20.2
Unknown	3	2.9
Effusion grade		
Small (1–2)	0	0
Moderate (3–4)	6	5.8
Large (5)	26	25
Massive (6)	72	69.2
Presenting symptom*		
Dyspnea	104	100
Chest pain	32	30.7
Cough	39	37.5
Chest pain and cough	24	23.1
Dyspnea score (NYHA)		
NYHA II	9	8.7
NYHA III	36	34.6
NYHA IV	59	56.7
Pleural fluid chemistry		
Exudate	104	100
Mean PH	7.14 ± 0.22	6.87–7.48
PH < 7.3	93	89.4
PH ≥ 7.3	11	10.6
Glucose (mg/dl)	73.3 ± 25.1	24–119
LDH (IU/L)	*1493* ± 294	586–2862
Pleural fluid cytology		
WBC (/μl)	*624.2* ± 58	300–2216
Mono (%)	*73.4* ± 3.6	65–87
Malignant (%)	*12.3* ± 5.2	4–28
RBC (/μl)	*19560* ± 58.7	1400–4800

Eastern Cooperative Oncology Group (ECOG) performance status score runs from 0 to 5, where 0 is fully active, 1 is restricted in physical strenuous activity, 2 is unable to carry out any work activities, 3 is only able to carry out limited self-care activities, 4 is completely disabled, and 5 is dead

Baseline effusion size was graded on chest radiograph immediately prior to trial intervention, using a validated grading system whereby grade 0 referred to no radiographic evidence of pleural fluid; grade 1, blunting of the costophrenic angle; grade 2 to 5, fluid occupying less than 25%, 25% to 50%, 51% to 75%, and more than 75% of the hemithorax, respectively

*The presenting symptoms are non-mutually exclusive

Table 3 Pathology of the primary tumor and different routes of delivery of 3 sclerosing agents for 104 cases with malignant pleural effusion

Pathology of the primary tumor	Bleomycin (n = 43)		Doxycycline (n = 36)		Betadine (n = 25)		Total
	Chest tube and bleomycin	Pig-tail and bleomycin	Chest tube and doxycycline	Pig-tail and doxycycline	Chest tube and betadine	Pig-tail and betadine	Total n (%)
Bronchogenic carcinoma	6	5	2	4	5	0	22 (21.2)
Hepatoma	4	2	1	3	2	0	12 (11.5)
Cancer breast	4	4	4	2	6	0	20 (19.2)
Osteosarcoma	3	0	0	3	0	0	6 (5.8)
Colorectal	3	0	0	3	3	0	9 (8.7)
Mesothelioma	3	0	0	2	1	0	6 (5.8)
Ovarian	3	0	1	2	2	0	8 (7.7)
Lymphoma	2	1	2	2	1	2	10 (9.6)
Kidney	1	0	0	2	0	0	3 (2.9)
Thymoma	1	0	1	0	0	1	3 (2.9)
Esophageal	0	0	1	0	1	0	2 (1.9)
Unknown primary	0	1	0	1	1	0	3 (2.9)
Total n(%)	30 (28.8)	13 (12.5)	12 (11.5)	24 (23.1)	22 (21.1)	3 (2.9)	104

demographic and clinical data of the patients are presented in Table 2. The primary tumor pathology of 104 patients is shown in Table 3.

We used three sclerosing agents. Their distribution and rate of success is shown in Tables 3 and 4.

Bleomycin, doxycycline, and betadine showed success rates of 79.1%, 80.6%, and 76%, respectively.

The route of instillation of the sclerosing agent into the pleural space was chest tube in 64 patients and small indwelling catheter in 40 patients.

Considering complications, 48.8% of bleomycin group patients suffered from pain in 9 patients (20.9%), fever in 8 patients (18.6%), encystation in 2 patients (4.7%), empyema in 1 patient (2.3%), and chest wall sinus in 1 patient (2.3%). In doxycycline group, 23 patients had complications (63.9%) in the form of: pain in 10 patients (27.8%), fever in 11 patients (30.6%), encystation in 1 (2.8%), empyema in 1 patient (2.8%), and chest wall sinus in 1 patient (2.8%).

Table 4. Distribution of the sclerosing agents among our patients

Result	Agent						χ^2	P
	Bleomycin (n = 43)		Doxycycline (n = 36)		Betadine (n = 25)			
	No	%	No	%	No	%		
Failure	9	20.9	7	19.4	6	24.0	0.186	0.911
Success	34	79.1	29	80.6	19	76.0		

All cases in betadine group had complications as 21 patients (84%) had pain, 10 patients had fever (40%), 2 patients (8%) developed hypotension, and 1 patient developed encystation. There were no great differences between the 3 groups apart from the highly significant post maneuver pain related to betadine (P value < 0.001). The degree of such betadine-related pain was mild to moderate and responded well to non-steroidal anti-inflammatory drugs (NSAID). So, such pain was non-limiting factor for betadine use (Table 5). The complications related to the route of delivery are mentioned in Table 6.

Discussion

In our study, the number of female patients is 54 (51.9%) which is slightly more than males (50 patients), but excluding 20 cases of cancer breast all of them are female plus 8 cases of ovarian tumors, male gender appears to predominate.

Most malignances predominate in old age; the mean age of our patients is 57.55 ± 9.02 years. Dye et al. [10] reported mean age 55.8 ± 7.7 years.

Johnston [11] conducted a mega study on 584 specimens from 472 patients found that nearly all neoplasms had been involved the pleura. However, bronchogenic carcinoma had been the most common neoplasm, accounting for approximately one-third of all malignant effusions followed by breast carcinoma and lymphomas. Tumors less commonly associated with malignant

Table 5 Complications related to the sclerosing agent

Complications	Agent						χ^2	P
	Bleomycin (n = 43)		Doxycycline (n = 36)		Betadine (n = 25)			
	No	%	No	%	No	%		
Negative	22	51.2	13	36.1	0	0.0	53.057	<0.001
Fever and pain	0	0.0	1	2.8	9	36.0		
Sinus	1	2.3	1	2.8	0	0.0		
Pain	9	20.9	9	25.0	12	48.0		
Fever	8	18.6	10	27.8	1	4.0		
Empyema	1	2.3	1	2.8	0	0.0		
Loculation	2	4.7	1	2.8	1	4.0		
Hypotension	0	0.0	0	0.0	2	8.0		

pleural effusions included ovarian and gastrointestinal carcinomas. In 5–10% of malignant effusions, no primary tumor was detected [12].

In our study bronchogenic carcinoma was the most encountered pathology (22 patients), followed by cancer breast in 20 patients (19.2%). Hepatocellular carcinoma is a major encounter in cases of malignant pleural effusion in Egypt as it is the end result of the endemic viral hepatitis [12].

The total success rate was 78.8% (82 patients) distributed as follows: 34 patients in the bleomycin group (79.1%), 29 patients in the doxycycline group (80.6%), and 19 patients in the betadine group (76%). There is no statistically significant difference between the three groups.

A study performed by Patz et al. [13] comparing doxycycline with bleomycin pleurodesis utilizing a small-bore catheter, demonstrated a success rate of 72% with bleomycin versus 79% with doxycycline.

Elayouty et al. [12] mentioned in their comparative study that bleomycin resulted in effective pleurodesis in 23/26 (89%). Povidone–iodine lead to effective pleurodesis in 22/25 (88%). As regards pain, 68% of povidone group developed pain versus 53% for bleomycin group. The incidence for fever was comparable being nearly one-third for each group.

Table 6 Complications related to the route of delivery

Complications	Route				$\chi2$	P
	Pig-tail catheter (n = 40)		Chest tube (n = 64)			
	No	%	No	%		
Negative	16	40.0	19	29.7	5.106	0.647
Fever and pain	2	5.0	8	12.5		
Sinus	0	0.0	2	3.1		
Pain	12	30.0	18	28.1		
Fever	7	17.5	12	18.8		
Empyema	0	0.0	2	3.1		
Loculation	2	5.0	2	3.1		
Hypotension	1	2.5	1	1.6		

Referring the success rate to the type of the primary tumor, there was no statistical difference between the various types, but 3 out of 6 patients with mesothelioma showed failure.

Shouman and colleagues [14] hypothesized that the lower rate of pleurodesis in patients with positive cytology is due to the fact that they have a larger tumor burden which covers a higher percentage of the pleural surfaces. Accordingly, the mesothelial cells are covered with the tumor and cannot respond to the pleurodesis agents in the usual manner.

Comparing the results between patients with either chest tube or small catheter, there was no significant statistical difference in success rate and occurrence of complications. But the four patients who developed either chest wall sinus (2) or empyema (2) were confined to chest tube cases.

As regards post maneuver pain, there was no significant difference between patients with either chest tube or catheter, but as regards quality of pain, patients with chest tube suffered extra pain related to the tube itself. This is not proved statistically as we did not perform the pain score analysis.

Kahrom et al. [15] from Iran in evaluated the efficacy of povidone–iodine, reported success rate 82.2% and occurrence of pain in 26.9% of their cases.

Shouman et al. [14] demonstrated that tetracycline, talc slurry, iodopovidone, and bleomycin, all resulted in comparable success rates of 80%, 80%, 66.6%, and 73.3% at 30 days.

Clementsen et al. [16] studied the effect of route size, either chest tube or small catheter, on the results of pleurodesis success and recurrence of effusion. No significant difference was found. But the larger tubes caused more discomfort.

This study showed insignificant complication rates among both routes as shown in Table 4.

Mager et al. [17] studied the effect of rolling after instillation of the agent, they found no significant effect. They recommended discontinuing this maneuver to simplify the practice.

Boland et al. [18] described the trapped lung after drainage by an air/fluid level and a lung that would not fully expand. It can cause failure simply due to the mechanical difficulty of getting the pleural surfaces apposition. Options for management this condition include pleurectomy, surgical decortication, a pleuroperitoneal shunt, and obligatory long-term drainage.

A recent Cochrane database systematic review and network meta-analysis [19] compared the results of 62 randomized trials and 3428 patients who underwent pleurodesis using different agents. They concluded that talc poudrage was a highly effective technique (ranked second of 16 (95% credible interval (Cr-I) 1 to 5)) and provided evidence that it caused fewer pleurodesis failures than eight other approaches. The projected ranks of other commonly used agents were: talc slurry (fourth; 95% Cr-I 2 to 8), mepacrine (fourth; 95% Cr-I 1 to 10), iodine (fifth; 95% Cr-I 1 to 12), bleomycin (eighth; 95% Cr-I 5 to 11), and doxycyline (tenth; 95% Cr-I 4 to 15).

Most of the secondary outcomes, including adverse events, were incoherently described by the involved studies. The reported adverse events were pain, fever, and mortality. The fever network was imprecise and showed considerable heterogeneity, but suggested placebo caused the least fever (ranked first of 11 (95% Cr-I 1 to 7)) and mepacrine and Corynebacterium parvum (C. parvum) seemed to be connected with the most fever (ranked tenth (95% Cr-I 6 to 11) and eleventh (95% Cr-I 7 to 11), respectively). No differences between interventions were revealed by the network meta-analysis of the pain data. The only potential difference in mortality was recognized in the mortality network was that those receiving tetracycline appeared to have a longer survival than those receiving mitoxantrone (OR 0.16 (95% confidence interval (CI) 0.03 to 0.72)). Indwelling pleural catheters were examined in two randomized studies, both of which reported improved breathlessness when compared to talc slurry pleurodesis, despite lower pleurodesis success rates.

The shortcomings and limitations of our study were a smaller sample that was unable to detect a significant difference between the different routes of delivery and the sclerosing agents and the lack of talc powder. There is agreement that Talc powder is the most effective agent but its side effects are dangerous as pneumonitis and acute respiratory distress syndrome, plus its unavailability in many countries including Egypt. Apart from talc powder, no one agent proved to be more efficient or less toxic up till now. The three agents we used showed similar results but doxycycline and betadine are more economic and available. We did not compare the visual analogue scores of patients due to unavailability of the pain charts in the records of these patients. A larger sample, longer study period, and larger fund are needed to determine if any statistical significance is present as regards effectiveness of different agents. This study does not stress on the association between pH and glucose levels in pleural fluid. Often in clinical situations, other disease-specific biomarkers would have better been used and contributed to the diagnostic procedure and may be an interesting issue for forthcoming studies.

Conclusions

Pleurodesis for recurrent malignant pleural effusion as a good palliative procedure with acceptable manageable complications. No significant differences between our agents and route used but one can consider price, availability, and patient's tolerance.

Abbreviations

MPE: Malignant pleural effusion; ECOG: Eastern Cooperative Oncology Group; CT: Computed tomography; CXR: Chest X-ray; NYHA: New York Heart Association; NSAID: Non-steroidal anti-inflammatory drugs; Cr-I: Credible interval

Acknowledgements

This trial would not be possible without the enthusiasm and commitment of clinicians, nurses, and our patients. The authors would like to thank Dr. Walid Mohammed, the lecturer of cardiothoracic surgery at Mansoura University Faculty of Medicine, Egypt, for his efforts in writing and revising the manuscript. The authors would like to thank Dr. Hatem Beshir https://orcid.org/0000-0003-1366-3949 from the Department of Cardiothoracic Surgery at Mansoura University for his efforts in analyzing the data and revision of this manuscript.

Ethical approval and consent to participate

We followed the Declaration of Helsinki regarding studies on human subjects [6]. Approvals of the institutional research board of Mansoura University Faculty of Medicine was obtained (MUIRB-201-16-11). Patients were informed and signed written consents for participation in the study, operation and publishing of clinical data.

Authors' contributions

All authors contributed equally in concepualization. MES, GA, and MS operated the cases. MES performed the literature review, obtained the medical records and participated in writing of the manuscript. GA introduced the idea of comparing different routes of delivery and participated in writing of the manuscript. MES performed literature review and wrote the manuscript with MS. MES and MS analyzed the results. All the authors have read and approved the manuscript in its currently submitted form.

References

1. Psallidas I, Kalomenidis I, Porcel JM, Robinson BW, Stathopoulos GT (2016) Malignant pleural effusion: from bench to bedside. European Respiratory Review. 25(140):189–198
2. Clive AO, Kahan BC, Hooper CE, Bhatnagar R, Morley AJ, Zahan-Evans N, Bintcliffe OJ, Boshuizen RC, Fysh ET, Tobin CL, Medford AR (2014 Dec 1) Predicting survival in malignant pleural effusion: development and validation of the LENT prognostic score. Thorax. 69(12):1098–1104
3. Estrada Saló G, Farina Ríos C, Fibla Alfara JJ, Gómez Sebastián G, Unzueta MC, León GC (2003) Spontaneous pneumothorax: Pleurodesis with an iodo-povidone hydroalcoholic solution. Arch Bronconeumol. 39:171–174
4. Olivares-Torres CA, Laniado-Laborín R, Chávez-García C, León-Gastelum C, Reyes-Escamilla A, Light RW (2002) Iodopovidone pleurodesis for recurrent pleural effusions. Chest. 122:581–583
5. Pamela B (1994) M. Leigh, A. Steven. Chemical pleurodesis for malignant pleural effusions. Ann. Intern. Med. 120:56–64
6. World Medical Association. World Medical Association Declaration of Helsinki. Ethical principles for medical research involving human subjects. Bull World Health Organ. 2001;79(4):373–374.
7. Smargiassi A, Inchingolo R, Zanforlin A, Valente S, Soldati G, Corbo GM (2013) Description of free-flowing pleural effusions in medical reports after echographic assessment. Respiration. 85(5):439
8. Rafei H, Jabak S, Mina A, Tfayli A (2015) Pleurodesis in malignant pleural effusions: Outcome and predictors of success. Integr Cancer Sci Therap. 2: 216–221
9. Davies HE, Lee YG (2013) Management of malignant pleural effusions: questions that need answers. Current opinion in pulmonary medicine. 19(4): 374–379
10. Dey A, Bhuniya S, Datta Chaudhuri A, Pandit S, Saha-Dutta Chowdhury M, Sengupta A, Saha I, De P (2010) Iodopovidone pleurodesis: experience of a tertiary hospital in Kolkata. Singapore Med J. 51(2):163–165

11. Johnston WW (1985) The malignant pleural effusion: a review of cytopathological diagnoses of 584 specimens from 472 consecutive patients. Cancer. 56:905–909
12. Elayouty HD, Hassan TM, Alhadad ZA (2012) Povidone- Iodine versus Bleomycin Pleurodesis for Malignant Effusion in Bronchogenic Cancer Guided by Thoracic Echography. J Cancer Sci Ther. 4:182–184
13. Patz EF, McAdams HP, Erasmus JJ (1998) Sclerotherapy for malignant pleural effusions: a prospective randomized trial of bleomycin vs doxycycline with small-bore catheter drainage. Chest. 113:1305–1311
14. Shouman W, Elgazzar A, Hussien R, ElShaaray M (2012) Chemical pleurodesis for malignant pleural effusion. Egyptian Journal of Chest Diseases and Tuberculosis. 61:115–120
15. Kahrom hadi, Manouchehr Aghajanzadeh, Mohammad Reza Asgari, Mahdi Kahrom Efficacy and safety of povidone-iodine pleurodesis in malignant pleural effusions. 2017;23:53-56
16. Clementsen P, Evald T, Grode G, Hansen M, Krag JG, Faurschou P (1998) Treatment of malignant pleural effusion: pleurodesis using a small percutaneous catheter. A prospective randomized study. Respir Med. 9(2): 593–596
17. Mager HJ, Maesen B, Verzijlbergen F, Schramel F (2002) Distribution of talc suspension during treatment of malignant pleural effusion with talc pleurodesis. Lung Cancer. 36:77–81
18. Boland GW, Gazelle GS, Girard MJ (1998) Mueller PR. Asymptomatic hydropneumothorax after therapeutic thoracentesis for malignant pleural effusions Am J Roentgenol. 170:943–946
19. Clive AO, Jones HE, Bhatnagar R, Preston NJ, Maskell N (2016) Interventions for the management of malignant pleural effusions: a network meta-analysis. Cochrane Database of Systematic Reviews. 5

Continuous paravertebral block by intraoperative direct access versus systemic analgesia for postthoracotomy pain relief

Ahmed Deebis[1*], Hala Elattar[2], Osama Saber[1], Kareem Elfakharany[1] and Nezar Elnahal[1]

Abstract

Background: Systemic analgesia with paracetamol and nonsteroidal anti-inflammatory drugs plus opioids as a rescue medication had reported to be better than that depend mainly on opioids for postoperative pain relief. Thoracic paravertebral block reported to provide a comparable postthoracotomy pain relief to epidural analgesia, with fewer side effects due to its unilateral effect. Thoracic paravertebral catheter can be inserted intraoperatively under direct vision during thoracic surgery (Sabanathan's technique). This prospective randomized study was designed to evaluate the safety and efficacy of this technique with continuous infusion of lidocaine compared to systemic analgesia for postthoracotomy pain relief.

Results: Sixty-three patients were randomized to receive a continuous infusion of lidocaine in the paravertebral catheter for 3 postoperative days (thoracic paravertebral group, $n = 32$) or systemic analgesia (systemic analgesia group, $n = 31$). All patients underwent standard posterolateral thoracotomy. There were no significant differences between both groups in age, sex, side, type, and duration of operation. Pain scores measured on visual analogue scale and morphine consumption were significantly lower in thoracic paravertebral group in all postoperative days. Spirometric pulmonary functions were not reaching the preoperative values in the third postoperative day in both groups, but restorations of pulmonary functions were superior in paravertebral group. No complications could be attributed to the paravertebral catheter. Side effects, mainly nausea and vomiting followed by urinary retention, were significantly more in systemic analgesia group ($P = 0.03$). Also, pulmonary complications were more in systemic analgesia group but not reaching statistical significance ($P = 0.14$).

Conclusion: Continuous paravertebral block by direct access to the paravertebral space using a catheter inserted by the surgeon is a simple technique, with low risk of complications, provides effective pain relief with fewer side effects, and reduces the early loss of postoperative pulmonary functions when compared to systemic analgesia.

Keywords: Paravertebral block, Postthoracotomy analgesia, Systemic analgesia, Sabanathan's technique, Lidocaine infusion

Background

Postthoracotomy pain is responsible for ineffective ventilation with inability to breathe deeply and mucous plugging leading to atelectasis, hypoxia, and ventilation perfusion mismatch predisposing to pulmonary infection and pulmonary complications [1, 2]. Multiple modalities were used to provide sufficient pain control with varying success: thoracic epidural, thoracic paravertebral, intrathecal, intercostal, interpleural analgesic techniques, and systemic analgesia [2–5]. Thoracic paravertebral block provides a comparable pain relief to epidural analgesia, with less side effects due to its unilateral effect [2, 6–9]. Recently, the group of procedure specific postoperative pain management (PROSPECT) of the European society

* Correspondence: ahmedeebis@gmail.com
[1]Cardiothoracic Surgery Department, Faculty of Medicine, Zagazig University, Zagazig, Sharkia Governorate, Egypt
Full list of author information is available at the end of the article

of regional anesthesia and pain therapy recommends thoracic paravertebral block (TPVB) with local anesthetics as a bolus preoperatively or at the end of the operation followed by continuous infusion as the first choice compared to thoracic epidural analgesia (TEA) as TPVB has a lower rate of complications [10]. The main disadvantage of TPVB technique is the lack of familiarity [11]. The conventional and the most commonly used technique for paravertebral block depends on loss of resistance to air technique for percutaneous insertion of the catheter that can be aided with ultrasound guidance or nerve stimulation, and this is usually done by the anesthetist [12, 13]. Thoracic paravertebral catheters can also be safely inserted with ease under direct vision during thoracic surgery by the surgeon (Sabanathan's technique) [14–16].

This study was designed to evaluate the safety and efficacy of TPVB by intraoperative insertion of the catheter directly into the paravertebral space with postoperative continuous infusion of lidocaine on postthoracotomy pain as compared to systemic analgesia.

Methods

This prospective study was conducted in our center after approval from our University Institutional Research Board (IRB) and written informed consent from all patients, in the period from June 2015 to January 2020. The study was registered in ClinicalTrials.gov (ID: NCT04482192).

Inclusion criteria were the adult patients scheduled to undergo elective posterolateral thoracotomy for pulmonary procedures with American Society of Anesthesiologists (ASA) physical status of II and III and body mass index (BMI) between 25 and 35 kg/m^2.

Exclusion criteria were patients younger than 18 years, emergency surgery, previous thoracotomy, drug addiction, allergy to paracetamol (acetaminophen) or ketorolac, allergy to local anesthetics used, coagulopathy, hepatic dysfunction, chronic renal failure, history of gastric ulcer or bronchial asthma, or lack of patient consent.

Randomization into two groups, thoracic paravertebral block (TPVB) group and systemic analgesia (SA) with 1:1 allocation, was done by sealed envelopes that were prepared with a computer-generated randomization.

Patient's sample

Based on a pilot study of 20 patients, 10 in each group, the mean visual analogue scores of pain at rest (VAS) ± SD at 6 h postoperatively for TPVB patients were 3.0 ± 1.4 and that for SA patients were 4.2 ± 1.6. The calculated significant sample size with a power of 0.85 and alpha error of 0.05 was 60 patients, with 1:1 allocation in each group.

Eighty-two patients were assessed for eligibility criteria to be included in the study, 18 patients were excluded pre-randomization, and one patient was excluded post-randomization due to re-exploration for bleeding. Sixty-three patients were analyzed in the study. Thoracic paravertebral block group (TPVB group) included 32 patients, and systemic analgesia group (SA group) included 31 patients (Fig. 1).

On the day before operation, patients were trained for the use of the paper-based visual analogue scale (VAS) for pain assessment. The VAS consists of a horizontal line of 10 cm long orientated from the right (0 = no pain) to the left (10 = worst pain imaginable). The patient places a mark on the line corresponding to intensity of pain. The distance between the starting point (the right end) to the patient mark, in centimeters, is recorded as his/her pain score.

Also, patients were instructed in the use of Microspiro HI-198 (Chest Corporation, Tokyo, Japan). After training, forced vital capacity (FVC), forced expiratory volume in 1 s (FEV_1), and peak expiratory flow rate (PEFR), in the sitting position, were recorded in the day before surgery.

Anesthesia

Anesthetic technique was standardized for all patients. Patients were premedicated with IV injection of glycopyrrolate 0.01 mg/kg. Anesthesia was induced with intravenous 1.5–2 mg/kg propofol and fentanyl 2 μg/kg. Intravenous atracurium 0.5 mg/kg was given to facilitate tracheal intubation. Anesthesia was maintained with isoflurane 0.8–1.2% in 100% oxygen, incremental doses (0.1 mg/kg) of atracurium, and mechanical ventilation. At the end of surgical operation, neuromuscular block was reversed using IV neostigmine 2.5 mg and glycopyrrolate 0.01 mg/kg.

Technique of intraoperative paravertebral catheter insertion

We used the technique that was described by Sabanathan et al. in 1988 [14] and modified by them in 1990 [15]. After completing the surgical pulmonary procedure and with the chest is still open, starting from the posterior end of the thoracotomy, parietal pleura is raised from the posterior chest wall to the vertebral body and for two spaces above and below the incision of thoracotomy creating a pouch. A 16-gauge disposable Tuohy needle is inserted percutaneously through a low posterior interspace. The needle is advanced until the tip appeared in the created pouch. The stylet is removed, and a 16-gauge side-holed epidural catheter is advanced into the created pouch, and the needle is withdrawn. Using a curved forceps, a small defect is done in the extrapleural fascia to be directly in the paravertebral space. The

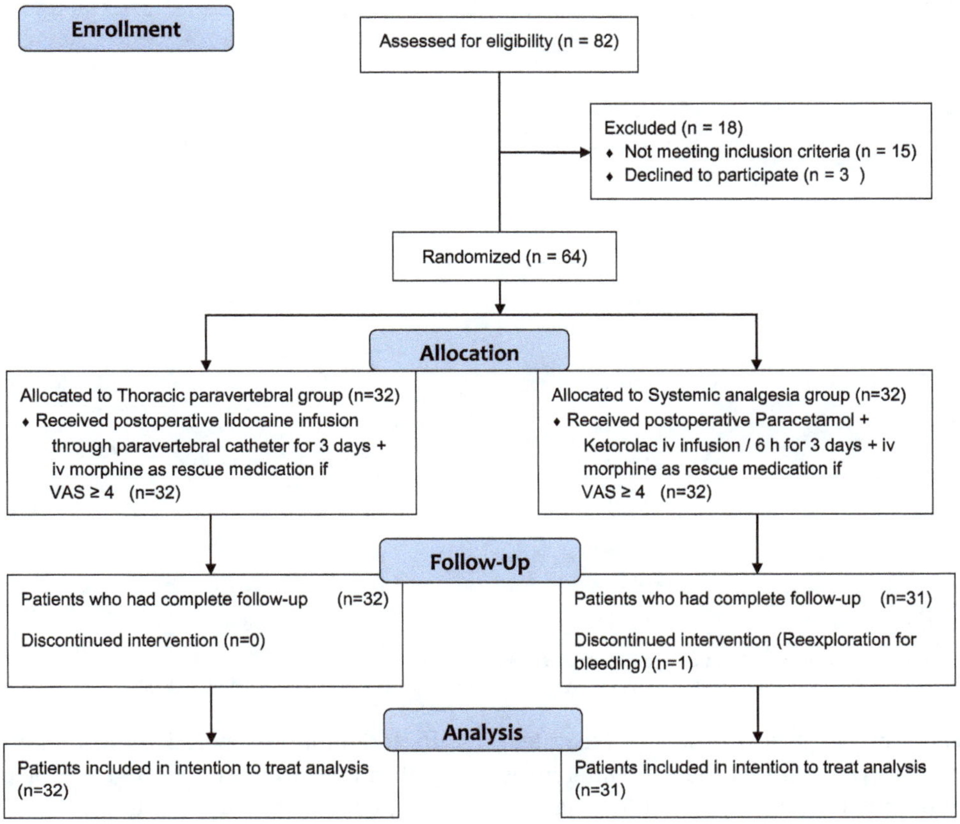

Fig. 1 CONSORT flow diagram

cannula is passed to the paravertebral space through the defect and advanced cranially for 2 to 3 cm. The parietal pleura is reattached to the posterior edge of the wound, and the catheter is secured. Then, a bolus dose 15–20 ml of 1% lidocaine is injected through the catheter, and the chest is closed as usual with one or two intercostal drainage tubes according to the surgical procedure.

Protocol of analgesia

All patients, in both groups, received intravenous analgesia with 1 g paracetamol and 30 mg ketorolac half an hour before the end of surgery.

Systemic analgesia (SA) group continues to receive 1 g paracetamol and 30 mg ketorolac by intravenous infusion every 6 h for 3 days. Thoracic paravertebral block (TPVB) group received continuous infusion of 0.1 ml/kg/h of 1.0% lidocaine (1 mg/kg/h) using infusion pump through the inserted paravertebral catheter for 3 days. Intravenous morphine sulfate (0.05 mg/kg) was given as a rescue medication if the VAS ≥ 4 for both groups. A senior nurse was responsible for handling the analgesia regimen, and another nurse was responsible for recording pain score on visual analogue scale (VAS) and morphine consumption, as scheduled.

Objective pulmonary function

Forced vital capacity (FVC), forced expiratory volume in 1 s (FEV_1), and peak expiratory flow rate (PEFR) were measured in the sitting position 24, 48, and 72 h postoperatively for all patients. Results were expressed as a percentage of the preoperative values that were done in the day before surgery.

End points

The primary end point was pain score on visual analogue scale (VAS) at rest and on coughing measured and recorded at 1, 6, 12, 24, 36, 48 h, and 72 h postoperatively. The secondary end points were total morphine consumption at the end of each postoperative day and pulmonary function tests at 24, 48, and 72 h postoperatively. Complications related to the catheter, postoperative pulmonary complications, respiratory depression (defined as respiratory rate less than 8 per min), nausea and vomiting, and urinary retention were recorded.

Statistical analysis

Continuous variables are presented as mean ± SD and categorical variables as number and percent. Continuous variables were compared using *t* test or Mann–Whitney test if not normally distributed, and categorical variables

Table 1 Characteristics of patients and surgical procedures

Characteristics	TPVB group (*n* = 32)	SA group (*n* = 31)	*P* value
Age (years)	48 ± 14	46 ± 11	0.53
Male	19 (59.4%)	17 (54.8%)	0.72
ASA II	22 (68.8%)	23 (74.2%)	0.62
ASA III	10 (31.2%)	8 (25.8%)	0.62
BMI (kg/m^2)	29 ± 5	28 ± 6	0.47
Type of surgery			
Wedge resection	6 (18.8%)	7 (22.5%)	0.71
Segmentectomy	3 (9.4%)	2 (6.5%)	0.81
Metastasectomy	2 (6.2%)	2 (6.5%)	0.71
Lobectomy	19 (59.4%)	18 (58%)	0.56
Pneumonectomy	2 (6.2%)	2 (6.5%)	0.71
Side of the procedure			
Left thoracotomy	18 (56.2%)	19 (61.3%)	0.68
Right thoracotomy	14 (43.8%)	12 (38.7%)	
Duration of surgery (min)	108 ± 44	98 ± 46	0.38

Continuous variables are presented as mean ± SD and categorical variables as number and percent
TPVB thoracic paravertebral block, *SA* systemic analgesia, *ASA* American Society of Anesthesiologists physical status, *BMI* body mass index

were compared using the chi^2 test or Fischer's Exact test if the frequency of the events is less than 5. Differences were accepted to be significant at $p < 0.05$. Analyses were done using IBM SPSS for Windows, Version 22.0 (IBM Corp., USA).

Results

Sixty-three adult patients included in the study, 32 in thoracic paravertebral block (TPVB) group and 31in systemic analgesia (SA) group, 36 males and 27 females. There were no significant differences between both groups regarding age, sex, ASA class, BMI, side, type, and duration of operation (Table 1).

Pain relief

Pain scores on visual analogue scale were significantly lower in TPVB group at rest and on coughing throughout the study period, indicating better pain relief in the TPVB group (Tables 2 and 3).

In addition, postoperative morphine consumption was significantly lower in TPVB group of patients in all the three postoperative days (Table 4).

Postoperative pulmonary function

In both groups, all pulmonary function tests (FVC, FEV_1, and PEFR) were reduced in first postoperative day (measured 24 h postoperatively) than the preoperative values and continue to increase in the second and third days but not reaching the preoperative values at 72 h postoperatively. But, all pulmonary function tests are significantly better in TPVB group in all days (Table 5).

Complications and side effects

No complications could be attributed to the paravertebral catheter or to lidocaine. Pulmonary complications were more in SA group but without statistical significance ($P = 0.14$) (Table 6). Side effects were significantly more in SA group ($P = 0.03$). The most frequent side

Table 2 Pain score on visual analogue scale at rest

	TPVB group (*n* = 32)	SA group (*n* = 31)	*P* value
VAS 1 h	4.1 ± 1.1	5.2 ± 1.3	< 0.001
VAS 6 h	3.0 ± 1.3	4.2 ± 1.5	0.001
VAS 12 h	2.9 ± 1.1	4.1 ± 1.3	< 0.001
VAS 24 h	2.0 ± 1.3	3.4 ± 2.0	0.002
VAS 36 h	1.8 ± 1.3	3.0 ± 2.0	0.008
VAS 48 h	1.6 ± 0.7	2.3 ± 0.8	< 0.001
VAS 72 h	1.1 ± 0.6	1.8 ± 0.8	< 0.001

TPVB thoracic paravertebral block, *SA* systemic analgesia, *VAS* visual analogue score of pain, presented as mean ± SD, *h* postoperative hour

Table 3 Pain score on visual analogue scale on coughing

	TPVB group (*n* = 32)	SA group (*n* = 31)	*P* value
VAS 1 h	6.0 ± 1.2	7.2 ± 1.5	0.001
VAS 6 h	4.0 ± 1.1	5.2 ± 1.3	< 0.001
VAS 12 h	3.9 ± 1.0	4.8 ± 1.4	0.006
VAS 24 h	3.7 ± 0.9	4.5 ± 1.3	0.008
VAS 36 h	3.3 ± 0.9	3.8 ± 1.0	0.041
VAS 48 h	2.0 ± 0.8	2.6 ± 0.9	0.007
VAS 72 h	1.7 ± 0.8	2.2 ± 0.8	0.016

TPVB thoracic paravertebral block, *SA* systemic analgesia, *VAS* visual analogue score of pain, presented as mean ± SD, *h* postoperative hour

Table 4 Postoperative morphine consumption daily for each group

	TPVB group (n = 32)	SA group (n = 31)	P value
Day 1 (mg/day)	20.1 ± 11.1	37.2 ± 19.1	< 0.001
Day 2 (mg/day)	12.2 ± 8.8	27.4 ± 18.4	< 0.001
Day 3 (mg/day)	9.7 ± 6.2	15.2 ± 11.8	0.028

Total morphine consumption every day presented as mean ± SD
TPVB thoracic paravertebral block, *SA* systemic analgesia

effects were nausea and vomiting (6 patients in SA group and 1 patient in TPVB group, P = 0.04). Urinary retentions were more in SA group but without statistical significance (P = 0.32) (Table 6).

Discussion

Postthoracotomy pain is reported as one of the most painful postoperative pain and frequently causes significant morbidity [1]. Combinations of analgesic drugs that have different mechanisms of action achieve a synergistic effect with better postoperative pain relief and fewer side effects [17]. A meta-analyses of randomized trials concluded that paracetamol (acetaminophen) in combination with a nonsteroidal anti-inflammatory drug for postoperative pain control achieved better pain relief than each drug alone, and this combination decreased opioid use [18]. According to the above concept, we used a multimodal systemic analgesia in the form paracetamol combined with ketorolac (nonsteroidal anti-inflammatory drug) plus morphine as a rescue medication for systemic (SA) analgesia group in this study.

Thoracic paravertebral space is a wedge-shaped space on both sides of vertebral column. Parietal pleura forms the anterolateral boundary of the space. Vertebrae and intervertebral foramina form its medial boundary. The space contains intercostal nerves (spinal nerves) and its posterior primary rami, the rami communicantes, and the sympathetic chain. The spinal nerves in the space formed from small bundles without enclosing fascial sheath making them highly susceptible for blockade with local anesthetics [11].. The injected local anesthetic drug in the paravertebral space diffuses cranially and caudally covering several segments resulting in unilateral somatic and sympathetic nerve block [13]. The conventional technique for TPVB is the percutaneous technique that may be aided with ultrasonic guidance or nerve stimulation with about 6 to 19% failure rate and a complication rate of 2.6 to 5% in the form of pneumothorax, vascular injury, Horner syndrome, and epidural or intrathecal spread [11]. Intraoperative insertion of the paravertebral catheter under direct vision into the paravertebral space is an alternative technique that can be done easily by the surgeon [14, 15]. Results of this study and that of many other studies [3, 14–16, 19–22] supported that this technique is an easy and safe and without complications related to catheter insertion.

The most commonly used local anesthetic drugs for continuous paravertebral block are bupivacaine, lidocaine, and ropivacaine. Bupivacaine and ropivacaine are long-acting local anesthetic drugs, while lidocaine is a short-acting one with a shorter half-life. So, for continuous infusion, lidocaine may be the better choice [20, 21, 23, 24]. Watson et al. [20] in a study comparing bupivacaine versus lidocaine for continuous paravertebral block after thoracotomy reported that their efficacy was equivalent with lesser risk of systemic toxicity for lidocaine. Also, Ghisi et al. [23] reported equal analgesic effect of lidocaine and ropivacaine for continuous paravertebral block, but they recommended the use of lidocaine because of its easier titratability and lower cost. As the results of this study, many investigators [16, 20, 21, 23, 24] used lidocaine for continuous paravertebral block without side effects related to the drug. Many studies [2, 4, 6, 9, 10] comparing postthoracotomy TPVB to epidural analgesia reported equivalent pain relief with lesser side effects of TPVB. TPVB is superior compared to pure intercostal nerve block in postthoracotomy pain relief as TPVB also blocks posterior primary rami and sympathetic fibers [22].

Table 5 Postoperative changes in pulmonary function tests (expressed as a percent of preoperative values)

Pulmonary function test	Time of test	TPVB group (n = 32)	SA group (n = 31)	P value
Forced vital capacity (FVC), mean ± SD	24 h	54 ± 9	26 ± 12	< 0.001
	48 h	65 ± 11	33 ± 13	< 0.001
	72 h	70 ± 12	46 ± 10	0.007
Forced expiratory volume in 1 s (FEV1), mean ± SD	24 h	60 ± 10	29 ± 12	< 0.001
	48 h	71 ± 12	36 ± 11	< 0.001
	72 h	76 ± 11	48 ± 10	0.003
Peak expiratory flow rate (PEFR), mean ± SD	24 h	58 ± 11	28 ± 11	< 0.001
	48 h	69 ± 14	38 ± 12	< 0.001
	72 h	75 ± 12	49 ± 13	0.001

Pulmonary function tests (expressed as a percent of preoperative values) presented as mean ± SD
TPVB thoracic paravertebral block, *SA* systemic analgesia

Table 6 Postoperative complications and side effects

	TPVB group (*n* = 32)	SA group (*n* = 31)	*P* value
Postop. pulmonary complications			
Prolonged air leak	1	2	0.49
Atelectasis	0	2	0.24
Pneumothorax	1	1	0.75
Bronchospasm	0	1	0.49
Pleural effusion	1	1	0.75
Total pulmonary complications	3 (9.4%)	7 (22.6%)	0.14
Postop. side effects			
Nausea and vomiting	1	6	0.04
Urinary retention	2	4	0.32
Respiratory depression	0	0	
Total side effects	3 (18.7%)	10 (54.8%)	0.03

Categorical variables are presented as number and percent
TPVB thoracic paravertebral block, *SA* systemic analgesia, *Postop.* postoperative

This study demonstrates significant pain relief in TPVB group compared to SA group supported by lower pain score on visual analogue scale at rest and on coughing and lesser morphine consumption. Marret et al. [25] comparing TPVB with ropivacaine to systemic analgesia and Fortier et al. [3] comparing 3 analgesic modalities (systemic analgesia, continuous wound catheter analgesia, and continuous thoracic paravertebral block with ropivacaine) demonstrated the superiority of TPVB for postthoracotomy pain relief with lesser morphine consumption as the results of our study. This study confirms the findings of other studies that there are marked alteration of pulmonary function following thoracotomy [11, 26, 27], and effective postoperative regional analgesia as thoracic paravertebral block and thoracic epidural block reduces this alteration and aids in its recovery [11, 16, 22, 24, 26]. This study recorded no significant difference in postoperative pulmonary complications between TPVB group and SA group. Nausea and vomiting were significantly more in SA group, and this is mostly due to increased morphine consumption in that group as postoperative nausea and vomiting are strongly influenced by postoperative opioid use in a dose-related manner [28, 29]. Many studies [8, 16, 22, 30] comparing TPVB with continuous local anesthetic perfusion versus intravenous or intramuscular opioids for postoperative analgesia reported better pain relief and lesser side effects in TPVB patients.

Limitations

As there were different routes of administration of analgesic drugs for each group of patients, it was very difficult to keep double blindness. Also, the number of patients can be considered as another limitation.

Conclusion

This study demonstrates that patients receiving continuous paravertebral block with lidocaine via a catheter inserted with direct access to the thoracic paravertebral space by the surgeon intraoperatively have significantly better pain relief with fewer side effects and better restoration of pulmonary functions compared to patients receiving systemic analgesia, and this technique (Sabanathan's technique) is safe and reliable as a method for postthoracotomy analgesia.

Abbreviations

PROSPECT: The group of procedure specific postoperative pain management; TPVB: Thoracic paravertebral block; TEA: Thoracic epidural analgesia; ASA: American Society of Anesthesiologists; BMI: Body mass index; SA: Systemic analgesia; VAS: Visual analogue score; CONSORT: Consolidated Standards of Reporting Trials; SD: Standard deviation

Acknowledgements

Not applicable.

Authors' contributions

AD designed the study, analysis, and interpretation of data; conducted the statistical analysis; drafted the manuscript; and supervised the study. HE involved in the study design, analyzed and interpreted the data, and drafted the manuscript. OS involved in the study design, analyzed and interpreted the data, and drafted the manuscript. KE involved in the study design, conducted the literature search, performed the data collection, and drafted the manuscript. NE conducted the review of data, involved in the study design, analyzed and interpreted the data, and drafted the manuscript. All authors have read and approved the final manuscript.

Author details

[1]Cardiothoracic Surgery Department, Faculty of Medicine, Zagazig University, Zagazig, Sharkia Governorate, Egypt. [2]Anesthesia and Intensive Care Department, Zagazig University, Zagazig, Egypt.

References

1. Kotze A, Scally A, Howell S (2009) Efficacy and safety of different techniques of paravertebral block for analgesia after thoracotomy: systematic review and metaregression. Br J Anaesth 103(5):626–636. https://doi.org/10.1093/bja/aep272
2. Joshi GP, Bonnet F, Shah R, Wilkinson RC, Camu F, Fischer B et al (2008) A systematic review of randomized trials evaluating regional techniques for postthoracotomy analgesia. Anesth Analg 107:1026–1040. https://doi.org/10.1213/ane.0b013e31817e7b40
3. Fortier S, Hanna HA, Bernard A, Girard C (2012) Comparison between systemic analgesia, continuous wound catheter analgesia and continuous thoracic paravertebral block: a randomised, controlled trial of postthoracotomy pain management. Eur J Anaesthesiol 29:524–530. https://doi.org/10.1097/EJA.0b013e328357e5a1
4. Wojtyś ME, Wąsikowski J, Wójcik N, Wójcik J, Wasilewski P, Lisowski P et al (2019) Assessment of postoperative pain management and comparison of effectiveness of pain relief treatment involving paravertebral block and thoracic epidural analgesia in patients undergoing posterolateral thoracotomy. J Cardiothorac Surg 14:78 https://doi.org/10.1186/s13019-019-0901-3
5. Kolettas A, Lazaridis G, Baka S, Mpoukovinas I, Karavasilis V, Kioumis I et al (2015) Postoperative pain management. J Thorac Dis 7:S62–S72. https://doi.org/10.3978/j.issn.2072-1439.2015.01.15
6. Krakowski JC, Arora H (2015) Con: thoracic epidural block is not superior to paravertebral blocks for open thoracic surgery. J Cardiothorac Vasc Anesth 29(6):1720-1722. https://doi.org/10.1053/j.jvca.2015.06.012. Epub 2015 Jun 10.
7. Casati A, Alessandrini P, Nuzzi M, Tosi M, Iotti E, Ampollini L et al (2006) A prospective, randomized, blinded comparison between continuous thoracic para-vertebral and epidural infusion of 0.2% ropivacaine after lung resection surgery. Eur J Anaesthesiol 23:999–1004. https://doi.org/10.1017/S0265021506001104
8. Davies RG, Myles PS, Graham JM (2006) A comparison of the analgesic efficacy and side-effects of paravertebral vs epidural blockade for thoracotomy–a systematic review and meta-analysis of randomized trials. Br J Anaesth 96:418–426. https://doi.org/10.1093/bja/ael020
9. Scarfe AJ, Schuhmann-Hingel S, Duncan JK, Ma N, Atukorale YN, Cameron AL (2016) Continuous paravertebral block for post-cardiothoracic surgery analgesia: a systematic review and meta-analysis. Eur J Cardiothorac Surg 50:1010–1018. https://doi.org/10.1093/ejcts/ezw168
10. Procedure specific postoperative pain management. (2015) Thoracotomy. http://www.esraeurope.org/prospect [Accessed 26 Jan 2020].
11. Rosenblatt MA, Lai Y. Thoracic nerve block techniques UpToDate Topic 100071 Version 24.0, last updated: Jun 10, 2019.https://www.uptodate.com/contents/thoracic-nerve-blocktechniques. [Accessed 23 Oct 2019]
12. Katz D, Khelemsky Y (2013) Paravertebral blockade techniques, clinical applications, and complications. Topics in Pain Management 28(11):1–7. https://doi.org/10.1097/01.TPM.0000431364.10401.ee
13. Batra RK, Krishnan K, Agarwal A (2011) Paravertebral block. J Anaesthesiol Clin Pharmacol 27(1):5–11 http://www.joacp.org/text.asp?2011/27/1/5/76608
14. Sabanathan S, Bickford-Smith PJ, Pradhan GN, Hashimi H, Eng JB, Mearns AJ (1988) Continuous intercostal nerve block for pain relief after thoracotomy. Ann Thorac Surg 46:425–426. https://doi.org/10.1016/s0003-4975(10)64657-7
15. Berrisford RG, Sabanathan SS (1990) Direct access to the paravertebral space at thoracotomy [Letter]. Ann Thorac Surg 49(5):854. https://doi.org/10.1016/0003-4975(90)90058-e
16. Deebis A, Abdel Sadek H (2001) Efficacy of extrapleural intercostal nerve block with continuous infusion of lidocaine on post-thoracotomy pain and pulmonary mechanics. Zagazig Med Assoc J 7(4):326–334
17. Maxwell C, Nicoara A (2014) New developments in the treatment of acute pain after thoracic surgery. Curr Opin Anaesthesiol 27(1):6–11. https://doi.org/10.1097/aco.0000000000000029
18. Elia N, Lysakoski C, Tramer MR (2005) Does multimodal analgesia with acetaminophen, nonsteroidal antiinflammatory drugs, or selective cyclooxygenase-2 inhibitors and patient-controlled analgesia morphine offer advantages over morphine alone? Meta-analyses of randomized trials. Anesthesiology 103:1296–1304. https://doi.org/10.1097/00000542-200512000-00025
19. Katayama T, Hirai S, Kobayashi R, Hamaishi M, Okada T, Mitsui N (2012) Safety of the paravertebral block in patients ineligible for epidural block undergoing pulmonary resection. Gen Thorac Cardiovasc Surg 60:811–814. https://doi.org/10.1007/s11748-012-0149-5
20. Watson DS, Panian S, Kendall V, Maher DP, Peters G (1999) Pain control after thoracotomy: bupivacaine versus lidocaine in continuous extrapleural intercostal nerve blockade. Ann Thorac Surg 67(3):825–528. https://doi.org/10.1016/s0003-4975(99)00086-7
21. Sullivan E, Grannis FW Jr, Ferrell B, Dunst M (1995) Continuous extrapleural intercostal nerve block with continuous infusion of lidocaine after thoracotomy. A descriptive pilot study. Chest 108(6):1718–1723. https://doi.org/10.1378/chest.108.6.1718
22. Sabanathan S, Mearns AJ, Bickford-Smith PJ, Eng J, Berrisford RG, Bibby SR, Majid MR (1990) Efficacy of continuous extrapleural intercostal nerve block on post-thoracotomy pain and pulmonary mechanics. Br J Surg 77:221–225. https://doi.org/10.1002/bjs.1800770229
23. Ghisi D, Fanelli A, Jouguelet-Lacoste J, La Colla L, Auroux AS, Chelly JE (2015) Lidocaine versus ropivacaine for postoperative continuous paravertebral nerve blocks in patients undergoing laparoscopic bowel surgery: a randomized, controlled, double-blinded, pilot study. Local Reg Anesth 8:71–77. https://doi.org/10.2147/LRA.S84476
24. Llevot JMR, Fayad MF, Pacheco MJB, Malo JMC, Gómez SN, Morales JO (2010) Continuous paravertebral block as an analgesic method in thoracotomy. Cir Esp 88(1):30–35. https://doi.org/10.1016/j.ciresp.2010.03.006
25. Marret E, Bazelly B, Taylor G, Lembert N, Deleuze A, Mazoit JX, Bonnet FJ (2005) Paravertebral block with ropivacaine 0.5% versus systemic analgesia for pain relief after thoracotomy. Ann Thorac Surg 79(6):2109–2113. https://doi.org/10.1016/j.athoracsur.2004.07.030
26. Sabanathan S, Eng J, Mearns AJ (1990) Alteration in respiratory mechanics following thoracotomy. JRColl Surg Edinb 35:144–150 PMID: 2203902
27. Borges-Santos E, Genz ICH, Longo AF, Hayahsi D, Goncalves G, Bellinetti LM et al (2012) Pulmonary function, respiratory muscle strength and quality of life in patients submitted to elective thoracotomies. Rev Col Bras Cir 39(1): 004–009. https://doi.org/10.1590/s0100-69912012000100003
28. Roberts GW, Bekker TB, Carlsen HH, Moffatt CH, Slattery PJ, McClure AF (2005) Postoperative nausea and vomiting are strongly influenced by postoperative opioid use in a dose-related manner. Anesth Analg 101:1343–1348. https://doi.org/10.1213/01.ANE.0000180204.64588.EC
29. Baldini G, Bagry H, Aprikian A, Carli F (2009) Postoperative urinary retention, anesthetic and perioperative considerations. Anesthesiology 110:1139–1157. https://doi.org/10.1097/ALN.0b013e31819f7aea
30. Asida SM, Ibrahim A, Youssef IA, Mohamad AK, Abdelrazik AN (2012) Post-thoracotomy pain relief: thoracic paravertebral block compared with systemic opioids. Egypt J Anaesth 28:55–60. https://doi.org/10.1016/j.egja.2011.10.004

A rare chest X-ray sign in the diagnosis of an intracardiac bullet

Mohamed Osman[1*], Reham Khalil[2], Ahmed Hany Abdalla[3], Azza Katta[4], Samer Nashef[5] and Sameh Elameen[1]

Abstract

Background: Gunshot injuries to the heart are often seen in cardiac surgical practice. Victims are usually investigated with various types of imaging modalities, including simple chest X-ray (CXR) which is a primary imaging modality that can easily locate a bullet and is useful in monitoring before surgical intervention as bullets may migrate.

Case presentation: A 32-year-old man was admitted as an emergency in a primary hospital after being injured by a gunshot to the chest. The bullet entry was over the back of the left shoulder with no exit point seen. The chest X-ray showed left pleural effusion and a retained intrathoracic bullet. A chest drain was inserted and drained 2200 ml of blood. Computed tomography (CT) scan showed an intracardiac bullet associated with left lower lobe contusion and left-sided hemothorax. He was urgently transferred to theater for exploration via left thoracotomy. The bullet could not be found so the inlet point in the left ventricle was sutured. After stabilizing the patient, he was referred to a specialized cardiac center for further management.

The patient arrived at our center 2 days after the injury, fully conscious and hemodynamically stable. On arrival, chest X-rays were obtained to rule out possible migration of the bullet and revealed that the retained bullet was still within the cardiac silhouette. The X-ray appearance of the bullet showed a characteristically double contour, strongly suggesting that the bullet had lodged in the heart muscle and was moving with each heartbeat.

The patient was transferred to the theater for median sternotomy. The aorta, superior vena cava, and inferior vena cava were cannulated, and cardiopulmonary bypass was initiated. The aorta was cross-clamped and the cardioplegia was given. Palpation of the still heart readily identified the bullet within the interventricular septum. The left ventricle was opened 1 cm from the left anterior descending artery just on top of the bullet. The bullet was successfully retrieved. The bullet was transfixing the septum causing a small ventricular septal defect which was closed using a Teflon patch and the ventricle was repaired.

Conclusion: The double contour appearance of the bullet indicates that the bullet is moving and strongly suggests an intramyocardial position.

Background

Gunshot injuries to the heart are often seen in cardiac surgical practice. In 2009, the World Health Organization reported 1217 cases of assault by guns and rifles in Egypt [1]. Victims are usually investigated with various types of imaging modalities, including simple chest X-ray (CXR). We report a rare CXR sign with a high diagnostic value in a case of an intracardiac bullet. This sign was described earlier by Demetrios and Jeffrey in 2000 [2].

Case presentation

A 32-year-old man was admitted as an emergency in a primary hospital after being accidentally injured by a gunshot to the chest from a distance. The bullet entry wound was over the back of the left shoulder with no exit point seen (Fig. 1a). CXR showed left pleural effusion and a retained intrathoracic bullet. A chest drain was inserted and drained 2200 ml of blood. The patient

* Correspondence: m.a.othman@gmail.com
[1]Cardiac Surgery Department, National Heart Institute, Cairo, Egypt
Full list of author information is available at the end of the article

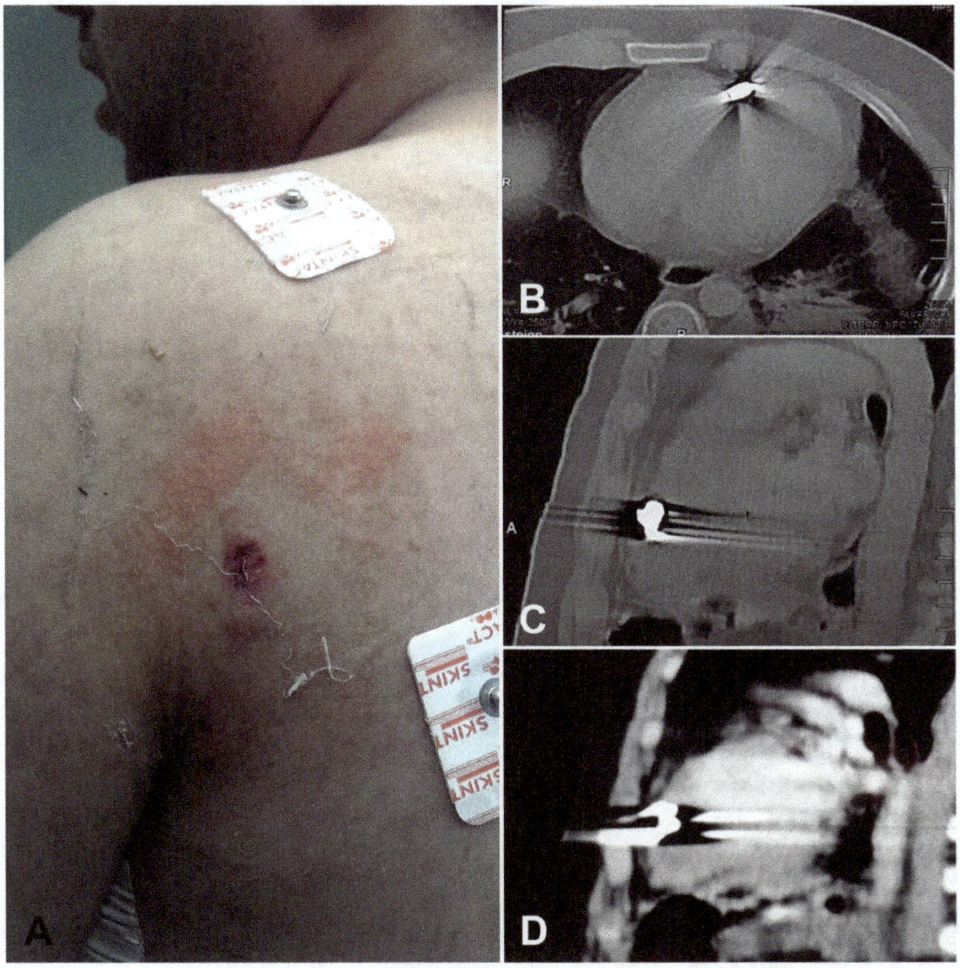

Fig. 1 a The bullet inlet at the left shoulder. **b–d** CT scan cuts show the bullet within the heart

received two units of blood and 3000 ml of crystalloids as resuscitative measures. Computed tomography (CT) scan showed an intracardiac bullet associated with left lower lobe contusion and left-sided hemothorax (Fig. 1b–d). He was urgently transferred to the operating room (OR) for exploration via left thoracotomy as he continued to bleed through chest drain. The aim of the exploration was to repair possible tear in the lung or the ventricle. There was minimal pericardial collection, the bullet could not be found so the inlet point in the left ventricle was sutured using a 4-0 Prolene. After stabilizing the patient, he was referred to a specialized cardiac center for further management.

The patient arrived at our center 2 days after the injury, fully conscious, well oriented, and hemodynamically stable with fair vital signs. On arrival, antero-posterior and lateral chest X-rays were obtained to rule out possible migration of the bullet and revealed that the retained bullet was still within the cardiac silhouette. The X-ray appearance of the bullet showed a characteristically double contour (Fig. 2a–c), strongly suggesting that the bullet had lodged in the heart muscle and was moving with each heartbeat, rather than mobile within the cardiac chambers as it had the same location in two sets of CXRs 2 days apart. Electrocardiography excluded ischemic changes and echocardiogram excluded septal defects or valve disruption; it also suggested the presence of the bullet in within the septum.

The patient was transferred to the theater for median sternotomy. The aorta, superior vena cava, and inferior vena cava were cannulated, and cardiopulmonary bypass was initiated. The aorta was cross-clamped and the heart arrested with cold crystalloid cardioplegia. This was done to minimize the chance of bullet embolization before manipulating the heart. The bullet inlet into the ventricle was inspected (lateral wall) (Fig. 3a), and palpation of the still heart readily identified the bullet within the interventricular septum. In the hope of reducing tissue damage, unsuccessful attempts were made to reach the bullet via both atria. Finally, the left ventricle was opened 1 cm from the left anterior descending artery midway between the apex and outflow tract just on top of the bullet (Fig. 3b). The bullet (9-mm ka pistol) was successfully retrieved (Fig. 3c–e). The bullet was

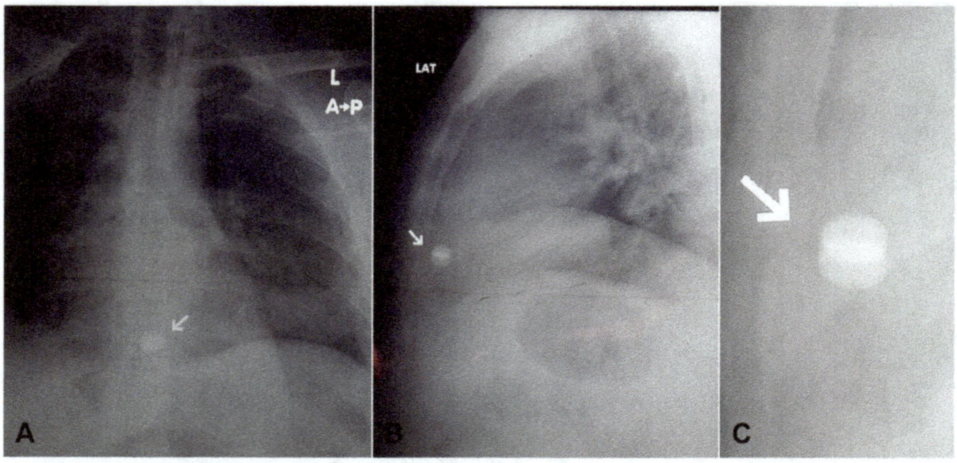

Fig. 2 a Antero-posterior CXR showing the bullet within the cardiac silhouette. **b**, **c** Lateral CXR showing the characteristic double contour of the bullet

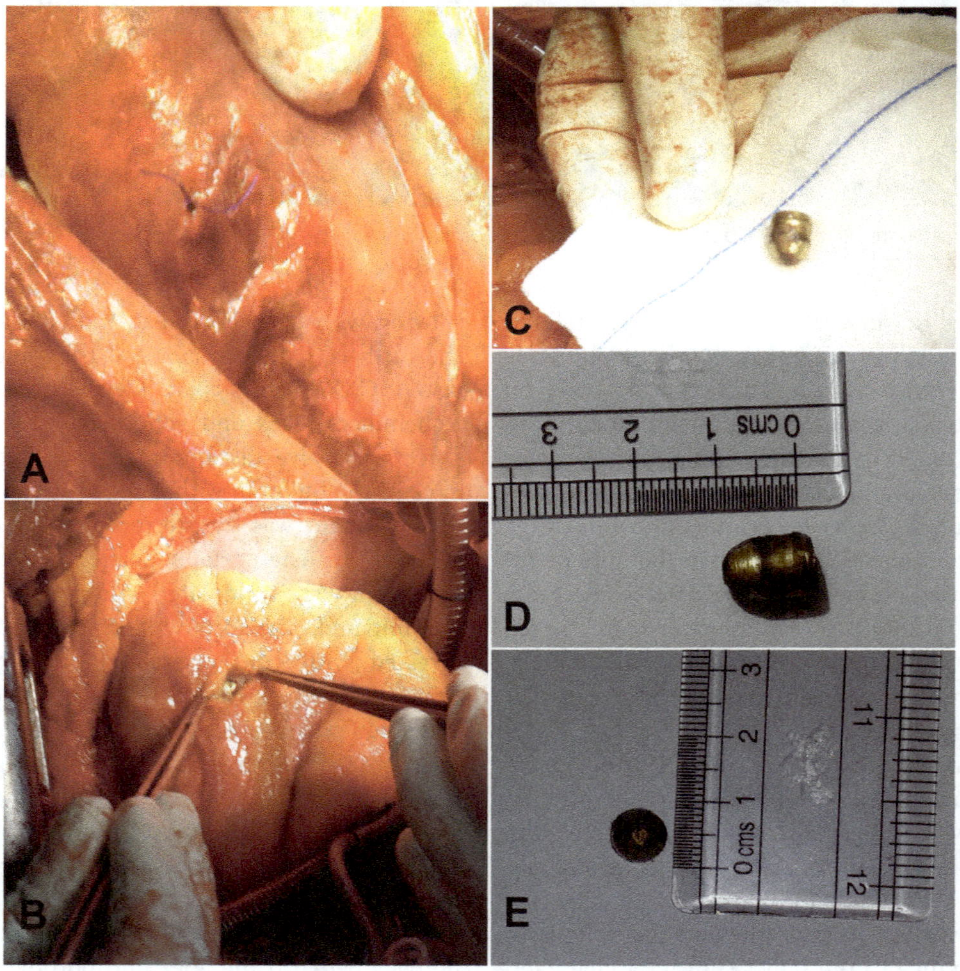

Fig. 3 a The bullet inlet point to the ventricle as seen during second exploration. **b** The bullet within the ventricle after ventriculotomy. **c–e** The bullet after extraction

transfixing the septum causing a small ventricular septal defect (VSD) which was occluded by the bullet itself. The VSD was closed using a Teflon patch and the ventricle was repaired. The patient was smoothly weaned from bypass after an ischemic time of 25 min and a bypass time of 45 min and made an uneventful recovery.

Discussion

The mortality of transmediastinal gunshot injuries is between 40 and 80% [3, 4]. Management depends on the stability of the patients and the time of presentation.

As a missile traverses the body, it causes injury by transferring some or all of its available energy, and this is manifested by lacerating and crushing tissues in its path and, in some cases, injury remote from the missile path. The resulting damage depends on the velocity (KE = ½ MV^2), injured organs, and the efficiency of first aid. KE = ½ M ($V1^2$ – $V2^2$), where KE is the available energy, M is the mass, and V1and V2 are the velocities at entry and at exit, respectively.

In general, bullets fired from handguns are propelled at a low velocity, have low available energy (100–500 J), and result in low-energy transfer wounds. Jonathan et al. recommended that exploration with treatment of the cardiac injury is warranted in the patient who presents with hemorrhage, great vessel injury, or tamponade. Missiles with low-risk characteristics (immobile right-sided, smooth, small [< 5 mm], or completely intramyocardial) that demonstrate no complications on initial and serial imaging may be managed non-operatively [5].

Patients with chest gunshot wounds should be investigated by different imaging modalities including CXR, CT scan, fluoroscopy, C-arm, and echocardiogram. The latter is important to exclude tamponade, VSD, and valve injury.

CXR is a simple primary imaging modality that can easily locate a bullet and is useful in monitoring before surgical intervention as bullets may migrate. The clue to diagnosis in this case was the double contour for the bullet on CXR, suggesting the bullet is intramyocardial, moving with each heartbeat during X-ray exposure. We report our case with this characteristic sign to draw attention to this sign in the diagnosis and management of bullet injuries. This feature was previously described by Demetrios and colleagues [2].

Fluoroscopy is a good tool to localize the bullet and to show its movement within the heart; however, it was not used in our case.

CT scan is particularly useful for delineating the trajectory of a bullet and detection of extra-cardiac associated injuries, thus directing subsequent examinations and treatment plan [6]. Additionally, CT angiography can be useful for the early diagnosis of vascular injuries of the great vessels and coronary arteries [3]. New technology as ECG-gated CT imaging has improved image quality and thus the diagnostic confidence in the preoperative localization of metallic foreign bodies in relatively rapid heart rates [6, 7].

We chose median sternotomy and the use of cardiopulmonary bypass (CPB) as we knew that the bullet is mostly intracardiac. Sternotomy gives excellent exposure of the heart with the option of using the CPB. We clamped the aorta before manipulating the heart to avoid bullet embolization. To retrieve the bullet, we started with the least invasive approaches first: right then left atrium, before ventriculotomy.

Conclusion

Bullet injuries to the chest should be investigated by recent CXR to confirm the position of the bullet before surgical intervention. The double contour appearance of the bullet indicates that the bullet is moving and strongly suggests an intramyocardial position.

Abbreviations

CT: Computed tomography; CXR: Chest X-ray; OR: Operating room; VSD: Ventricular septal defect; KE: Kinetic energy

Acknowledgments

Not applicable.

Authors' contributions

All authors contributed equally in the case report as follows: MO operated on the patient as the first surgeon and wrote the draft copy of the case report; RH analyzed and reported the CT scan and the chest X-ray; AH anesthetized the case and searched the literature and collected the data to write the case report; AK performed and reported the Echo; SN wrote and revised the manuscript and the discussion; and SA operated in the case and prepared and revised the manuscript. All authors have read and approved the manuscript.

Author details

[1]Cardiac Surgery Department, National Heart Institute, Cairo, Egypt. [2]Radiology Department, Ain Shams University, Cairo, Egypt. [3]Anaesthesia Department, National Heart Institute, Cairo, Egypt. [4]Cardiology Department, National Heart Institute, Cairo, Egypt. [5]Cardiothoracic Surgery Department, Royal Papworth Hospital, Cambridge, UK.

References

1. Injury surveillance: a tool for decision-making: annual injury surveillance report, Egypt, 2009
2. Jeffrey K, Demetrios D (2000) Retained cardiac missile: an unusual case report. J Trauma Injury Infec Crit Care 48(2):312
3. Burack JH, Kandil E, Sawas A et al (2007) Triage and outcome of patients with mediastinal penetrating trauma. Ann Thorac Surg 83(2):377e82
4. Okoye OT, Talving P, Teixeira PG et al (2013) Transmediastinal gunshot wounds in a mature trauma centre: changing perspectives. Injury 44(9): 1198e203
5. Jonathan B, Eric K, Jason M et al (2009) Conservative management of retained cardiac missiles: case report and literature review. J Surg Educ 66(4):228–235
6. Ibirogba S, Nicol AJ, Navsaria PH (2007) Screening helical computed tomographic scanning in haemodynamic stable patients with transmediastinal gunshot wounds. Injury 38(1):48e52
7. Hachulla A-L, Ronot M, Noble S et al (2016) ECG-triggered high-pitch CT for simultaneous assessment of the aorta and coronary arteries. J Cardiovasc Comput Tomogr 10(5):407e13

25

Short-term outcomes of surgical myocardial revascularization on health-related quality of life: a validation of the Arabic MacNew heart disease questionnaire

Mohammad Abdallah[1,2*], Shymaa Mamdouh[3], Abdel-Hady El-Gilany[3], Wael Abdel-Aziz[4], Olfat Farag[3] and Noha ElAdawy[3]

Abstract

Background: Impaired quality of life (QOL) is common in coronary heart disease and is the major indications for coronary artery bypass graft (CABG) operations. This study aims to compare the QOL of patients with coronary heart disease before and after CABG surgery.

Results: A translated Arabic version of the Mac-New health-related QOL questionnaire was used to evaluate QOL improvement in 446 patients who benefited from elective CABG at Nasser Institute for Research and Treatment. There was a statistically significant improvement in physical, emotional, social, and global domains of QOL, as evaluated 3 and 6 months after surgery. Follow-up was 90.4% complete. At 3 months, multiple linear regression has shown that male patients ($\beta = 0.48$, $p \leq 0.001$) and rural residence ($\beta = 0.39$, $p \leq 0.001$) were significant independent predictors of improvement in physical QOL domain. While hypercholesterolemia ($\beta = -0.20, -0.49, -0.37, -0.46$, $p \leq 0.001$), hypertension ($\beta = -0.29, -0.39$, $p \leq 0.001$, $\beta = -0.35$, $-\beta = 0.35$, $p = 0.001$), and smoking ($\beta = -0.79$, $p \leq 0.001$, $\beta = -0.33$, $p = 0.04$, $\beta = -0.69$, $p \leq 0.001$, $\beta = -0.47$, $p = 0.005$) were significant predictors of worsening in physical, emotional, social, and global domains, respectively. At 6 months, low preoperative ejection fraction (EF) ≤ 40% was the strongest predictor of improvement ($\beta = 0.54$, 0.49, 0.44, and 0.52, $p \leq 0.001$) in physical, emotional, social, and global domains of QOL, respectively. But, peripheral vascular disease (PVD) ($\beta = -0.53$, $p = 0.05$, $\beta = -0.81$, $p = 0.005$, $\beta = -0.62$, $p = 0.03$, $\beta = -0.76$, $p = 0.008$) and smoking ($\beta = -0.53$, $p = 0.001$, $\beta = -0.42$, $p = 0.01$, $\beta = -0.42$, $p = 0.01$, $\beta = -0.41$, $p = 0.02$) were significant predictors of worsening in physical, emotional, social, and global domains of QOL, respectively.

Conclusions: CABG surgery improved in all domains of QOL. Further studies are required to evaluate changes in QOL at longer period intervals.

Keywords: Quality of life, Coronary artery disease, Coronary artery bypass graft surgery

* Correspondence: dr.mohamedd84@gmail.com
[1]Department of Cardiothoracic Surgery, National Heart Institute, Cairo, Egypt
[2]Department of Cardiothoracic Surgery, Shebein Elkom Teaching Hospital, Shebein Elkom, Egypt
Full list of author information is available at the end of the article

Background

Coronary heart disease (CHD) has many adverse effects on different aspects of physical, psychological, social, and spiritual health [1]. Coronary artery bypass grafting (CABG) is the treatment of choice for patients with atherosclerotic CHD. The benefits include relief of angina, improvement in the quality of life (QOL), and an increase in life expectancy in high-risk patients [2]. QOL is a multidimensional concept that includes an individual's physical, psychological, and social status; it is a sense of well-being which is due to satisfaction or dissatisfaction with different aspects of life which are important for an individual. Change in patients' QOL is one of the essential outcomes of CABG surgery [3]. The dimensions or subscales yield summary scores that constitute a profile of QOL and is a subjective patients' perception of their health and treatment and is a core concept "patient-reported outcomes" (PROs) of the patient's perspectives in epidemiological, health economics, clinical, and health services research [3]. Consequently, assessing the QOL is one of the debatable topics of recent decades in clinical research [4].

Generic QOL measurements include the Short Form Health Survey (SF-36), Sickness Impact Profile, and Nottingham Health Profile (NHP). The SF-36 and the NHP appear to have better content validity in the field of cardiac surgery because each covers energy/vitality and bodily pain, and appropriate if not essential aspect of cardiac surgery recovery for ischemic heart diseases and procedures. Disease-specific QOL measures include Duke Activity Status Index, MacNew Heart Disease Quality-of-Life Measure, Seattle Angina Questionnaire, Minnesota Living with Heart Failure Questionnaire; Heart-QOL [5]. MacNew Heart Disease QOL questionnaire was the most commonly used in different cardiac patients and was translated and validated into many languages [6].

There is a dearth of knowledge about the effect of CABG surgery on patients QOL in Egypt. The study objectives were to (1) validate a translated Arabic version of the Mac-New health-related quality of life questionnaire; (2) assess changes in QOL after 3 and 6 months of CABG surgery; and (3) identify factors related to QOL changes after CABG.

Methods

Setting and participants

The study followed the STROBE cross-sectional reporting guidelines [7]. This is a descriptive follow-up study on CHD patients who underwent CABG surgery. It was carried out at the Outpatient Clinic of the Cardiac Surgery Unit of Nasser Institute Hospital for Research and Treatment, Cairo, Egypt, during the period from May 2017 to July 2018.

A convenience sample (based on the time frame) of 446 patients underwent elective CABG surgery and fulfilling the legibility criteria during the study period were included. Only 43 patients (9.6%) of patients were dropped out from follow-up at 6 months (11 deaths, 9 wrong mobile and/or address, and 23 did not reply after three calls in three consecutive days).

Legibility criteria

Eligible patients were all adult aged ≥ 18 years diagnosed with ischemic heart disease (IHD) who underwent isolated elective CABG in patients. Patients should be fully conscious and accepting to participate in the study. Excluded patients were those in critical preoperative state, impaired consciousness, patients who were unable to complete the study tools (e.g., hearing impairment), and other concomitant surgeries (e.g., valvular surgery, CABG with valvular surgery, aortic aneurysm surgery).

The patients were interviewed during the study period at 3 months after CABG surgery and followed-up at 6 months postoperatively.

Data collection

Data were collected at 3 months with direct patients' interviews, from medical records and 6 months after surgery through telecommunications of patients via mobile phones to highlight further QOL changes. The Mac New Heart Disease HRQOL questionnaire is a self-administered modification of the original quality of life after myocardial infarction [8]. It comprises 27 items which fall into 3 domains emotional (14 questions), physical (14 questions), and social (13 questions) dimensions. The score of every question was modified to be 3 Likert scale (1 to 3) instead of 7 Likert scales to be easier and understandable in our culture. Three are the best present conditions of QOL and one is the minimum score (the worst present conditions of QOL). The higher score in every domain means higher QOL. Each domain score is calculated as the average of the responses in that domain, and the tool also has a global HRQOL score which calculated as the average overall scored items. The questionnaire was forward translated into the Arabic language by two different translators and back translated to English to ensure linguistic validity. The questionnaire was validated by three experts in public health and two experts in cardiothoracic surgery. The content validity index for relevance and clarity of different items varied from 0.72 to 1.0 (a copy of the study questionnaire is available upon request from the corresponding author).

A pilot study was done on 10 patients (not included in the full-scale study) to test the reliability of the translated Mac-New Heart Disease HRQOL questionnaire. The Cronbach's alphas of emotional, physical, social, and total scale were found to be 0.87, 0.96, 0.92, and 0.96, respectively. The interclass correlation was 0.96. There were no missing items. The ceiling effects of different items ranged from 0 to 20%, while the floor effects varied from 0 to 30% for different items.

Data collection approach

Data were collected 3 months after CABG surgery by direct interviews with patients to include illiterate patients. However, at 6 months was collected by telecommunications as most the patients do not keep in the follow-up.

Ethical consideration

The study proposal was approved by IRB, authors' institution. Patients gave informed consent to participate in the study after assurance of data confidentiality and they have the right to withdraw from the study at any time.

Statistical analysis

The data were collected and analyzed using Statistical Package for Social Sciences (SPSS for Windows program version 22; SPSS Inc., Chicago, Il, USA). Cronbach's alpha was used to test the internal consistency of the construct. The floor effects, ceiling effects, interclass correlation were calculated. The change in QOL was calculated by the difference between score post-surgery and pre-surgical scores for each domain. Kolmogorov-Smirnov one-sample test was used to assess the distribution of quantitative data and found to be non-parametric. The quantitative data were presented as the median (maximum-minimum). Non-parametric tests (Friedman's test and Wilcoxon's sign test) were used whenever appropriate. Scores were long transformed through two steps: first QOL scores were ranked and then transformed through inverse distribution function. Normal (IDF. Normal) to have normalized ones [9]. Correlation coefficients were calculated using the parametric Pearson rank correlation coefficient. Significant correlations were entered into a linear regression model to evaluate the contribution of factors found to be significant in bivariate analysis in predicting the normalized QOL difference scores after 3 and 6 months of CABG surgery. $P \leq 0.05$ was considered statistically significant.

Results

Table 1 shows statistically significant improvement in all domains of QOL after 3 and 6 months of CABG surgery ($p \leq 0.001$). More improvement was noticed in the physical and social domains than the emotional domain 6 months after CABG surgery (median scores were 3.0 and 3.0 vs. 2.93, respectively).

Multiple linear regression after 3 months of CABG surgery shows that male sex ($p \leq 0.001$) and rural residence ($p \leq 0.001$) are significant independent predictors of physical QOL improvement. Education was a significant independent predictor for QOL improvement in emotional ($p = 0.005$), social domain ($p = 0.03$), and global domain ($p \leq 0.001$), respectively. Hypercholesterolemia, hypertension, smoking, and gastrointestinal disease ($p \leq 0.001$) were independent significant predictors for QOL worsening in all domains of QOL ($p \leq 0.001$). While renal disease ($p = 0.02$) and cerebrovascular disease ($p = 0.03$) were significant independent predictors of worsening social domain of QOL (Table 2).

Multiple linear regression after 6 months of CABG surgery shows that low EF ≤ 40% ($p \leq 0.001$) was a significant independent predictor of higher median difference scores of all QOL domains. However, peripheral vascular disease (PVD) was a significant independent predictor of lower median difference scores of all domains of QOL ($p \leq 0.05$) (Table 3).

Discussion

The Arabic version of the MacNew heart disease questionnaire is both valid and reliable. The overall Cronbach's alpha is 0.96. This is comparable to its version in other languages, e.g., 0.94 for French version [10], 0.90 to 0.94 for Danish, Norwegian, and Swedish versions, respectively [11], 0.93 for Korean version [12], and 0.95%

Table 1 Comparison of scores of domains of quality of life before and after CABG

Domain	QOL before CABG (446) median (minimum-maximum)	QOL after 3 month of CABG (446) median (minimum-maximum)	QOL after 6 month of CABG (403) Median (minimum-maximum)	Significance (Friedman's test)
Physical	1.64 (1.00-2.07)^{A,B}	2.93 (1.00-3.00)^{A,C}	3.00 (2.29-3.00)^{B,C}	$\chi^2 = 712.35, p \leq 0.001$
Emotional	1.71 (1.00-2.07)^{A,B}	2.79 (1.00-3.00)^{A,C}	2.93 (2.00-3.00)^{B,C}	$\chi^2 = 676.09, p \leq 0.001$
Social	1.77 (1.00-2.15)^{A,B}	3.00 (1.00-3.00)^{A,C}	3.00 (2.00-3.00)^{B,C}	$\chi^2 = 724.71, p \leq 0.001$
Global	1.74 (1.00-2.15)^{A,B}	2.81 (1.00-3.00)^{A,C}	2.96 (2.15-3.00)^{B,C}	$\chi^2 = 676.12, p \leq 0.001$

^{A,B,C}Significant difference between the corresponding times by Wilcoxon's test for paired comparison

Table 2 Multiple linear regression analysis of independent predictors of physical, emotional, social, and global QOL-normalized difference score after 3 months of CABG surgery

Predictors	Physical domain difference score		Emotional domain difference score		Social domain difference score		Global domain difference score	
	B	*p*	*B*	*p*	*B*	*p*	*B*	*p*
Gender	0.48	≤ 0.001	0.50	≤ 0.001	0.43	≤ 0.001	0.49	≤ 0.001
Age			0.01	0.04				
Residence	0.39	≤ 0.001	0.30	0.001	0.37	≤ 0.001	0.36	≤ 0.001
Education			0.36	0.005	0.29	0.02	0.02	0.03
Diabetes	−0.20	0.05						
Dyspnea grade					0.51	0.003		
Hypercholestermia	−0.20	≤ 0.001	−0.49	≤ 0.001	−0.37	≤ 0.001	−0.46	≤ 0.001
Hypertension	−0.29	≤ 0.001	−0.39	≤ 0.001	−0.35	≤ 0.001	−0.35	0.001
Smoking	−0.79	≤ 0.001	−0.33	0.04	−0.69	≤ 0.001	−0.47	0.005
Gastrointestinal disease	−0.44	0.003	−0.63	≤ 0.001	−0.51	0.001	−0.59	≤ 0.001
Renal disease	−0.66	0.03			−0.66	0.02		
Cerebrovascular disease	−0.63	0.006			−0.50	0.03	−0.54	0.02
Constant	0.145		0.759		0.121		0.287	
R^2	0.23		0.24		0.22		0.22	
F	7.406		8.063		7.274		7.157	
P	≤ 0.001		≤ 0.001		≤ 0.001		≤ 0.001	

Coding of variables included in the model
0 was given for female, urban residence, low education, no diabetes, no hypercholestermia, no smoking, no hypertension, no gastrointestinal disease, no renal disease, no cerebrovascular disease, and low dyspnea grade (NYHA1- NYHA 2)
1 was given for male, rural residence, high education, diabetes hypercholestermia, hypertension, renal disease, gastrointestinal disease, smoking, high dyspnea grade (NYHA3-NYHA4)

Table 3 Multiple linear regression analysis of follow-up independent predictors of physical, emotional, social, and global QOL-normalized difference score after 6 months of CABG surgery

Predictors	Physical domain difference score		Emotional domain difference score		Social domain difference score		Global domain difference score	
	B	*p*	*B*	*p*	*B*	*p*	*B*	*p*
Preoperative EF	0.54	≤ 0.001	0.49	≤ 0.001	0.44	≤ 0.001	0.52	≤ 0.001
Occupation	0.31	0.02			0.32	0.02	0.29	0.02
Diabetes	−0.25	0.03					−0.24	0.03
Hypertension	−0.28	0.009	−0.33	0.004	−0.31	0.005	−0.31	0.006
Smoking	−0.53	0.001	−0.42	0.01	−0.42	0.01	−0.41	0.02
Peripheral vascular disease (PVD)	−0.53	0.05	−0.81	0.005	−0.62	0.03	−0.76	0.008
Gastrointestinal disease			−0.39	0.02				
Angina grade							0.20	0.02
Constant	0.445		0.179		0.123		0.316	
R^2	0.21		0.19		0.17		0.20	
F	6.094		5.461		4.694		5.676	
P	≤ 0.001		≤ 0.001		≤ 0.001		≤ 0.001	

Coding of variables included in the model:
0 was given for not working, no PVD, no smoking, no diabetes, no gastrointestinal disease, low angina class (CCS1-CCS2), and EF ≥ 40%
1 was given for working, PVD, smoking, diabetes, presence of gastrointestinal disease, high angina class (CCS3-CCS4), and EF < 40%

for German version [13]. But much higher than 0.80 of the Turkish version [14].

The present study found a statistically significant improvement in all domains of QOL after 3 and 6 months of CABG. Physical and social domains exhibited the greatest improvement with the smallest improvement in the emotional one after 6 months of surgery. This is in agreement with a previous study reported in Greece [15]. This may be due to CABG has a greater influence on physical functioning as well as a decrease of symptoms, and consequently, a better living with this condition. But in contrast, a study conducted in Holland showed a decline in HRQOL 6 months after CABG surgery [16]. This could be explained by the effect of anxiety and depression in CABG patients.

The current finding indicated that male patients were one of the significant predictors of all domains of QOL post 3 months of surgery. The reason for that result is that the majority of female patients were older age, not working, had multiple diseased vessels, lower preoperative scores in all domains of QOL, and had multiple comorbidities. This is in line with previous findings reported in Pakistan and Belgrade [17, 18]. But, two Iranian studies found no significant association between sex and change in QOL scores [19, 20]. Also, the rural residence was an independent predictor of all domains of QOL post 3 months of surgery. Similarly, a previous study in France found the same results [21]. This could be attributed to more physical activity, less life stress, or a better lifestyle of rural patients compared to urban inhabitants.

The present study showed that education and occupation were one of the independent predictors for higher social QOL domains after 3 and 6 months of surgery, respectively. Such results agree with a previous study conducted in France [21]. This might be explained by that educated persons maintain their lifestyle, health-related behavior, and consider the essence of their illness and surgery complications. Also, strong financial security may help patients to survive more easily after surgery and get better QOL by avoiding negative feelings and self-criticism that their physical, mental, and social health could be seriously impacted. However, an Iranian study [22] contradicts such results.

The present study found that severe angina (CCS3-CCS4) after 6 months of surgery was one of the independent predictors of improving QOL in the global domain. That result was consistent with a Belgrade study [18]. While a French study [23] disagreed with that finding.

The current study found high-grade dyspnea class (NYHA3-NYHA4) after 3 months of surgery was one of the independent predictors of increasing QOL in the social domain. This is in line with research conducted in Serbia [24]. This may be clarified by the fact that CABG has a stronger effect on dyspnea relief. Also, the current study showed that hypercholesterolemia and hypertension were significant predictors of QOL worsening after 3 months of CABGs in all domains of QOL. This agrees with a study conducted in Serbia [24] and the USA [25]. This could be explained that hypertensive patients might be controlled with drugs that could influence QOL after surgery and complicated by other chronic diseases.

The current study showed that diabetes was one of the significant independent predictors of QOL worsening in the physical domain after 6 months of surgery. This is concordant with a study reported in France [21]. On the other hand, a previous study in Iran [22] found higher QOL in diabetic patients than non-diabetic ones.

The present study showed that smoking was one of the significant predictors of QOL worsening in all domains after 3 and 6 months of surgery. This is in harmony with previous studies in the UK [26] and the USA [25]. It could be explained that smoking is potentially modifiable and related to a broad spectrum of an undesirable outcomes.

The present study found that peripheral vascular disease (PVD) significantly impaired QOL after 6 months of surgery in all domains of QOL. This finding agrees with a previous study in the USA [25].

The present finding showed that cerebrovascular disease and renal disease were one of the significant predictors of QOL worsening in the social domain of QOL after 3 months of surgery. Similarly, previous studies reported in the USA [25, 27], respectively.

The present study indicated that patients with gastric problems were one of the independent predictors of all domains of QOL after 3 months of surgery and only emotional domain after 6 months of surgery. This agrees with a previous study in the UK [28].

The current study showed a significantly higher improvement in all QOL domains after 6 months of surgery in patients with low EF < 40%. This is consistent with a study conducted in Finland [29]. This could be explained that patients regained their QOL, and relieved from their physical, emotional, and social difficulties due to enhanced function of the left ventricle. On the other hand, previous researches in the USA [25] and Belgrade [18] disagreed with these results.

The present study found that increasing age was a significant independent predictor of improving emotional difference QOL domain after 3 months of surgery. This is similar to studies conducted in the USA [25] and Finland [29]. The possible explanation is that old patients suffer from severe physical, emotional, and social constraints before surgery, and CABG surgery could be performed with tolerable morbidity, mortality, and with a significant enhancement in functional, emotional, and social status of elderly.

Study limitations and strengths

Although this study is a prospective single-center one and its results cannot be generalized at the national level, it contains patients from a high-volume referral cardiac center, which is a major advantage. The study is one of the very few QOL studies reported in Egypt and the Arab world in the cardiac surgery spectrum. It covers a research gap that an important limitation in the current use of HRQOL tools in cardiac surgery and it has a prospective nature. The patients were followed up for 6 months postoperatively by telecommunications using mobile phones, which are the major advantage. This study is the first Arabic and Egyptian study to construct and validate the MacNew heart disease questionnaire in its newly translated Arabic form. Also, it will change the practice in cardiac surgery. This study will give a background to the cardiac surgeons on how to choose their patients in a good way before the operation, including this will reflect on reducing mortality and morbidity rates and increasing focus on QOL.

Conclusion

CABG surgery has a positive effect on QOL with significant improvement in all domains of QOL after surgery, especially the physical and social scores. Male sex, rural residence hypercholesterolemia, and hypertension are significant independent predictors of QOL in all domains of QOL 3 months after surgery. Low EF < 40% is the strongest predictor of QOL improvement in all domains after 6 months of surgery.

The Arabic version of the MacNew questionnaire is recommended for assessing health-related quality of life in Arabic-speaking patients with IHD or patients undergoing CABG. Nationwide longitudinal studies are needed to assess changes in QOL after CABG over longer intervals.

Supplementary information

Additional file 1. Arabic version of McNew Questionaire

Additional file 2. Modified MacNew QLMI (Valenti etal., 1996)

Abbreviations

CABG: Coronary artery bypass graft surgery; CHD: Coronary heart disease; COP: Cardiac output; ECHO: Echocardiography; EF: Ejection fraction; HRQOL: Health-related quality of life; ICU: Intensive care unit; IDF. Normal: Inverse distribution function. Normal.; IHD: Ischemic heart disease; IRB: Institutional Research Board; LITA: Left internal thoracic artery; LVED D: Left ventricular end diastolic diameter; LVESD: Left ventricular end systolic diameter; NYHA: New York Heart Association; PVD: Peripheral vascular disease; PROs: Patient-reported outcomes; QOL: Quality of life; SPSS: Statistical package of social sciences; SVG: Saphenous vein graft; USA: Unites States of America

Acknowledgements

We would like to thank the patients, staff members of the Institute for their cooperation and the director of the Institute for accepting this work.

Authors' contributions

MA conducted the literature search, performed the data collection and interpretation of the data, and drafted the manuscript. WA, AG, and OF supervised the study and conducted the review of data, involved in the study design, analyzed and interpreted the data, and drafted the manuscript. SM designed the study, analyzed and interpreted the data, and drafted the manuscript. NA was one of the supervisors of the research. All authors have read and approved the final manuscript.

Author details

[1]Department of Cardiothoracic Surgery, National Heart Institute, Cairo, Egypt. [2]Department of Cardiothoracic Surgery, Shebein Elkom Teaching Hospital, Shebein Elkom, Egypt. [3]Department of Public Health and Preventive Medicine, Faculty of Medicine, Mansoura University, Mansoura, Egypt. [4]Department of Cardiothoracic Surgery, Faculty of Medicine, Mansoura University, Mansoura, Egypt.

References

1. Barzin M, Mirmiran P, Afghan M, Azizi F (2011) Distribution of 10-year risk for coronary heart disease and eligibility for therapeutic approaches among Tehranian adults. Public Health 125(6):338–344
2. Hillis LD, Smith PK, Anderson JL, Bittl JA, Bridges CR, Byrne JG et al (2011) 2011 ACCF/AHA guideline for coronary artery bypass graft surgery: a report of the American College of Cardiology Foundation/American Heart Association task force on practice guidelines developed in collaboration with the American Association for Thoracic Surgery, Society of Cardiovascular Anesthesiologists, and Society of Thoracic Surgeons. J Am Coll Cardiol 58(24):e123–e210
3. Haraldstad K, Wahl A, Anden R, Andersen JR, Andersen MH, Beisland E et al (2019) A systematic review of quality of life research in medicine and health sciences. Qual Life Res 28:2641–2650
4. Higginson IJ, Carr AJ (2001) Measuring quality of life: using quality of life measures in the clinical setting. BMJ 322(7297):1297–1300
5. Tully PJ (2013) Quality-of-life measures for cardiac surgery practice and research: a review and primer. J Extra Corpor Technol 45(1):8–15
6. Hofer S, Saleem A, Stone J, Thomas R, Tulloch H, Oldridge N (2012) The MacNew heart disease health-related quality of life questionnaire in patients with angina and patients with ischemic heart failure. Value Health 15:143–150
7. Von Elm E, Altman DG, Egger M, Pocock SJ, Gøtzsche PC, Vandenbroucke JP et al (2014) The strengthening the reporting of observational studies in epidemiology (STROBE) statement: guidelines for reporting observational studies. Inter J Surg 12(12):1495–1499
8. Valenti L, Lim L, Heller RF, Knapp J (1996) An improved questionnaire for assessing quality of life after acute myocardial infarction. Quality of Life Res 5(1):151–161
9. Templeton GF (2011) A two-step approach for transforming continuous variables to normal: implications and recommendations for IS research. Commun Assoc Inf Syst 28(1):4. https://aisel.aisnet.org/cais/vol28/iss1/4. https://doi.org/10.17705/1CAIS.02804
10. Pavya B, Iliou M, Höferc S, Vergès-Patois B, Coronee S, Aeberhard P et al (2015) Validation of the French version of the MacNew heart disease health-related quality of life questionnaire. Arch Cardiovasc Dis 108:107–117
11. Alphin S, Hofer S, Perk J, Slørdahl S, Zwisler AO, Oldridge N (2015) The MacNew heart disease health-related quality of life questionnaire: a Scandinavian validation study. Soc Indic Res 122:519–537
12. Kang K, Gholizadeh L, Inglis SC, Han HR (2019) Validation of the Korean version of the MacNew heart disease health-related quality of life questionnaire. J Nurs Res 27(2):e11. https://doi.org/10.1097/jnr.0000000000000274

13. Gramm L, Farin E, Jaeckel WH (2012) Psychometric properties of the German version of the MacNew heart disease health-related quality of life questionnaire. Health Qual Life Outcomes 10:83
14. Daskapan A, Höfer S, Oldridge N, Alkan N, Muderrisoglu H, Tuzun EH (2008) The validity and reliability of the Turkish version of the MacNew heart disease questionnaire in patients with angina. J Eval Clin Pract 14:209–213
15. Merkouris A, Apostolakis E, Pistolas D, Papagiannaki V, Diakomopoulou E, Patiraki E (2009) Quality of life after coronary artery bypass graft surgery in the elderly. Eur J Cardiovasc Nurs 8(1):74–81
16. Middel B, El Baz N, Pedersen SS, van Dijk JP, Wynia K, Reijneveld SA (2014) Decline in health-related quality of life 6 months after coronary artery bypass graft surgery: the influence of anxiety, depression, and personality traits. J Cardiovasc Nurs 29(6):544–554
17. Barolia R, Ali F, Jaffar S, Sami S (2012) Coronary artery bypass grafting: quality of life of patients in Karachi. British J Nursing 21(6):349–355
18. Peric V, Stolic R, Jovanovic A, Grbic R, Lazic B, Sovtic S, Borzanovic M (2017) Predictors of quality of life improvement after 2 years of coronary artery bypass surgery. Ann Thorac Cardiovasc Surg 23(5):233–238
19. Rankin S (1990) Differences in recovery from cardiac surgery: a profile of male and female patients. Heart Lung 19:481–448
20. King KM, Collins-Nakai RL (1998) Short term recovery from cardiac surgery in women: suggestions for practice. Can J Cardiol 14:1367–1371
21. Perrotti A, Ecarnot F, Monaco F, Dorigo E, Monteleone P, Besch G et al (2019) Quality of life 10 years after cardiac surgery in adults: a long-term follow-up study. Health Qual Life Outcomes 17(1):88
22. Najafi M, Sheikhvatan M, Montazeri A (2009) Quality of life-associated factors among patients undergoing coronary artery bypass surgery as measured using the WHOQOL-BREF. Cardiovasc J Africa 20(5):284
23. Falcoz PE, Chocron S, Stoica L, Kaili D, Puyraveau M, Mercier M et al (2003) Open heart surgery: one-year self-assessment of quality of life and functional outcome. Ann Thorac Surg 76(5):1598–1604
24. Peric V, Borzanovic M, Stolic R, Jovanovic A, Sovtic S, Dimkovic S et al (2008) Predictors of worsening of patients' quality of life six months after coronary artery bypass surgery. J Card Surg 23(6):648–654
25. Rumsfeld JS, Ho PM, Magid DJ, McCarthy M Jr, Shroyer ALW, MaWhinney S et al (2004) Predictors of health-related quality of life after coronary artery bypass surgery. Ann Thorac Surg 77(5):1508–1513
26. Lindsay GM, Hanlon P, Smith LN, Wheatley DJ (2000) Assessment of changes in general health status using the short-form 36 questionnaire 1 year following coronary artery bypass grafting. Eur J Cardio Thoracic Surg 18(5):557–564
27. Parikh CR, Coca SG, Smith GL, Vaccarino V, Krumholz HM (2006) Impact of chronic kidney disease on health-related quality-of-life improvement after coronary artery bypass surgery. Arch Internal Med 166(18):2014–2019
28. Al-Ruzzeh S, Athanasiou T, Mangoush O, Wray J, Modine T, George S et al (2005) Predictors of poor mid-term health related quality of life after primary isolated coronary artery bypass grafting surgery. Heart 91(12):1557–1562
29. Järvinen O, Saarinen T, Julkunen J, Huhtala H, Tarkka MR (2003) Changes in health-related quality of life and functional capacity following coronary artery bypass graft surgery. Eur J Cardio Thorac Surg 24(5):750–756

26

Primary cardiac tumors: a spectrum of pathologies and scenarios

Mohammed Sanad[1,2,3*], Sherif Arafa[4], Mohammed Adel Hegazy[5] and Wael Abdel Aziz Abdel Hamid[1,2]

Abstract

Background: Cardiac tumors are rare, and their diagnosis is challenging. The level of evidence for the management of cardiac tumors came from case reports or small case series. We aim to present our multicenter experience in the diagnosis and management of cardiac tumors.

Results: We performed a prospective study, including 82 cases of cardiac tumors encountered at three centers in 5 years. The mean age was 62 ± 5.8 years old (range 2 months–74 years), and 91.4% were females constituted. The median EuroSCORE II was 4.27%. All cases underwent radical excision of the tumor. Five cases underwent additional mitral valve replacement and one case underwent coronary bypass grafting. Pathological diagnoses were left atrial myxomas ($n = 65$, 79.3%), right atrial myxomas ($n = 5$, 6.1%), bi-atrial myxomas ($n = 2$, 2.4%), right ventricular outflow tract myxoma ($n = 1$, 1.2%), myxosarcoma ($n = 1$, 1.2%), thymoma ($n = 1$, 1.2%), recurrent hemangioendothelioma ($n = 1$, 1.2%), round cell tumor ($n = 1$, 1.2%), cardiac lymphoma ($n = 1$, 1.2%), rhabdomyomas ($n = 2$, 2.4%), and renal cell carcinomas ($n = 2$, 2.4%). Two patients (2.4%) had re-exploration for bleeding. One patient (1.2%) with right atrial thymoma experienced a severe vasoplegia with unstable hemodynamics. Two patients had operative mortality (2.4%), one with recurrent cardiac hemangioendothelioma. During 1-year follow-up, one patient (1.2%) died because of metastatic myosarcoma. Recurrence was reported in 2 patients (2.4%).

Conclusions: The clinical scenario of cardiac tumors depends mainly on tumor location and size rather than the histopathology. Surgical resection is feasible in benign tumors while very challenging in malignant tumors.

Keywords: Cardiac tumor, Malignancy, Cardiac lesion, Survival

Background

Cardiac tumors are rare, with an incidence of less than 0.33% [1]. They are categorized as primary and secondary, depending on the origin of the tumors. Primary cardiac tumors present 5% of all cardiac tumors and originate primarily from the heart. In contrast, secondary cardiac tumors are the most common cardiac tumors, and they present metastasis to the heart from other organs [1].

Around 75% of primary tumors are benign, and 75% of these are atrial myxomas [1, 2].

Myxomas commonly originate from the left atrium, and ventricular myxomas were rarely reported. Additionally, infantile myxoma was not frequently reported in the literature [3].

Surgical excision is usually curative in primary cardiac tumors, and it is the main treatment modality. In secondary tumors, surgery has a palliative role in symptoms relief [2, 3].

Currently, the level of evidence for the management of cardiac tumors is derived from case reports or small case series, and specific tumors were rarely presented in the literature. This study aims to review our multicenter experience in the diagnosis and management of primary cardiac tumors.

* Correspondence: mohamedsanad2008@yahoo.com; mams@mans.edu.eg
[1]Department of Cardiothoracic Surgery, Faculty of Medicine, Mansoura University, Mansoura, Dakahlia, Egypt
[2]Department of Cardiothoracic Surgery, Nasser Institute for Research and Treatment, Egypt Ministry of Health and Population, Cairo, Egypt
Full list of author information is available at the end of the article

Methods

Study design and setting

This prospective multicentric cohort study included a total of 82 consecutive patients operated for primary cardiac tumors at three referral centers from 2013 to 2018. All cases had a 1-year follow-up.

Inclusion and exclusion criteria

All cases with primary cardiac tumors with no evidence of metastasis at the different age groups were included in our study. Cases with secondary cardiac tumors were excluded.

One hundred seven patients with cardiac tumors were examined for eligibility criteria. We excluded 25 patients with secondary cardiac tumors, and a total of 82 eligible patients diagnosed with primary cardiac tumors were enrolled.

Ethical considerations

We conducted the study according to the declaration of Helsinki. Approvals of the Institutional Research Boards were obtained. Informed written consent was obtained from all cases after the explanation of the details and possible complications of the surgical intervention. All patients signed written consent for publishing the medical data without identification.

Surgical workup and approach

All cases were subjected to complete history taking, thorough physical examination, and routine preoperative laboratory investigations. Besides, radiological investigations including chest X-ray and echocardiography (transthoracic and/or transesophageal) were performed to assess the site, size, and tumor extension. In all malignant tumors, a metastatic workup was performed preoperatively.

All cases presenting with cardiac tumors were operated on emergency basis for fear of complications of the intracardiac mass as per policy of our centers.

The cardiac anesthesia team performed full invasive monitoring, and general anesthesia was used in all cases as per standard of care.

Following tailored surgical planning, all cases were operated immediately after diagnosis through a full median sternotomy. Cardiopulmonary bypass was conducted using aortic and bicaval cannulation with moderate hypothermia, and intermittent antegrade cold blood cardioplegia was used in all cases. The incision depends on the location of the tumor, and care was taken to prevent the fragmentation of the masses. Concomitant mitral valve replacement was performed in five cases. Irrigation and suctioning of the atria and ventricles were performed to ensure no residual fragmentations. Following cardiac reconstruction, weaning off bypass was performed, and the surgery was completed as standard.

Postoperative management

Following the operation, the cases were transferred to the cardiac surgery intensive care unit (ICU) under full invasive monitoring, then to the ward unless complications occurred. Early ambulation and chest physiotherapy were encouraged. Pain control was achieved using non-steroidal anti-inflammatory drugs (NSAIDs) and opioids accordingly. Immediate postoperative echocardiography was performed to all patients.

All cases were reviewed for the need for postoperative adjuvant therapy by the multidisciplinary team (MDT). At the regular follow-up visits, cases were assessed clinically and radiologically for the outcome of resection.

Study outcomes

We reported the histological types of the resected specimens and the postoperative morbidity and mortality.

Statistical analysis

The data were tabulated and analyzed using the IBM SPSS software version 22.0 (IBM Inc., Chicago, IL, USA). Qualitative data were described using the number and percent. Quantitative variables were reported as mean and standard deviation (SD).

Results

Demographic data and surgical findings

The mean age was 62 ± 5.8 years old (range 2 months–74 years), and 75 patients were females (91.4%). All cases underwent radical excision of the tumors. Five cases underwent concomitant mitral valve replacement with a hemangioendothelioma, a myxosarcoma, and three myxomas excisions. One case was operated for left atrial myxoma, single-vessel coronary artery bypass grafting, along with mitral valve replacement and tricuspid valve annuloplasty. The preoperative demographic and clinical data are mentioned in Table 1. The operative data are presented in Table 2. The pathology of the operated cases is shown in Table 3.

Morbidity and mortality

Two patients had re-exploration for bleeding. One patient with chronic viral hepatitis experienced high drainage that was controlled with blood product transfusion. No patient had complete heart block, and one patient with infiltrating cardiac hemangioendothelioma had an incomplete heart block that was managed with temporary epicardial pacing and was weaned on the second postoperative day. One patient was diagnosed with right atrial thymoma and experienced severe vasoplegia and unstable hemodynamics.

Table 1 Preoperative characteristics of the study patients

Variables		$n = 82$
Age (years)		62 ± 5.8 (2 months–74 years)
Females		75 (91.46)
Body mass index (kg/m^2)		27.8 ± 4.3 (16.6–44.1)
Smoking status (ex-smoker or current smoking)		12 (14.63)
EuroSCORE II		4.27 (2.39–56.37)
Extracardiac arteriopathy		0
Poor mobility		0
Diabetes mellitus (insulin-dependent)		24 (29.26)
Hypertension		38 (46.34)
Dyslipidemia		24 (29.27)
Viral hepatitis C		12 (14.63)
Ischemic heart disease		2 (2.44)
Active endocarditis		0
Prior cardiac surgery		0
Chronic lung disease		16 (19.52)
Critical preoperative condition		6 (7.3)
Functional classification	NYHA I	5 (6.1)
	NYHA II	3 (3.65)
	NYHA III	68 (82.92)
	NYHA IV	6 (7.3)
Left ventricular function	EF > 50%	79 (96.34)
	EF 31–50%	2 (2.44)
	EF 21–30%	1 (1.22)
	EF < 21%	0
Pulmonary hypertension		38 (46.43)
Presenting symptom	Asymptomatic	10 (12.19)
	Syncopal attacks	16 (19.52)
	Shortness of breath	72 (87.8)
	Embolic complications	3 (3.65)

SD standard deviation, *n* number of patients, *EuroSCORE* European system for cardiac operative risk evaluation, *NYHA* New York Heart Association, *EF* ejection fraction, *CHD* coronary heart disease. (Continuous data are presented as mean and standard deviation and categorical data as number and percent)

Two patients had operative mortality, and one had late postoperative morality. One patient was a 35-year-old male with recurrent cardiac hemangioendothelioma with chest wall invasion and mediastinal lymphadenopathy, and mortality was encountered on the 2nd postoperative day.

The second case was a 52-year-old female with ischemic heart disease (IHD), left atrial myxoma with severe mitral valve stenosis (MS), severe tricuspid valve regurgitation (TR), and poor biventricular function with 25% ejection fraction. She underwent radical excision of the mass, mitral valve replacement (MVR), De-Vega tricuspid valve annuloplasty (TVR), and single-vessel coronary artery bypass grafting (CABG) (saphenous vein graft to an obtuse marginal artery). The patient had long cross-clamp (150 min) and bypass times (260 min). Weaning off bypass failed. Pathology confirmed the diagnosis of myxoma.

The third was late postoperative mortality in a 42-year-old female patient who underwent resection for myxosarcoma. She presented 3 months later with recurrence in the chest wall, and she died after 1 week in the oncology department. No other mortalities were recorded upon a during 1-year follow-up.

Scenarios of rare cases

Recurrent cardiac hemangioendothelioma

A 35-year-old male patient presented with a 3-month history of progressive dyspnea.

Table 2 Intraoperative characteristics of the study patients

Variables		n = 82
Priority of surgery	Elective	3 (3.66)
	Urgent	7 (8.54)
	Emergency	71 (86.58)
	Salvage	1 (1.2)
Site of the tumor	Left atrium	68 (82.92)
	Right atrium	11 (13.41)
	Biatrial	2 (2.44)
	Right ventricular outflow tract	1 (1.22)
	Inferior vena cava	2 (2.44)
Surgical approach	Biatriotomy	34 (41.46)
	Left atriotomy	20 (24.39)
	Right atriotomy	26 (31.71)
	Right ventriculotomy	1 (1.22)
	Aortotomy	1 (1.22)
Complexity of procedure	Isolated	76 (92.69)
	Two procedures	5 (6.09)
	Three procedures	1 (1.22)
Type of surgery	Tumor excision	76 (92.69)
	Excision and MVR	5 (6.09)
	Excision, single vessel CABG, MVR, TVR	1 (1.22)

CABG coronary artery bypass grafting, *MVR* mitral valve replacement, *TVR* tricuspid valve repair. (categorical data as number and percent)

Transesophageal echocardiography (TEE) (Fig. 1a, b) revealed an intracardiac mass measuring 2.2 × 5 cm, infiltrating the lower 1/3 of the interatrial septum (IAS), with direct extension to the atrial surface of the anterior mitral leaflet (AML) till its tips for 5.5 cm distance with proper differentiation between the mass and the chordal tissue with good biventricular function.

Intraoperatively, left atriotomy revealed a large tumor that was not separable from the mitral valve. The tumor was extending through the mitral valve annulus.

Table 3 Pathological diagnoses of the studied patients

Pathology	n (%)
Right atrial myxoma	5 (6.1)
Left atrial myxoma	65 (79.27)
Biatrial myxoma	2 (2.44)
RVOT myxoma	1 (1.22)
Myxosarcoma	1 (1.22)
Thymoma	1 (1.22)
Hemangioendothelioma	1 (1.22)
Round cell tumor	1 (1.22)
Cardiac lymphoma	1 (1.22)
Rhabdomyoma	2 (2.44)
Tumor extension from RCC	2 (2.44)

RVOT right ventricular outflow tract, *RCC* renal cell carcinoma. (Categorical data as number and percent)

The decision was radical excision. The fossa ovalis was excised with all the tumor tissue, which was extending into the lower part of the septum till the IVC and till the muscular apical part of the IAS. The AML with the tumor was excised totally except a tiny small part near the site of the left circumflex (LCX) artery. MVR was performed after creating a new mitral valve annulus using polypropylene suture 4/0. A mechanical valve of size 25 was inserted. IAS was closed using a pericardial patch, and TV repair was done using DeVaga semicircular tricuspid annuloplasty. The patient had an incomplete heart block that was managed using temporary pacing. ICU stay was 5 days, and the hospital stay was 7 days.

Histopathological sections revealed a vascular tumor, and the vessels were arranged in hemangiopericytoma pattern. Immunohistochemistry was positive for CD34 and negative for CD99, desmin, and myogenin. The diagnosis was consistent with hemangioendothelioma.

The oncologist recommended no adjuvant chemo/radiotherapy. Upon close follow-up, the patient presented 10 months later with a recurrence of symptoms. A workup was done including echocardiography, contrast computed tomography (CT), cardiac magnetic resonance imaging (CMRI), and ^{18}F-FDG positron emission tomography (PET-CT) (Fig. 1c, d).

Workup revealed a large, irregular, heterogeneous, lobulated intracardiac mass involving the IAS, creeping

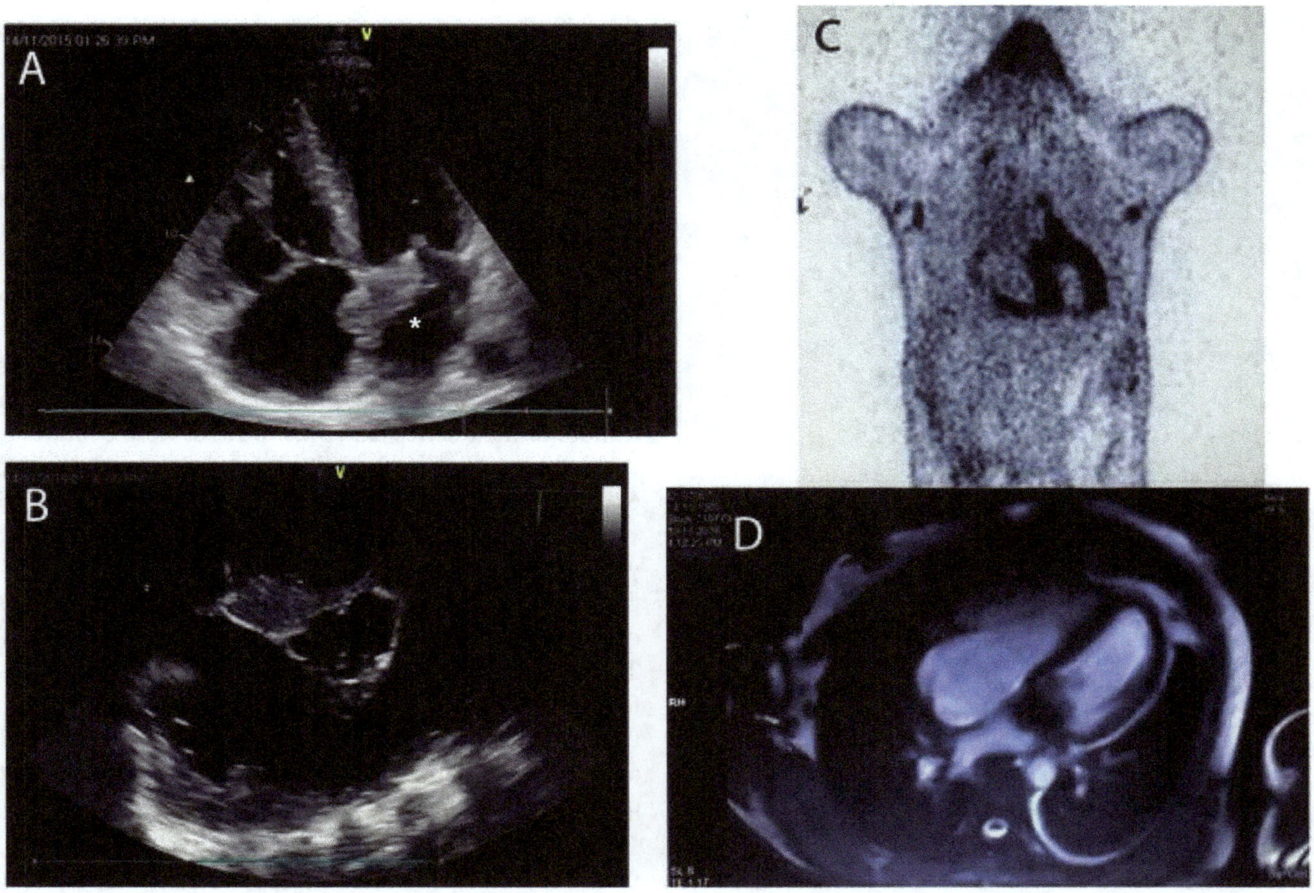

Fig. 1 Cardiac hemangioendothelioma. **a** and **b** Transesophageal echocardiography images showing the mass infiltrating the IAS and the aortomitral continuity. **c** PET CT scan showing the recurrence of the resected mass along with multiple pleural deposits. **d** Cardiac MRI showing recurrence

through the mitral inflow towards the left ventricular outflow tract (LVOT) and the aortic root. The lesion was protruding through the left atrium (LA) and left ventricular (LV) lumens. It measured 6.2 cm and had a maximum standard uptake value (SUVmax of 14.3). The lesion was expanding bilaterally to the costochondral junctions. Multiple axillary and superior mediastinal, prevascular, para-tracheal, and aortopulmonary lymphadenopathy were noted. Bilateral parietal pleural nodules were seen with SUVmax of 2.9. The right internal mammary artery was involved with a 1.4-cm lesion with a SUVmax of 5.8.

The patient underwent a re-operative surgery for recurrence. The tumor was attached to the annulus and the interventricular septum (IVS) and obstructing the LVOT; therefore, a biopsy was taken. Mortality occurred on the 2nd postoperative day.

Right atrial thymoma

A 70-year-old male had right atrial mass measuring 10 × 6 cm by echocardiography. Radical resection of the mass was performed. The specimen is exhibited in (Fig. 2). Histopathological assessment was consistent with right atrial thymoma. The postoperative course was stormy, and the patient developed vasoplegia postoperatively that was managed with intravenous (IV) methylene blue injection. The patient was discharged on the 10th postoperative day. No recurrence was recorded upon 1 year of follow-up.

Infantile right atrial myxoma

A 2-month-old boy presented with cyanosis, tachypnea, and systemic congestion. Echocardiography showed a mass in the right atrium obstructing the tricuspid valve. The excision of the mass was done along with the right atrial wall attachment (Fig. 3). Reconstruction of the IAS and the right atrial wall was done using autologous pericardium. Histopathology was consistent with right atrial myxoma. No recurrence was recorded upon 1 year of follow-up.

Left atrial lymphoma

A 65-year-old female patient presented with dyspnea NYHA functional class III for 3 months. Echocardiography revealed a left atrial mass. Upon left atriotomy, the mass was attached to the free will of the left atrium

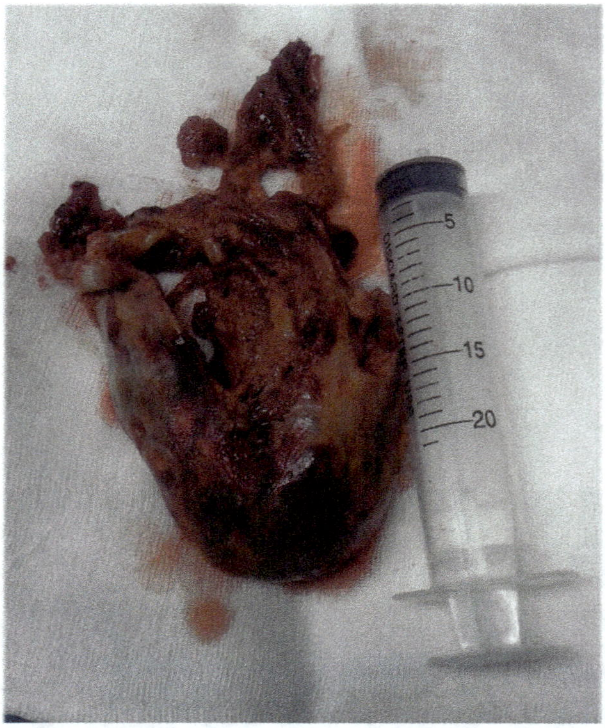

Fig. 2 Right atrial thymoma

near the mitral annulus, and radical excision was performed. Gross examination exhibited a tan-colored fleshy tissue mass measuring about 4.5 × 3 × 5 cm (Fig. 4). Histopathology revealed extensive necrotic tumor tissue with viable areas of malignant tumor infiltration. Immunohistochemistry (IHC) showed positive diffuse membranous staining of malignant cells for LCA, CD20& cytoplasmic stain for vimentin and negative for desmin, S100, CD34, CD3, and CD99. The diagnosis was consistent with intracardiac left atrial non-Hodgkin's lymphoma, diffuse large beta-cell lymphoma (NHL-DLBCL) proved by positivity for MUM1, BCL6, and BCL2 and negativity for CD10.

Following the decision of the MDT, the patient received postoperative chemotherapy. She was followed up for 1 year without recurrence before she was lost to follow up.

Right ventricular outflow tract (RVOT) myxoma

A 41-year-old female presented with lower limb edema and systemic congestion symptoms. Echocardiography showed a right ventricular mass obstructing the RVOT. Right atriotomy and right ventriculotomy were done to excise the mass attached to the interventricular septum (IVS) obstructing the RVOT (Fig. 5a, b, c). An 8-cm right ventriculotomy incision was performed at the infundibulum of the RVOT 2 cm lateral to the left anterior descending coronary artery near to the apex. The mass was assessed through the right ventriculotomy incision. The basal attachment was found originating from the IVS. The specimen was dissected and then excised from the IVS. Pathology was consistent with RVOT myxoma.

Discussion

The incidence of primary cardiac tumors varies between 0.001 and 0.03%, and 0.3–0.85% of all open-heart surgeries are for cardiac tumor resections [4, 5]. Twenty-five percent of primary cardiac tumors are malignant, with sarcoma accounting for a majority of the reported cases [6]. Most of the primary cardiac tumors reported in our series of 82 patients were benign (91%), and atrial myxoma was the most common type (87%). Kumar and associates reported a 98% prevalence of primary cardiac tumors in their series, and 92% of them were benign [4].

Nomoto and coworkers [7] reported a prevalence of 64% for primary cardiac tumors in 61 patients in a 15-year prospective study. The reported mean age was 65 years. Benign tumors were found in 30 cases out of 41 patients who had surgery. Myxoma (67%) was the most common type, followed by papillary fibroelastoma (23%). The most common site was the left atrium (35%), followed by the right atrium (25%). Primary malignant tumors were diagnosed in 10 cases (24%), including six angiosarcomas, three lymphomas, and one leiomyosarcoma [7]..

Cardiac tumors yield symptoms through any of 4 mechanisms: obstruction of blood flow, local invasion inducing arrhythmias, systemic or pulmonary embolization [2, 5, 7], and systemic or constitutional symptoms [5, 7].

Embolization was reported in 30–43% of these patients [5]. None of our cases had thromboembolism postoperatively, which could be attributed to the rapid intervention once the diagnosis is established. However, three patients presented with a prior history of thromboembolism, two right-sided strokes, and one right-sided lower limb ischemia.

Our patients presented mainly with dyspnea (87.8%), followed by syncopal attacks (19.52%) in cases with left atrial masses causing mitral valve obstruction. Ten patients (12.19%) were asymptomatic. Chest pain proposes malignancy in nearly all cases, but angina can result from coronary artery tumor embolism in either benign or malignant tumors [7]. All patients in our series were operated upon on an emergency basis once the diagnosis has been established.

Echocardiography was the first diagnostic modality, and further imaging was rarely required in our patients. 18F-fluorodeoxyglucose positron emission tomography/computed tomography (FDG-PET/CT) has a sensitivity of over 90% in differentiating benign and malignant processes [8]. In our study, one case with a recurrent hemangioendothelioma required both FDG-PET/CT and CMR to assess the extent of recurrence and metastasis.

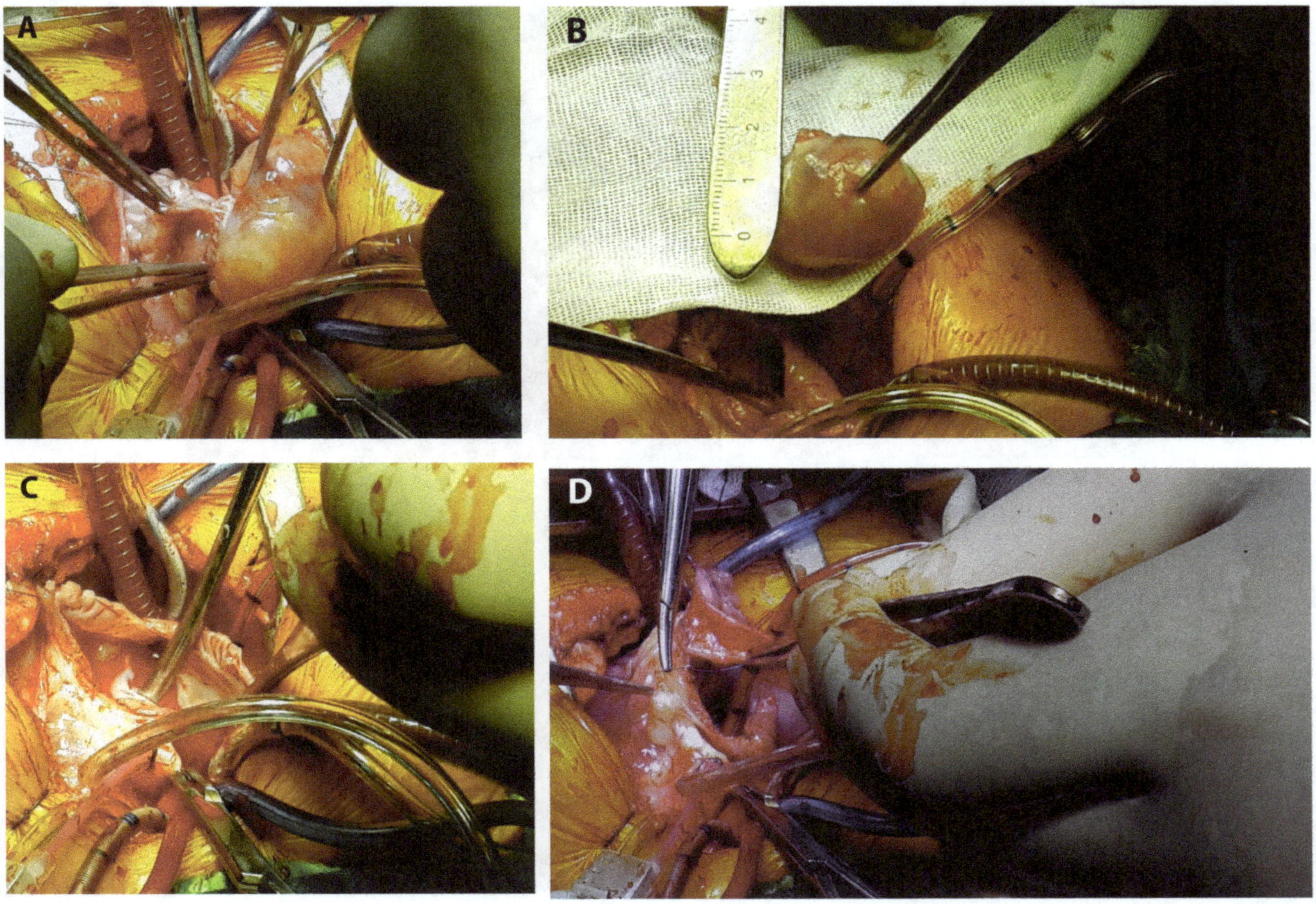

Fig. 3 Infantile right atrial myxoma. **a** The mass is observed attached to the IAS and excised with a free margin of the IAS and the right atrial wall. **b** Specimen after excision showing a mass of size 4 × 2 cm. **c** The defect in the IAS. **D** Reconstruction of the IAS using autologous pericardium and closure of the right atrial wall

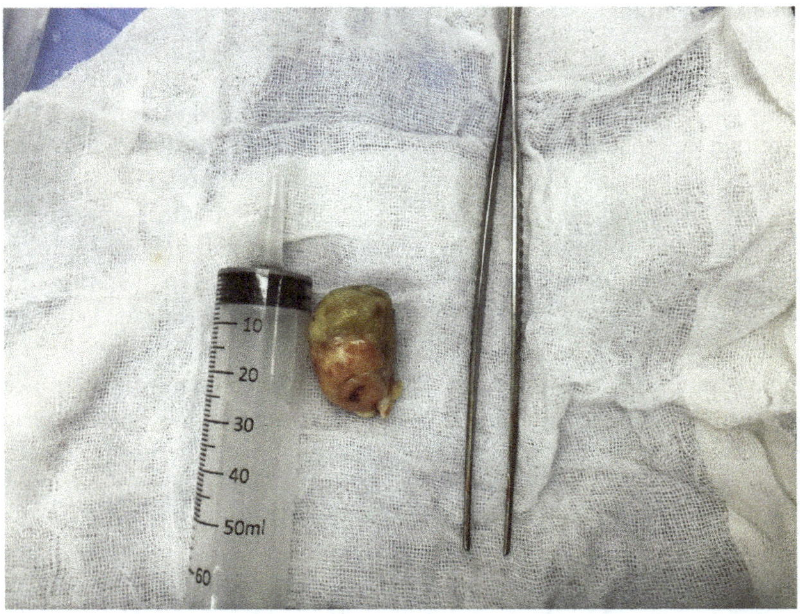

Fig. 4 Intracardiac lymphoma

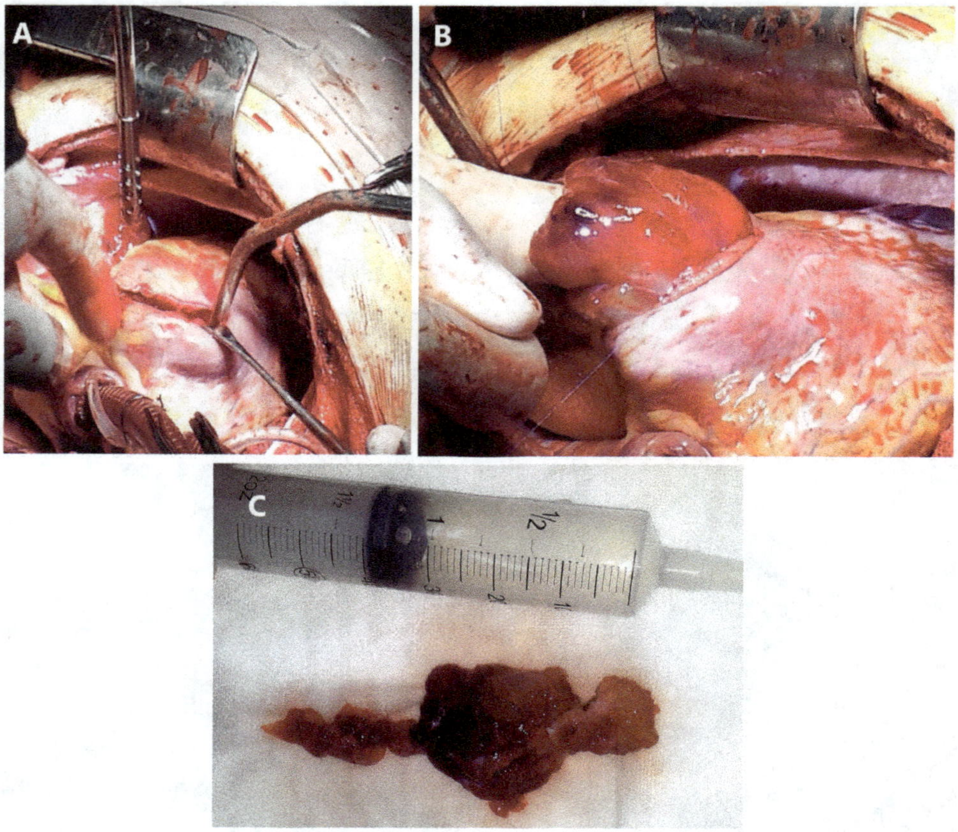

Fig. 5 Myxoma of the right ventricular outflow tract. **a** An 8-cm right ventriculotomy incision was at the infundibulum of the RVOT 2 cm lateral to the left anterior descending coronary artery. **b** The mass is shown out of the right ventriculotomy incision with its basal attachment to the IVS. **c** The specimen after excision from the IVS

Seventy-five percent of myxomas arise in the left atrium, 18% in the right atrium [2]. They rarely occur in the ventricles with a reported incidence of (3–4%) [2].

Myxomas are pedicled in most cases and extend into the affected chamber. In life-threatening cases, the cavity can be filled by the tumor mass, and the tumor may prolapse to the ventricle during diastole, especially in late-presenting cases [2].

We presented a rare case that originated from the IVS that was obstructing the RVOT. Cardiac myxoma extending into the RVOT is rare, especially in early childhood. Symptoms and signs include peripheral edema, ascites, and shortness of breath as a result of RVOT obstruction [3, 7, 9].

According to previous reports, LV myxomas usually arise from the septal endocardium [10], and there are a few case reports of growth from the LV free wall [8, 11]. Cardiac myxomas related to the Carney complex (CNC) more frequently occur in the left ventricle, compared with sporadic myxomas [11].

Hemangioendothelioma is a rare vascular tumor that has unpredictable behavior [12, 13]. To our best knowledge, the number of reported cases worldwide does not exceed 20 [12–15]. Mitral valve involvement in primary cardiac hemangioendothelioma is extremely rare, with three cases reported in the literature [12, 13].

Based on the WHO classification, hemangioendothelioma is classified into benign, intermediate (locally aggressive), or malignant tumors [16, 17].

Hemangioendothelioma occurs in nearly all age groups and shows no sex predilection [16]. However, tumors developing within the heart of infants are extremely rare. To date, there is one infant reported in the literature by Seo, and associates [16] for a half monozygotic twin [16] who presented with an upper respiratory tract infection.

The reported sites of hemangioendothelioma are the left atrium [12–15, 18, 19], mitral valve [12, 13], right atrium with or without extension to the superior vena-cava [13, 16, 20, 21]. Both local invasion and distant metastasis were reported in some cases [21].

Treatment of this type of tumor includes wide surgical resection, radiotherapy, and chemotherapy, and the reported survival was up to 3 years [12, 13, 15]. Studies have reported difficulty in achieving complete resection of tumors with negative margins. In cases in which complete resection is possible, patients commonly experience local recurrence [12, 15, 19]. Our study presented a case of hemangioendothelioma who was managed with complete resection and had a recurrence after 1 year.

Timely detection and a radical surgical resection is, so far, the more acceptable management, given the limited experience for handling this type of tumor [12–19]. Our experience suggests an aggressive clinical approach and surgical removal within the first hours of the suspected diagnosis for the greatest chance of complete resection and reducing the risk of recurrence.

Primary cardiac lymphoma (PCL) is one of the rarest tumors of the heart. It belongs to extranodal non-Hodgkin's lymphomas [22]. It composes 1.3% of all cardiac tumors and 0.5% of all extranodal lymphomas [22]. The most common type of tumor is diffuse large B cell lymphoma [23].

The right atrium [24] and ventricle are usually involved [25], and biatrial cases were reported [26]. Rare sporadic PCLs were reported in the left ventricle [27]. Treatment is a combination of surgery and chemotherapy [23]. We report a case of primary cardiac lymphoma of the left atrium.

Post-treatment surveillance for PCL should include FDG-PET/CT scanning because relapses are common [22].

A review by Petrich and coworkers [28], including 197 cases of PCL published between 1947 and 2009, found that it is more common in the elderly age (median age 63 years). Ermann and coworkers [29] reported a series of 309 patients diagnosed with PCL between 2004 and 2015, and the median survival was 49.5 months. The majority of PCL patients were male (54.7%) and white (81.2%), with a mean age of 68.3 years.

Chen and associates [23] reported 101 cases in a systematic review of literature from 2009 to 2019. They concluded that surgery alone did not improve patients' long-term prognosis or reduce the risk of death within 1 month [23].

Pediatric primary cardiac tumors in children are mostly benign, while approximately 10% are malignant [3]. Cardiac rhabdomyoma is the most common cardiac tumor during fetal life and childhood (40–60%). Myxoma is exceedingly rare in fetuses and neonates [3]. We present three cases of pediatric cardiac tumors: an extremely rare case of infantile right atrial myxoma in a 2-month-old infant and 2 cases of intracardiac rhabdomyoma aged 3 months and 1 year.

Surgical modalities vary according to the site and the size of the tumor. Cardiac tumors are challenging for cardiac surgeons because countless adaptability is vital. The heart team must be highly experienced in adult, pediatric, and rhythm surgery, as well as transplantation and artificial heart implantation [2].

Simple resection is the treatment of choice for benign tumors such as myxomas. Attention is crucial in cannulation and bypass to circumvent dislodging fragment. We open both atria from the right superior pulmonary vein without injuring the tumor. The tumor and its root can then be removed from the septum en block. All the chambers of the heart should be inspected to exclude the presence of further tumors.

Complex tumor resection is conceivable, providing the mass is limited to the heart and, if the malignant tumor has not infiltrated the adjacent tissues.

In advanced tumors, including the right side of the heart, the whole right half can be resected, and pulmonary blood flow is secured utilizing Fontan circulation; however, right heart failure may result [18].

Our results designate that the results of surgical treatment of benign cardiac tumors are excellent in all age groups, with a meager rate of recurrence. The long-term outcomes are favorable. For malignant cardiac tumors, however, the literature reports a dismal prognosis [8]. Survival rates vary from 7 months to a maximum of 2 years from diagnosis [6, 8]. On long-term follow-up, the majority of patients die of distant metastases. The median survival time of patients treated conventionally with chemotherapy and radiotherapy alone is less than a year [8, 15, 30].

Simple, incomplete resection (debulking) outspreads survival by only a few months [5]. Radical resection combined with postoperative chemotherapy improves the long-term outcome [9]. Heart transplantation remains an option for extensive cardiac tumors with better survival rates [30].

Study limitations

Although the study is prospective multicenter research, myxomas were the main bulk of cases encountered. Mid-term and long-term survival are lacking. Left ventricular assist devices are not available at our centers nor heart transplantation. A larger sample is needed to include more pathologies, and mid-term follow-up is required to assess morbidity and mortality.

Conclusions

The diagnosis of cardiac tumors is challenging. The clinical scenario depends mainly on tumor location and size rather than the histopathology. Advanced imaging modalities are rarely required in primary cases, and echocardiography is the main diagnostic modality. Surgical resection has a good prognosis in benign tumors, while it is very challenging in malignant tumors, and multimodal therapy is required.

Abbreviations

MRI: Magnetic resonance imaging; CT: Computed tomography; IVC: Inferior vena cava; RA: Right atrium; NYHA: New York Heart Association Dyspnea Classification; TEE: Transesophageal echocardiography; TTE: Transthoracic echocardiography; IAS: Interatrial septum; AML: Anterior mitral leaflet; LCA: Left Circumflex Artery; MVR: Mitral valve replacement; ICU: Intensive care unit; CMRI: Cardiac magnetic resonance imaging; FDG-PET-CCT: 18Ffluorodeoxyglucose positron emission tomography (PET-CT); LVEF: Left ventricular function; SUVmax: Maximum standard uptake value; LVOT: Left ventricular outflow tract; LA: Left atrium; LV: Left ventricle; IV: Intravenous; RVOT: Right ventricular outflow tract; IVS: Interventricular septum; LAD: Left anterior descending coronary artery; MDT: Multidisciplinary team; CNC: Carney complex; PCL: Primary cardiac lymphoma; NHL-DLBCL: Non-Hodgkin's lymphoma, diffuse large beta-cell lymphoma

Acknowledgements
This trial would not be possible without the enthusiasm and commitment of clinicians, nurses, and our patients. The authors would like to thank Dr. Hatem Beshir https://orcid.org/0000-0003-1366-3949 from the department of cardiothoracic surgery at Mansoura University for his tremendous efforts in literature review, analyzing the data, writing, and revision of this manuscript.

Previous presentations
Early results were presented as an oral presentation during the proceedings of the 25th annual meeting of the Egyptian Society of Cardiothoracic Surgery, April 2018 in Cairo, Egypt.
Presented as a poster presentation #470 during the proceedings of the 26th annual meeting of the Asian Society for Thoracic and Cardiovascular Surgery (ASCVTS 18), May 2018 in Moscow, Russia.
Results presented orally at the 15th annual congress of update in cardiology and cardiovascular surgery (UCCVS 2019), March 2019 in Antalya, Turkey. (conference abstract only was published in American Heart journal).
One case scenario was presented as an independent manuscript.
Arafa S, Sanad M. Primary cardiac hemangioendothelioma of the mitral valve. Egypt Heart J. 2018 Sep;70(3):229-232. doi: 10.1016/j.ehj.2018.06.002. Epub 2018 Jul 7. PMID: 30190651; PMCID: PMC6123280.

Authors' contributions
All authors contributed equally in conceptualization. MS, WA, and MAH operated the cases. MS, WA, and MAH performed the literature review. SA performed echocardiographic assessment for all cases and participated in writing of the manuscript with MS and WA. MS and WA analyzed the results. All the authors have read and approved the manuscript in its currently submitted form.

Author details
[1]Department of Cardiothoracic Surgery, Faculty of Medicine, Mansoura University, Mansoura, Dakahlia, Egypt. [2]Department of Cardiothoracic Surgery, Nasser Institute for Research and Treatment, Egypt Ministry of Health and Population, Cairo, Egypt. [3]Department of Cardiothoracic Surgery, Mansoura International Hospital, Egypt Ministry of Health and Population, Mansoura, Dakahlia, Egypt. [4]Department of Cardiology and Angiology, Faculty of Medicine, Mansoura University, Mansoura, Dakahlia, Egypt. [5]Department of Anesthesia and Surgical intensive care, Faculty of Medicine, Mansoura University, Mansoura, Dakahlia, Egypt.

References
1. Ren DY, Fuller ND, Gilbert SAB, Zhang Y (2017) Cardiac tumors: clinical perspective and therapeutic considerations. Curr Drug Targets 18(15):1805–1809
2. He DK, Zhang YF, Liang Y, Ye SX, Wang C, Kang B, Wang ZN (2015) Risk factors for embolism in cardiac myxoma: a retrospective analysis. Med Sci Monit 21:1146
3. Uzun O, Wilson DG, Vujanic GM, Parsons JM, De Giovanni JV (2007) Cardiac tumours in children. Orphan J Rare Dis 2(1):11
4. Kumar N, Agarwal S, Ahuja A, Das P, Airon B, Ray R (2011) Spectrum of cardiac tumors excluding myxoma: experience of a tertiary center with review of the literature. Pathol Res Pract 207:769–774
5. Wang Z, Chen S, Zhu M, Zhang W, Zhang H, Li H, Yuan G, Zou C (2016) Risk prediction for emboli and recurrence of primary cardiac myxomas after resection. J Cardiothorac Surg 11(1):22
6. Li S, Gao C (2017) Surgical experience of primary cardiac tumor: single-institution 23-year report. Med Sci Monit 23:2111
7. Nomoto N, Tani T, Konda T, Kim K, Kitai T, Ota M, Kaji S, Imai Y, Okada Y, Furukawa Y (2017) Primary and metastatic cardiac tumors: echocardiographic diagnosis, treatment and prognosis in a 15-years single center study. J Cardiothorac Surg 12(1):103
8. Mahmoud HM, Moursi I (2014) A rare case of a big left ventricular myxoma presenting with a cerebrovascular stroke. Egypt Heart J 66(4):375–377
9. Hoffmeier A, Sindermann JR, Scheld HH, Martens S (2014) Cardiac tumors—diagnosis and surgical treatment. Dtsch Arztebl Int 111(12):205
10. Fakhari S, Bilehjani E (2016) A large left ventricle myxoma: presenting with epigastric pain and weight loss. Case Rep Cardiol 2016
11. Kuyama N, Hamatani Y, Fukushima S, Ikeda Y, Nakai E, Okada A, Takahama H, Amaki M, Hasegawa T, Sugano Y, Kanzaki H, Fujita T, Ishibashi-Ueda H, Yasuda S, Anzai T, Kobayashi J (2018) Left ventricular myxoma with carney complex. ESC Heart Fail 5(4):713–715
12. Arafa S, Sanad M (2018) Primary cardiac hemangioendothelioma of the mitral valve. Egypt Heart J 70(3):229–232
13. Ellouze M, Dami M, Beaulieu Y, Perrault LP, Romeo P (2015) Resection of a right atrial epithelioid hemangioendothelioma. Cardiovasc Pathol 24(6):401–404
14. Cottini M, Lappa A, Donfrancesco S. Primary cardiac hemangioendothelioma in the adult and cardiac involvement in patient with non-cardiac hemangioendothelioma. Review of the Literature. Cancer Stud Ther J Volume. 2017;2(5):1–6.
15. Safirstein J, Aksenov S, Smith F (2007) Cardiac epithelioid hemangioendothelioma with 8-year follow-up. Cardiovasc Pathol 16(3):183–186
16. Seo JW, Song MK, Park SH, Park HE, Park SA (2019) Primary cardiac hemangioendothelioma in an infant: a case report. Clin Pediatr Hematol Oncol 26:60–65
17. Bartsch H, Haugen A, Risch A. World Health Organization classification of tumours. Pathology and Genetics of Tumours of the Lung, Pleura, Thymus and Heart. Chapter 1, Tumours of the Lung. 2004:24Ǧ25. [Online]: available from Url: https://patologi.com/who%20lunge.pdf
18. Lisy M, Beierlein W, Müller H, Bültmann B, Ziemer G (2007) Left atrial epithelioid hemangioendothelioma. J Thorac Cardiovasc Surg 133(3):803–804
19. Marchiano D, Fisher F, Hofstetter S (1993) Epithelioid hemangioendothelioma of the heart with distant metastases. A case report and literature review. J Cardiovasc Surg 34(6):529–533
20. Allain G, Hajj-Chahine J, Lacroix C, Tomasi J, Corbi P, Jayle C (2014 Nov) Surgical management of an epithelioid hemangioendothelioma of the superior vena cava protruding into the right atrium. J Card Surg 29(6):779–781
21. Ishibashi H, Takasaki C, Akashi T, Okubo K. Successful excision of epithelioid hemangioendothelioma of the superior vena cava. The Annals of thoracic surgery. 2020 Apr(4):e271-e273. [svc}
22. Jonavicius K, Salcius K, Meskauskas R, Valeviciene N, Tarutis V, Sirvydis V (2015) Primary cardiac lymphoma: two cases and a review of literature. J Cardiothorac Surg 10(1):138
23. Chen H, Qian S, Shi P, Liu L, Yang F (2020) A presentation, treatment, and survival analysis of primary cardiac lymphoma cases reported from 2009 to 2019. Int J Hematol 13:1–9
24. Yousif P, Kotecha A, Thakur A, Ismail HM (2019) A rare case of diffuse large B cell lymphoma presenting as a cardiac mass. Am J Case Rep 20:1821
25. Tabbah R, Nohra E, Rachoin R, Saroufim K, Harb B (2020) Lymphoma involving the heart: a case report. Front Cardiovasc Med 7:27
26. Li Y, Zhou Z, Xin F, Zhang C, Zhang R, Sun D, Liu W (2019) Primary cardiac lymphoma in both atria: a case report. J Clin Ultrasound 47(9):561–563
27. Matsunaga K, Kobayashi T, Takahashi M, Gohra H. A huge primary cardiac malignant lymphoma in the left ventricle. The Annals of Thoracic Surgery. 2020.
28. Petrich A, Cho SI, Billett H (2011) Primary cardiac lymphoma. Cancer. 117: 581–589
29. Ermann DA, Noble W, Parekh JD, Kapoor V, Latif A, Silberstein PT. Primary cardiac lymphoma: characteristics, treatment, and survival utilizing the National Cancer Database (NCDB). InB69. THORACIC ONCOLOGY: OPTIMIZING DIAGNOSIS AND MANAGEMENT 2019 May (pp. A3990-A3990). American Thoracic Society.
30. Hoffmeier A, Deiters S, Schmidt C, Tjan TD, Schmid C, Drees G, Fallenberg EM, Scheld HH (2004) Radical resection of cardiac sarcoma. Thorac Cardiovasc Surg 52(02):77–81

27

Index of deterioration of patients with mechanical prosthetic heart valve thrombosis

Ahmed Hassouna, Mohamed El-Ghanam*, Hasan Moftah, Khaled Samir and Khaled Refaat

Abstract

Background: Mechanical prosthetic heart valves are known for their durability; however, a malfunctioning prosthesis can deteriorate rapidly to become a life-threatening complication. Our aim was to calculate a numerical index to express the rate of clinical deterioration of patients presenting with a mechanical prosthetic heart valve thrombosis (PVT), called the index of deterioration (ID), and to evaluate its usefulness in predicting hospital outcomes.

Results: The median ID and range were (0.43, 0.03-3) NYHA class/day. A higher ID was significantly related to early development of PVT after native valve replacement, younger age, female gender, pregnancy, non-compliance to oral anticoagulation (OAC), low LVEF%, high mean pressure gradient across a mitral prosthesis, raised serum creatinine, and SGOT on admission ($P < 0.05$). Independent predictors were early presentation after native valve replacement, female gender, and non-compliance to OAC ($P < 0.05$).

ID correlated positively with the need for urgent/emergency surgery, and the durations of cardiopulmonary bypass, postoperative mechanical ventilation, and positive inotropes. ID correlated negatively with the postoperative LVEF% ($P < 0.05$). Median ID of the 21 mortalities (0.75, 0.1-3) was > 2.1 times that of survivors (0.35: 0.03^{-2}; $P = 0.002$), and the median ID of the 29 cases with postoperative complications (0.5, 0.1-1.5) was 2.5 times that of the 39 uneventful cases (0.2, 0.03-2; $P = 0.011$). The ID significantly predicted both mortality (odds ratio 3.87; 1.33-1.29; $P = 0.013$) and mortality and hospital complications (odds ratio 4.77; 1.49-15.2; $P = 0.008$). The respective discriminating abilities were AUC 0.734 (0.616-0.852; $P = 0.002$) and 0.724 (0.61-0.835; $P < 0.001$). EuroScore II correlated positively with ID ($r = 0.571$; $P < 0.001$) but showed better discriminative abilities.

Conclusion: The simple index of deterioration was useful in monitoring deterioration and predicting hospital progression and outcomes in patients presenting with PVT.

Keywords: Prosthetic valve malfunction, Prosthetic valve thrombosis, Mechanical valve thrombosis, Scoring systems, EuroScore II

Background

In our experience, mitral valve repair is not always feasible in the young rheumatic population and valve replacement with a mechanical valve is preferred over the use of a bioprosthesis, which is likely to degenerate over time and require reintervention [1]. Although mechanical valves have long term durability, yet the incidence of malfunction is not negligible (0.1-6%) and mechanical prosthetic valve thrombosis (PVT) is one of those serious complications, where patients often deteriorate rapidly, compromising management outcomes. The aim of this study was to express the rate by which those patients deteriorate clinically by a simple numerical index and to test its value in monitoring hospital progression and predicting outcomes of surgery.

* Correspondence: mohamedelghanam@yahoo.com
Cardiothoracic Surgery Department, AinShams University, Cairo, Egypt

Methods

This prospective study included 86 patients with PVT who were operated upon in our hospital between January 2016 and October 2019. Written informed consent was obtained from all participants in this study. Inclusion criteria were patients of both sexes presenting with symptoms and or signs suggesting PVT that was documented by transthoracic as well as transesophageal echocardiography on hospital admission. We have excluded cases with recurrent PVT as well as the subset of patients who presented within a short period (1-2 weeks) of the development of mild symptoms (NYHA class I or II), had a small thrombus on echocardiography (< 1 cm) and who responded positively after a short period (1-2 days) of continuous IV heparinotherapy or fibrinolytic therapy.

History intake included date of native valve replacement type and size of implanted prosthesis and any history of valve or anticoagulant related complications. We suggested that every prosthesis is doomed to become malfunctioning 1 day or another and hence, the period that elapsed between the date of implantation of the prosthesis and the appearance of the signs and or symptoms suggesting PVT was recorded in months and was called the latent period of malfunction (LPM). The usually much shorter period that follows afterward and till the patient is reoperated was recorded in days and it was called the manifest period of malfunction (MPM). The patient's medications were reviewed, especially his compliance to oral anticoagulation therapy (OAC). Noncompliance was defined as a patient skipping > 2 successive doses, changing dose, stopping intake, or shifting to another anticoagulation regimen, without cardiological consultation. In order to calculate the index of deterioration (ID), we assigned the numbers 1, 2, 3, and 4 to the patient's NYHA class I, II, III, and IV respectively. The change in NYHA class for a particular patient (delta NYHA) was calculated by subtracting the baseline numerical NYHA class value before the event form the numerical NYHA class value of the patient at presentation. The patient's ID was then calculated by dividing the delta NYHA by the duration of the MPM in days.

Once admitted, all patients benefited from routine preoperative preparation. Female patients were assessed for their pregnancy state and pregnant cases received immediate obstetric evaluation. Based on the clinical and echocardiographic findings, the timing of surgery was decided by the attending surgeon. Surgery was performed through median sternotomy under cardiopulmonary bypass, moderate hypothermia, and antegrade cold blood cardioplegia. The prosthesis was inspected, with the primary intention to be replaced by a mechanical prosthesis in most of the cases. The use of a bioprosthesis or limited thrombectomy was left to the personal surgeon's judgment and patient preference. Operative survivors were transported to the ICU and managed routinely till discharge.

Statistical analysis

Qualitative variables were presented as numbers and percentages, and the significance of their association was tested by chi-square or Fisher's exact test, as indicated. Shapiro-Wilk test showed a significant deviation of normality and calculated ID scores were hence expressed as medians and range. The significance of their association was tested by Spearman's correlation rank test and groups were compared by Mann and Whitney test or Kruskal and Wallace test, as indicated.

To evaluate the discriminative ability of ID, we have calculated EuroScore II for our patients and both scores were subjected to the receiver-operating characteristic analyses, calculating the area under the curve (AUC) for hospital mortality as well as both hospital mortality and complications. In addition, univariate logistic regression analyses were run to evaluate the predicted probability of ID and EuroScore or hospital mortality as well as model calibration by the Hosmer-Lemeshow test for the lack of "goodness of fit."

In order to detect the independent preoperative predictors of clinical deterioration (ID), variables that were significantly related to ID on univariate analysis were introduced in a multiple linear regression model. The dependent variable was the normalized values of ID, calculated by the 2 steps approach described by Templeton GF, which involves ranking cases followed by normalization of ranks with the inverse distribution function using fractional rank, mean, and standard deviation [2]. Normality was then rechecked by the Shapiro-Wilk test. All tests were bilateral, and a P value of 5% was the limit of statistical significance. The analysis was performed by the statistical package software IBM-SPSS version 25 (IBM Corp, Chicago, IL, USA).

Results

Table 1 shows the patients demographics. The median age was 49 (16-74) years, with a female predominance and a majority of patients having a single mechanical bileaflet prosthesis implanted in the mitral position (67 cases, 78%). The main presenting symptom was dyspnea and palpitation and 96.5% of cases presented with NYHA class III or IV. Two-thirds of patients were not compliant to OAC regimen on admission, including all the 16 pregnant cases included in our study. Eight of those cases (75%) reduced their recommended warfarin dose or completely stopped the intake for fear of warfarin-related embryopathy. The other 4 cases were shifted to inadequate heparin therapy by their attending obstetrician, without cardiological consultation. There

Table 1 Patients' demographics (n = 86)

Variable	
Age (years)	40 (16-74)
Female gender	52 (60.5%)
Pregnancy	16 (18.6%)
Number of implanted prostheses	91
Mechanical bileaflet	85 (93.4%)
Mechanical mono-leaflet	4 (4.4%)
Additional tricuspid bioprosthesis*	2 (2.2%)
Position of implantation	
Mitral	68 (79.1%)
Aortic	13 (15.1%)
Mitral and aortic	3 (3.5%)
Mitral + tricuspid bioprosthesis*	2 (2.3%)
Non-compliance to OAC	53 (61.6%)
Main presenting symptom:	
Dyspnea and palpitation	70 (81.4%)
Thromboembolic event	12 (14%)
Threatened abortion	4 (4.6%)
NYHA class at presentation	
Class IV	47 (54.7%)
Class III	36 (41.9%)
Class II	3 (3.5%)
Numerical NYHA class	3.5 (2-4)
LVEF%	57.5 (22-73)
Mean pressure gradient across mitral prosthesis (mm Hg)	12 (9-20)
Mean pressure gradient across aortic prosthesis (mm Hg)	54 (5-80)
INR on admission	1.55 (0.7-4.2)
Serum creatinine (mg/dl)	1.37 (0.6-4.2)
SGOT (units/liter)	45 (15-150)
Latent period** (months)	44.6 (0.77-365)
Index of deterioration (ID)	0.43 (0.03-3)
EuroScore II	6.75 (1.69-26.5)

Values are presented as number (%) or median and range
n number of patients, *PVT* prosthetic valve thrombosis, *LVEF%* left ventricular ejection fraction percentage
*Well-functioning bioprosthesis
**Time between implantation of mechanical prosthesis and development of symptoms and/or signs suggesting PVT

was a statistically significant negative correlation between the index of deterioration and the time elapsed between native valve replacement and LPM (Fig. 1). The earlier the patient developed the malfunction, the faster he deteriorated ($r = -0.489$; $P < 0.001$).

Table 2 shows selected operative and postoperative outcomes. Only 2 patients were operated upon electively after presenting with progressive dyspnea and echocardiographic data showing a small thrombus, 60 and 180 months after mitral valve replacement with a SJ bileaflet mechanical prosthesis. The 2 patients were operated upon after failure to improve from a brief 2-days trial of heparin therapy followed by fibrinolytic therapy. Out of the 91 implanted prostheses, 86 were malfunctioning (94.5%), 80% of which were replaced with a bileaflet mechanical prosthesis. The use of a bioprosthesis was limited to the 16 cases (18.6%) who either preferred to avoid the life-long OAC regimen, as well as those patients having a history of repeated non-compliance to OAC. On the other hand, management was limited to thrombectomy and careful cleaning of the valve housing in one case presenting with a small recent thrombus and a low INR of 1.4 on admission. Unfortunately, the patient died postoperatively from persistent low cardiac output, with an apparently well-functioning prosthesis on transesophageal echocardiography. Our overall hospital mortality was high (21%) and 29 patients had non-fatal in-hospital complications (33.7%). A total of 49 complications were recorded in those cases including significant postoperative bleeding in 8 patients (16.3%), which necessitated reoperation in 2 cases (4%), prolonged mechanical ventilation in 7 cases (14.3%), need for reintubation in 4 cases (8.2%), temporary heart block in 6 cases (12.2%), low cardiac output in 5 cases (10.2%), cerebrovascular stroke in 2 cases (4%), septic shock in 2 cases (4%), multiorgan failure in 2 cases (4%), and acute renal failure necessitating dialysis in another case (2%). Ten adverse fetal outcomes were recorded among the 16 pregnant patients (20.4%), included 4 cases of abortion (8.2%), and 6 fetal losses (12.2%).

Table 3 shows the ID values for patients' subgroups and their correlation with the patients' demographics, associated risk factors, and hospital outcomes. Younger age on admission, female gender, pregnancy, and non-compliance to OAC were all significantly associated with a high ID. A high ID significantly correlated with increased mean pressure gradient across a malfunctioning mitral prosthesis, need for urgent or emergency surgery, and prolonged durations of cardiopulmonary bypass, postoperative mechanical ventilation, and inotropic support. A high ID was significantly associated with hospital mortality as well as the development of complications among survivors.

Table 3 also shows the calculated EuroScore II values that nearly followed the same pathway as the ID, with a statistically significant positive correlation between both indices ($r = 0.571$; $P < 0.001$; Fig. 2). EuroScore II correlated negatively with LPM and MPM and positively with NYHA class at presentation as well as the need for emergency surgery. A high EuroScore II was also significantly related to mortality and to the development of complications among hospital survivors. Unlike the

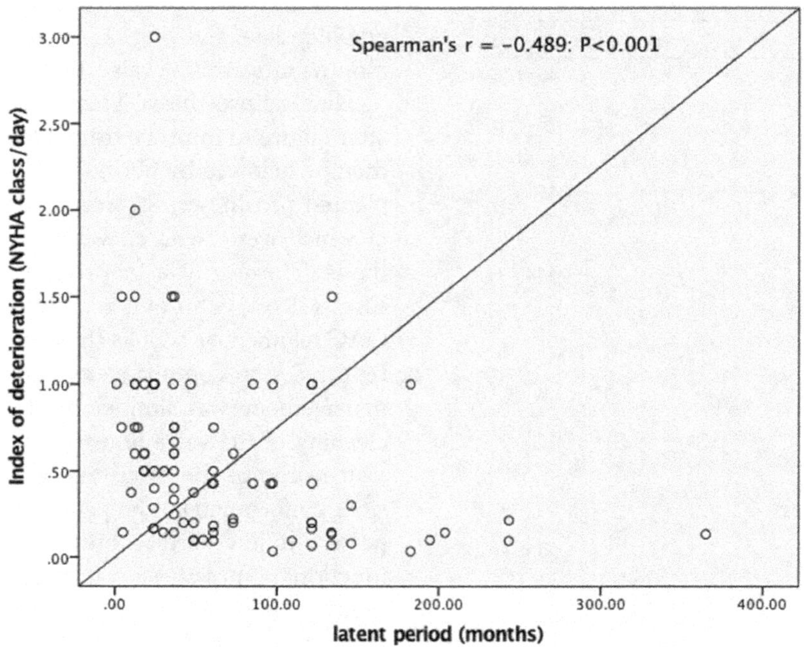

Fig. 1 Correlation between index of deterioration and latent period

index of deterioration, EuroScore II did not significantly correlate with the patient's demographics at presentation, namely, age, gender, pregnancy status, and non-compliance to OAC.

Preoperative variables that were statistically significant on univariate analysis were introduced in a linear regression model to detect the independent preoperative predictors of ID, using the normalized ID as the dependent variable. The mean normalized ID ± standard deviation was 0.56 ± 0.48, the normalized ID of mortalities (0.82 ± 0.33) was significantly higher than that calculated for survivors (0.5 ± 0.49; P = 0.003). Out of the nine statistically significant variables shown in Table 3, only six were introduced in the model, namely, age on admission, gender, pregnancy state, non-compliance to OAC, mean pressure gradient across the prosthesis, and LPM. Both NYHA class and MPM were excluded for the high co-linearity due to their use in the direct calculation of the dependent variable itself. The urgency of the operation was not used for being the result rather than being the predictor of the deterioration. The model significantly explained ID, R^2 = 0.33; P < 0,001. The independent predictors of high ID were female gender (B = 0.236: 0.042-0.43; P = 0.018), non-compliance to OAC (0.215, 0.031-0.4; P = 0.023), and early presentation of PVT as indicated by a short latent period of malfunction (−0.003: −0.004 to −0.002; P < 0.001).

Table 4 shows variables that were significantly related to hospital mortalities in univariate analysis. In order to detect the independent preoperative predictors of mortality variables that were statistically significant on univariate analysis were introduced in a logistic regression model. The model predicted mortality (sensitivity 96.4%, specificity 57.1%, and Negelkerke R square 0.577; P < 0.001); data fitted the model (Hosmer-Lemeshow test; P = 0.7) and the only independent predictor was low LVEF% on admission (odds ratio 0.85, 0.75-0.96; P = 0.008). The model was not improved by the introduction of either ID or EuroScore or both and none of them significantly predicted mortality.

Although our observed 21% hospital mortality was nearly triple that expected by EuroScore II (mean, 7.3%, median, 6.7%, range, 1.69-26.5, and 95% interval of confidence of median, 4-84-6.89); P < 0.001, yet the discriminative ability of the later (AUC 0.799, 0.69-0.9; P < 0.001) was better than that calculated with ID (AUC 0.734, 0.62-0.75; P = 0.002), as shown in Fig. 3. Univariate logistic regression analysis showed that both scores significantly predicted mortality but the EuroScore odds ratio 1.35 (1.13-1.61); P = 0.001 and Hosmer and Lemeshow test; P = 0.345; demonstrated more accurate predictive ability than those calculated for ID: odds ratio, 3.87 (1.3-11.3); P = 0.013; and Hosmer and Lemeshow test P = 0.07. As shown in Fig. 4, better discriminative ability for hospital mortality and complications was also recorded with EuroScore II (AUC 0.799: 0.69-0.9; P < 0.001) than with ID (AUC 0.734, 0.62-0.85; P < 0.002). Univariate logistic regression analysis showed that both scores significantly predicted mortality but the EuroScore odds ratio 1.36 (1.15-1.62); P < 0.001 and Hosmer and Lemeshow test; P = 0.08; demonstrated more accurate predictive ability than that calculated for ID:

Table 2 Selected operative and postoperative outcomes

Variable	
Schedule of surgery	
Emergency	51 (59.3%)
Urgent	33 (38.4%)
Elective	2 (2.3%)
Management of malfunctioning prosthesis*	
Replacement with mechanical prosthesis	69 (80.2%)
Replacement with bioprosthesis	16 (18.6%)
Thrombectomy alone	1 (1.2%)
Aortic cross clamp time (min)	61 (37-200)
Cardiopulmonary bypass time (min)	110 (55-360)
Difficulty to wean from bypass	25 (29.1%)
Duration of mechanical ventilation (h)	24 (6-168)
Duration of inotropes (h)	48 (0-216)
Transfused blood products (l)	4 (2-12)
ICU stay (days)	4 (1-39)
Total hospital stay (days)	10 (1-40)
Postoperative LVEF%	54 (22-70)
Postoperative pressure gradient across prosthesis (mm Hg)	
Mitral	5 (3-10)
Aortic	20 (15-50)
Hospital mortality	18 (21%)
Low cardiac output	–8 (44.4%)
Multi organ failure	–4 (22.2%)
Septic shock	–6 (33.3%)
Uneventful cases	39 (45.3%)

Values are presented as numbers (%) or median (range)
LVEF% left ventricular ejection fraction percentage
*Out of the 91 implanted prostheses, only 86 were malfunctioning (94.5%)

odds ratio, 3.87 (1.5-15.2); P = 0.008; and Hosmer and Lemeshow test P = 0.05.

Discussion

Every foreign material implanted in the circulation invites thrombosis and hence, PVT is expected to remain an inherent complication of heart valve replacement. Put it another way, every mechanical prosthesis is assumed to develop PVT 1 day or another, which is why we have termed the period extending from the implantation of the prosthesis and till the development of the signs and/or the symptoms suggesting PVT as the latent period of malfunction (LPM). In a study that included 680 consecutive patients undergoing mechanical mitral valve replacement, routine transesophageal echocardiography performed at day 9 identified thrombus in as much as 9.4% of patients. Although 97% of those patients were successfully managed by anticoagulant therapy, yet 2 cases of PVT needed intervention [3].

Pathologically, the formation of a thrombus on the prosthetic structures reduces the effective orifice area and increases the trans-valvular gradient, producing a variety of symptoms starting from progressive shortness of breath and palpitation and up to a fulminating congestive heart failure. In addition, the hemodynamic disturbance involves the creation of areas of turbulence that increases shear stress and endothelial injury, and adjacent areas of stasis that increases blood coagulability (both inviting more thrombosis [4]) and can generate thromboembolic events [5, 6].

There are several mechanisms by which PVT occur, varying from a fast process commencing early after implantation, to the generation of vegetation during the process of endocarditis or the formation of thrombi with the slow ingrowth of a fibrotic pannus over the years [5, 7]. Blackstone and Kirklin have shown that prosthetic valve-related adverse outcomes are not only dependent upon the underlying pathology but also on the timing of presentation [8]. In consequence, we expected that the different pace of those mechanisms will be reflected on the pattern of clinical presentation, especially the length of the period that starts with the patient developing symptoms and/or signs suggesting PVT and ends by reoperation: the manifest period of malfunction (MPM). We expected that the number of NYHA classes the patient loses during this period will objectively reflect the ongoing pathology and, hopefully, may be useful in predicting hospital outcomes. We can easily note that the operative risk of a patient who progresses slowly to reach NYHA class IV over a relatively long period of time is in many times different from another NYHA class IV patient whose prosthesis was catastrophically obstructed by a large thrombus. In fact, the importance of both deterioration in NYHA class and the rate by which it occurs was previously noted by Husebey and colleagues who suggested that advanced NYHA functional class and need for emergency (rapid rate of progression) have to be treated separately [9]. Our suggested ID overcomes this separation as it expresses both the size of deterioration (advancement in NYHA class) and its rate (MPM) in a single numerical value.

The annual rate of PVT is estimated to be between 0.1 and 5.7%, with higher rates being observed in the early perioperative period [10, 11], with prosthesis implanted in the mitral and tricuspid position [5, 12], in association with subtherapeutic anticoagulation [11–15] or interruption of oral anticoagulants for anticipated non-cardiac surgery [16] or during pregnancy [15, 17]. Predominance of female gender was reported in 2 large series [8, 11]. Blackstone and Kirklin identified female gender as the only risk factor that was significantly associated with acute prosthetic thrombosis [8].

Table 3 Index of deterioration versus EuroScore values

Variable	Index of deterioration (ID) Effect size	P value	EuroScore II Effect size	P value
A-Preoperative (on admission)				
Age (years)	$r = -0.245$	0.023	$r = 0.039$	0.73
Gender				
Females versus males	0.55 (0.07-3) vs. 0.21 (0.03-1.5)	0.003	8.4 (2.9-26.5) vs. 5 (1.69-15)	0.13
Non-pregnant females vs. males*	0.46 (0.07-1.5) vs. 0.23 (0.03-1.5)	0.05	8.4 (2.9-26.5) vs. 5 (1.69-15)	0.27
Pregnancy: pregnant vs. other cases	0.87 (0.3-3) vs. 0.39 (0.03-1.5)	0.003	8.4 (3.4-11.2) vs. 6.5 (1.7-26.5)	0.13
Position				
Mitral + tricuspid	2 (2-2)		11.5 (7.9-15)	
Mitral + aorta	1 (0.07-1)		6.6 (6.4-10.5)	
Single mitral	0.46 (0.07-3)		6.9 (2.8-18)	
Single aortic	0.3 (0.03-1)	0.43	6.4 (1.7-26.5)	0.47
Non-compliance to OAC: yes vs. no	0.5 (0.1-3) vs. 0.33 (0.03-1.5)	0.03	6.9 (2.8-18) vs. 6.4 (1.7-26.5)	0.36
Thromboembolic events: yes vs. no	0.29 (1-1.5) vs. 0.5 (0.03-3)	0.35	8.4(2.9-11.4) vs. 6.6 (1.7-26.5)	0.99
LVEF% at presentation	$r = -0.155$	0.155	$r = -0.44$	< 0.001
Mean gradient across prosthesis				
Mitral	$r = 0.52$	< 0.001	$r = 0.325$	0.007
Aortic (mm Hg)**	$r = -0.44$	0.129	$r = -0.53$	0.061
NYHA functional class				
Class II	0.1 (0.03-0.14)		2.86 (1.69-3.7)	
Class III	0.17 (0.03-2)		3.7 (2.77-11.95)	
Class IV	0.75 (0.14-3)	< 0.001	8.44 (3.72-26.5)	< 0.001
Latent period (months)	$r = -0.489$	< 0.001	$r = -0.228$	0.035
Manifest period (days)	$r = -0.974$	< 0.001	$r = -0.478$	< 0.001
Schedule of surgery				
Emergency ($n = 50$)	0.6 (0.1-3)		8.44 (3.72-26.5)	
Urgent ($n = 45$)	0.17 (0.03-1)		3.73 (2.77-10.65)	
Elective ($n = 5$)	0.088 (0.03-0.14)	< 0.001	2.53 (1.69-3.38)	< 0.001
B-Operative and postoperative				
Aortic cross clamp time (min)	$r = 0.17$	0.12	$r = 0.204$	0.06
Cardiopulmonary bypass time (min)	$r = 0.66$	0.013	$r = 0.35$	0.001
Mechanical ventilation	$r = 0.31$	0.004	$r = 0.219$	0.043
Inotropes duration (h)	$r = 0.23$	0.031	$r = 0.165$	0.128
ICU stay (days)	$r = 0.18$	0.09	$r = 0.17$	0.12
Total hospital stay (days)	$r = 0.035$	0.75	$r = 0.03$	0.79
Postoperative LVEF%	$r = -0.252$	0.019	$r = -0.424$	< 0.001
Mean gradient across prosthesis				
Mitral	$r = 0.33$	< 0.006	$r = -0.308$	0.011
Aortic (mm Hg)*	$r = -0.511$	0.075	$r = -0.302$	0.316
Mortality				
Mortalities ($n = 18$)	0.75 (0.1-3)		8.5 (4.2-26.5)	
Survivors ($n = 68$)	0.35 (0.03-2)	0.002	6.27 (1.69-13.84)	< 0.001
Hospital survivors:				
Complicated ($n = 29$)	0.5 (0.1-1.5)		6.89 (2.86-13.84)	

Table 3 Index of deterioration versus EuroScore values *(Continued)*

	Index of deterioration (ID)		EuroScore II	
Variable	Effect size	*P* value	Effect size	*P* value
Uneventful cases (n = 39)	0.2 (0.03-2)	0.011	4.4 (1.69-13.84)	0.006

Values are calculated on admission or during hospitalization and are expressed as median (range) or as Spearman's correlation coefficient *r*
vs. versus, *PVT* prosthetic valve thrombosis, *n* number of patients, *LVEF* left ventricular ejection fraction
*36 females, 34 males
**Excluding 5 patients with more than one prosthesis

In our study, the median LPM that extended up to 30 years after native valve replacement was as early as 44.6 months, 85% of thrombosed prostheses were implanted in the mitral position, 60% of patients were females and two-thirds of cases had a positive history of non-compliance to OAC. Comparable results noting the timing of presentation (39± 42 months), 85% female predominance, 85% mechanical prosthesis implanted in the mitral position, and 26% non-compliance to OAC were reported by Durrleman and colleagues [11]. Our 61.6% rate of non-compliance is even higher than the 45% rate reported by Buttard and colleagues [13] but can be attributed to our series including 16 non-compliant pregnant patients. In fact, the ID was able to identify every one of those risk factors, being significantly higher in those patients who were older, of female gender, pregnant, having a history of non-compliance to OAC, or who developed PVT early after native valve replacement, compared to the other patients who were privileged by the absence of those risk factors. In concordance to others, the female gender [8, 11], early PVT after native valve replacement [11, 12], and non-compliance to OAC [11–13, 17] were associated with worsening of outcomes and those were the factors that independently predicted a high ID in our study. In practice, a female presenting with PVT is expected to deteriorate 2 times faster than a male companion; this deterioration will unfortunately be doubled in case she was pregnant. Playing the same tune, a patient who is non-compliant to OAC is expected to deteriorate 50% faster than a compliant patient, with all other parameters being equal. As such, the ID may be useful to schedule patients for surgery and, in fact, the median ID of our emergency cases was 0.6, which was 3.5 times that of urgent cases and nearly 7 times that calculated in patients who were operated upon electively.

On the other hand, the ID correlated positively with major adverse operative and postoperative outcomes, such as the durations of cardiopulmonary bypass, mechanical ventilation, and need for inotropes. A high ID was an indicator of a limited improvement of LVEF% after surgery, development of non-fatal complications, and mortality. The median ID of patients who developed non-fatal hospital complications was 2.5 times that

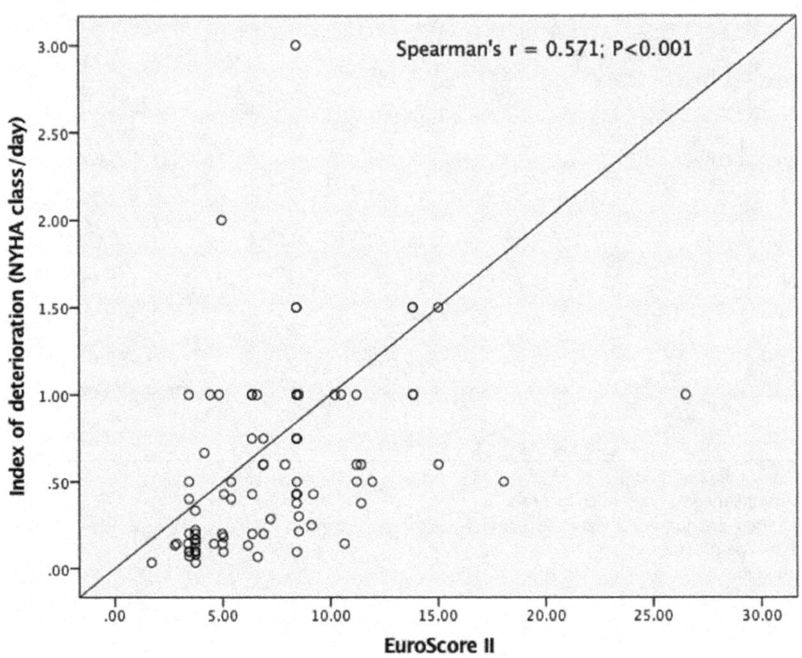

Fig. 2 Correlation between Index of deterioration and EuroScore II

Table 4 Analysis of mortality

Variable	Hospital survivors (*n* = 68)	Hospital mortalities (*n* = 18)	*P* value
A-Preoperative			
Age (years)	39 (24-74)	49.5 (16-64)	0.21
Female gender	40 (58.8%)	11 (61.1%)	0.86
Pregnant patients	12 (17.6%)	4 (22.3%)	0.9
Position of malfunctioning prosthesis			
Mitral	58 (85.3%)	15 (83.3%)	
Aortic	10 (14.7%)	3 (16.7%)	0.86
NC-OAC (*n* = 47)	40 (50.6%)	13 (61.9%)	0.36
Thromboembolic events	8 (11.8%)	4 (22.2%)	0.26
NYHA class on admission			
Class II	3 (4.4%)	0	
Class III	34 (50%)	2 (11.1%)	0.004
Class IV	31 (45.6%)	16 (88.9%)	0.003
Numerical NYHA class*	3 (2-4)	4 (2-4)	
LPM (months)	48 (4-365)	36 (0.8-121.7)	0.225
MPM (days)	8.5 (2-60)	3.5 (2-21)	0.006
LVEF% at presentation	60 (40-73)	44.5 (22-66)	0.007
Mean pressure gradient across mitral prosthesis (mm Hg)**	15 (9-43)	21 (12-30)	0.027
Mean pressure gradient across aortic prosthesis (mm Hg)**	67 (45-80)	35 (25-50)	0.018
INR on admission	1.5 (0.7-3.4)	1.8 (1-4.4)	0.078
Serum creatinine on admission (mg/dl)	1.35 (0.8-4.2)	1.55 (1-3.4)	0.026
SGOT on admission (units/liter)	40 (15-120)	72.5 (24-150)	0.002
Schedule of surgery			
Emergency (*n* = 50)	37 (54.4%)	14 (77.8%)	
Urgent (*n* = 45)	29 (42.6%)	4 (22.2%)	
Elective (*n* = 5)	2 (2.9%)	0	0.18
B-Operative and postoperative			
Operative procedure			
Replacement with a mechanical valve	55 (80.9%)	14 (77.8%)	
Replacement with a tissue valve	13 (19.1%)	3 (16.7%)	
Limited procedure without replacement	0	1 (5.6%)	0.37
Aortic cross clamp time (min)	60 (37-140)	87.5 (50-200)	0.02
Cardiopulmonary bypass time (min)	102 (55-205)	160 (100-360)	< 0.001
Mechanical ventilation duration (h)**	24 (8-120)	33.5 (6-168)	0.54
Inotropes duration (h)***	48 (6-168)	33.5 (12-216)	0.031
Postoperative LVEF%***	55 (40-70)	37.5 (15-45)	< 0.001
ICU stay (days)***	4 (1.5-14)	2.5 (2-39)	0.025
Total hospital stay (days)***	10 (6-21)	3.5 (1-40)	< 0.001

Values are presented as numbers (%) or median (range)
n number of patients, *NC-OAC* non-compliance to oral anticoagulants
*NYHA classes: II, III, and IV were assigned the numerical values 2, 3, and 4
**Excluding 5 patients with more than one prosthesis
***Calculated for the 68 operative survivors

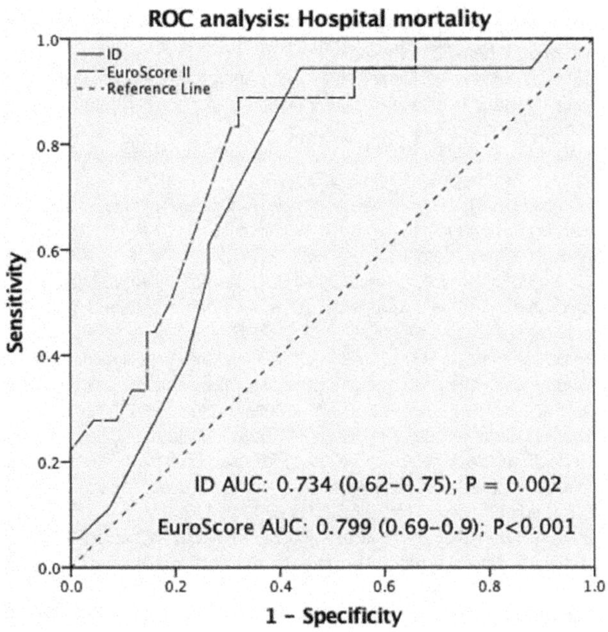

Fig. 3 ROC analysis: hospital mortality: index of deterioration versus EuroScore II

calculated for uneventful cases (P = 0.011) and the median ID of the 18 hospital mortalities was more than double that of the 68 survivors (P = 0.002). In practice, a patient, whose ID is 0.35 NYHA class/day or higher, is expected to develop non-fatal complications and mortality, with a sensitivity of 78.7% and specificity of 64.1%. An ID $\geq$ 0.46 or higher is expected to unfortunately join mortality, with a sensitivity of 81% and specificity of

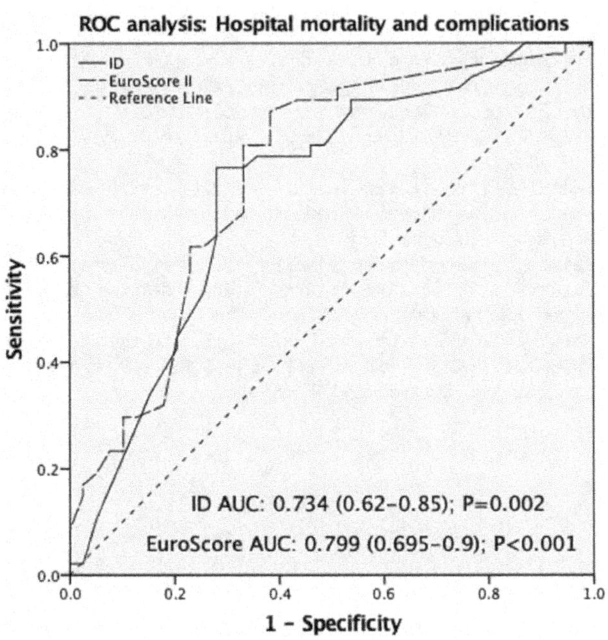

Fig. 4 ROC analysis: hospital mortality and complications: index of deterioration versus EuroScore II

62%. We have previously tested the ID in a group of 75 patients presenting with different types of prosthetic malfunctions including PVT, prosthetic valve endocarditis, severe prosthetic dehiscence, and primary bioprosthetic failure. Due to the inclusion of a large number of patients with slowly progressive valve dehiscence, it was more suitable to calculate LPM in months rather than in days, giving larger crude ID values than the ones calculated in the actual study [18]. The ID calculated for different valve malfunctions also correlated positively and significantly with the early presentation of the malfunction, need for emergency, and longer durations of bypass and positive inotropes as well as hospital mortality [18].

Although the hospital mortality in our study was as heavy as 21%, yet it was within the widely variable range reported to be as low as 5% in a small selected series of 20 patients [15] to 20.6% in a large series of 63 patients who developed mainly PVT due to pannus formation [14] to as much as 41% in a Canadian series of 39 patients [11]. Many risk factors have been identified to influence outcomes of surgery including early presentation [8, 11] myocardial depression, as indicated by low EF [14], and increased left ventricular diameter [14, 19], advanced NYHA class [20], prolonged cardiopulmonary bypass time [21], non-compliance to oral anticoagulation (OAC) regimen [11, 13], and need for any additional procedure [20] Our study has shown that low LVEF% on admission was the only independent predictor of hospital mortality and not the ID or the EuroScore II.

Although the STS risk score has been found to be highly effective for determining numerous outcomes such as short and long-term mortality, stroke, length of hospital stay and renal failure, prolonged ventilation, infection, and reoperation, yet it was modeled to fit specific surgical cases: isolated coronary artery bypass grafting (CABG), isolated aortic valve replacement (AVR), isolated mitral valve replacement (MVR), mitral valve repair (MV repair), CABG + AVR, CABG + MVR, and CABG + MV repair [22]. Because of this limitation, the STS risk scoring system cannot be used to study other types of cardiac surgery that are not yet included. On the other hand, the other most commonly used scoring system (the EuroScore II) that was designed to expect mortality in various surgical cases showed poor clinical relevance in the segment of patients where it is needed the most, i.e., the high risk and emergency cases [23–25]. Many studies have shown a significant discrepancy between observed and expected mortality in those patients when calculated by EuroScore II which sometimes overestimates [24] and in other times underestimates mortality [23] in high-risk patients [23, 24] as well as in emergency surgery [25]. In our study, the observed mortality was triple that expected by EuroScore II. Although it discriminated mortality and complications better than the ID, yet the wide gap between observed and expected values may be due to EuroScore II totally disregarding the important effect of time factor on outcome, whether the time delay between the implantation and the development of PVT [8, 10, 11]: the LPM or the speed by which the patient deteriorates: the MPM; which is the basis upon which the ID was founded [18]. Another important forgotten factor is the patient's compliance to OAC [11–15, 17]which is an independent predictor of deterioration, as expressed in terms of ID.

Conclusion

The simple two-factors based ID (NYHA deterioration and time) was never thought as a replacement for the well-known multifactorial scoring systems, but as a useful numeric index to monitor deterioration and predicting hospital progression and outcomes in patients presenting with PVT. It raised questions about the need to include the time factor and non-compliance to OAC in predicting outcomes in those patients. However, larger studies are needed to show if the index of deterioration can be helpful to take decisions during the course of management of those patients.

Abbreviations

AUC: Area under the curve; AVR: Aortic valve replacement; CABG: Coronary artery bypass grafts; ID: Index of deterioration; LPM: Latent period of malfunction; LVEF %: Left ventricular ejection fraction %; MPM: Manifest period of malfunction; MVR: Mitral valve replacement; NYHA: New York Heart Association Classification; OAC: Oral anticoagulant; PVT: Prosthetic valve thrombosis; SJ: St Jude

Acknowledgements

Not applicable

Authors' contributions

All the authors shared in the study design, collecting data, and calculating the results. AH, MG, and KR were the main persons in writing and revising this manuscript. AH was also responsible for the statistical analysis of the results. MG is the corresponding author; HM and KS were the surgeons operating on the included patients. All the authors have read and approved the submitted version of the manuscript.

References

1. Yau TM, El-Ghoneimi YA, Armstrong S, Ivanov J, David TE (2000) Mitral valve repair and replacement for rheumatic disease. J Thorac Cardiovasc Surg. 119:53–60
2. Templeton GF. The two-steps approach for transforming continuous variables to normal: implications and recommendations for IS research. Communications of the association for information systems: vol 28, Article 4: DOI: https://doi.org/10.17705/1CAIS.02804. Available at: https://aisel.aisnet.org/cais/vol28/iss1/4
3. Laplace G, Lafitte S, Labèque JN et al (2004) Clinical significance of early thrombosis after prosthetic mitral valve replacement: a postoperative mono- centric study of 680 patients. J Am Coll Cardiol 43:1283–1290
4. Wolberg AS, Aleman MM, Leiderman K et al (2012) Procoagulant activity in hemostasis and thrombosis: Virchow's triad revisited. Anesth Analg 114:275–285
5. Roudaut R, Serri K, Lafitte S (2007) Thrombosis of prosthetic heart valves: diagnosis and therapeutic considerations. Heart 93:137–142
6. Zoghbi WA, Chambers JB, Dumesnil JG et al (2009) Recommendations for evaluation of prosthetic valves with echocardiography and Doppler ultrasound. J Am Soc Echocardiogr 22:975–1014
7. Sun JC, Davidson MJ, Lamy A et al (2009) Antithrombotic management of patients with prosthetic heart valves: current evidence and future trends. Lancet 374:565–576
8. Blackstone EH, Kirklin JW (1985) Death and other time - related events after valve replacement. Circulation 72:753–767
9. Husebey DG, Pluth JR, Pielher JM, Schaff HV, Orzulak TA,Puga FY et al. Reoperation on prosthetic heart valves: an analysis of risk factors in 552 patients. JThorac Cardivasc Surg 1983; 86:543-552.
10. Lin SS, Tiong IY, Asher CR et al (2000) Prediction of thrombus-related mechanical prosthetic valve dysfunction using transesophageal echocardiog- raphy. J Am Coll Cardiol 86:1097–1101
11. Nicolas Dürrleman, Michel Pellerin, Denis Bouchard, Yves Hébert, Raymond Cartier, Louis P Perrault, Arsène Basmadjian, Michel Carrier. Prosthetic valve thrombosis: twenty-year experience at the Montreal Heart institute, J Thoracic Cardiovascular Surgery 2004; 127, 5: 1388-1392.
12. Lin SS, Tiong IY, Asher CR et al (2000) Prediction of thrombus-related mechanical prosthetic valve dysfunction using transesophageal echocardiog- raphy. J Am Coll Cardiol 86:1097–1101
13. Buttard P, Bonnefoy E, Chevalier P, Marcaz PB, Robin J, Obadia JF et al (1997) Mechanical cardiac valve thrombosis in patients in critical hemodynamic compromise. Eur J Cardiothorac Surg. 11:710–713
14. Toker ME, Eren E, Balkanay M, Kirali K, Yanartas M, Çaliskan A et al (2006) Multivariate analysis for operative mortality in obstructive prosthetic valve dysfunction due to pannus and thrombus formation. Int Heart J 47:237–245
15. Ahn H, Kim KH, Kim KC, Kim CY (2008) Surgical management of mechanical valve thrombosis: twenty-six years' experience. J Korean Med Sci 23:378–382
16. Gohlke-Bärwolf C (2000) Anticoagulation in valvar heart disease: new aspects and management during non-cardiac surgery. Heart 84:567–572
17. Sahnoun-Trabelsi I, Jimenez M, Choussat A et al (2004) Thromboses de prothèses valvulaires cardiaques chez la femme enceinte. Archives des maladies du coeur et des vaisseaux. 97:305–310
18. A. Hassouna. Index of deterioration of patients with prosthetic valve malfunctions. The Bulletin of the Egyptian Society of Cardiothoracic Surgery 1995; 3: 75 - 87.
19. Bortolotti U, Milano A, Mossuto E, Mazzaro E, Thiene G, Casarotto D (1994) Early and late outcome after reoperation for prosthetic valve dysfunction: analysis of 549 patients during a 26-year period. J Heart Valve Dis 3:81–87
20. Muhammad Sharoz Rabbani, Irfan Qadir, Yasir Ahmed, Marrium Gul, Hasanat Sharif Heart valve surgery: EuroSCORE vs. EuroSCORE II vs. Society of Thoracic Surgeons score Heart International 2014; 9(2):53-58.
21. Carlos Manuel de Almeida Branda˜o, Pablo Maria Alberto Pomerantzeff, Luciano Rapold Souza, Flavio Tarasoutchi, Max Grimberg, Jose' Antonio Franchini Ramires, Se'rgio Almeida de Oliveira. Multivariate analysis of risk factors for hospital mortality in valvular reoperations for prosthetic valve dysfunction. Euro J Cardio-thoracic Surgery 2002; 22: 922–926.
22. Online STS risk calculator. http://riskcalc.sts.org/stswebriskcalc/. Accessed 10 June 2020.
23. Ranucci M, Di Dedda U, Castelvecchio S et al (2016) In search of the ideal risk-scoring system for very high-risk cardiac surgical patients: a two-stage approach. J Cardiothorac Surg 11:13
24. Casalino S, Stelian E, Mangia F, Novelli E, Renzi L, Alessi C, Diena M (2007) Evaluation of the EuroSCORE in high risk patients undergoing cardiac surgery. Euro J Anaesthesiol 24:20
25. Grant SW, Hickey GL, Dimarakis L, Cooper G, Jenkins DP, Uppal R, Buchan L, Bridgewater B (2013) Performance of the EuroSCORE models in emergency cardiac surgery. Circulation 6(2):178–185

28

Outcome of MC3 ring annuloplasty for moderate and severe functional tricuspid regurgitation associated with rheumatic mitral valve disease

Shady Eid Al-Elwany, Yasser Shaban Mubarak and Yasser Ali Kamal*

Abstract

Background: To evaluate early and midterm outcomes of tricuspid ring annuloplasty using three-dimensional (3D) MC3 ring for treatment of functional tricuspid regurgitation (FTR) during mitral valve replacement for rheumatic valve disease.

Results: This prospective study included 105 patients who underwent repair for ≥ moderate tricuspid regurgitation (TR) during mitral valve replacement for rheumatic valve disease. Between January 2016 and December 2018, a group of 23 patients who underwent ring annuloplasty with Edward MC3 rings was compared to another group of 82 patients who underwent standard suture (DeVega) repair. The primary outcome was residual TR (≥ moderate TR). During an average follow-up period of 18.84 ± 9.90 months (range 3–33 months), the preoperative grade of TR improved significantly in both groups. The postoperative mean of TR in the MC3 group was significantly lower than that in the DeVega group (0.17 ± 0.49 versus 0.77 ± 0.93, $P = 0.004$). The rate of TR recurrence (≥ 2+ TR) was significantly higher after MC3 ring annuloplasty (4.3% versus 23.1%, $P = 0.03$). Freedom from mild TR was 30.5% in the DeVega group and 61% in the ring annuloplasty group ($P = 0.007$). Freedom from residual TR was 76.8% in the DeVega group and 95.7% in the ring annuloplasty group ($P = 0.04$).

Conclusions: The use of MC3 rings is a safe and effective alternative to DeVega repair for the management of FTR. However, further evaluation of long-term durability is recommended.

Keywords: Tricuspid valve, Functional tricuspid regurgitation, Suture annuloplasty, Ring annuloplasty

Background

Functional tricuspid regurgitation (FTR) is a common consequence with mitral valve disease (rheumatic, ischemic, degenerative, or dilated cardiomyopathy), secondary to dilation or dysfunction of the right ventricle, tricuspid annular dilatation, leaflet tethering, atrial fibrillation (AF), or pulmonary hypertension [1]. In patients with rheumatic heart disease (RHD), leaflet thickening and restriction of the tricuspid valve (TV) can result in FTR, but the incidence of organic TV involvement may be higher [2].

The available guidelines recommend the surgical treatment of severe FTR during valve surgery regardless of the presence of symptoms. However, in less than severe FTR, the decision for surgery is controversial, with a preference for surgery if there is a significant annular dilatation [1, 3].

Currently, the surgical techniques for FTR vary from suture repair to implantation of prosthetic rings. Since the first introduction of prosthetic rings for tricuspid annuloplasty in 1971, multiple ring designs have been developed to reinforce the tricuspid annulus by fixing the annulus during systole, restoring the physiologic valve geometry, reducing the annular dilatation, or restoring the 3D morphology [4]. The prosthetic rings for tricuspid annuloplasty have been categorized in

* Correspondence: Yasser.Ali@mu.edu.eg; yaser_ali_kamal@yahoo.com
Department of Cardiothoracic Surgery, Faculty of Medicine, Minia University, El-Minya 61519, Egypt

accordance with the degree of rigidity, the completeness of the circularity, and the dimensionality. Therefore, the prosthetic ring may be rigid or flexible, complete or incomplete, and planar or three dimensional (3D) [5, 6].

The MC3 ring (Edwards LifeScience, Irvine, CA, USA), the first 3D ring, was introduced to restore the geometry of the tricuspid annulus relying on the advantage of accommodating the 3D aspect of the tricuspid annulus [7]. In literature, some studies have reported favorable early outcomes of MC3 rings for the management of FTR during surgery for left-valve disease [8, 9].

Generally, there is good evidence supporting ring annuloplasty over De Vega's annuloplasty supporting its use for moderate to severe TR [6]. However, the data still limited regarding the specification of outcomes to the pathology of the heart valve disease and type of prosthetic ring. Therefore, this study aimed to evaluate our own experience with the early and midterm outcomes of tricuspid annuloplasty using MC3 ring for repair of FTR associated with rheumatic mitral valve disease, in comparison to outcomes of suture repair.

Methods

This prospective study evaluated early and midterm outcomes after operations for TV repair which were performed at our institution, between January 2016 and December 2018. The mean follow-up duration was 18.84 ± 9.90 months (range 3–33 months). The study included 105 patients who underwent repair for FTR during mitral valve replacement for rheumatic valve disease. There were 82 patients who underwent suture (DeVega) repair and 23 patients underwent ring annuloplasty using Edward MC3 incomplete 3D ring. The indications of surgery for FTR were (1) severe TR or (2) moderate TR with annular dilatation greater than 40 mm and/or preoperative systolic pulmonary artery pressure (SPAP) > 50 mmHg. We excluded patients with non-rheumatic mitral disease, combined mitral and aortic valve replacement, mitral valve repair, concomitant coronary artery or aortic surgery, mild or organic tricuspid regurgitation, emergency surgery, reoperations, or missed data. Based on echocardiographic data, the severity of TR was graded as 0 (no TR), 1+ (mild TR), 2+ (mild to moderate TR), 3+ (moderately severe TR), or 4+ (severe).

The type of tricuspid valve repair was chosen according to the surgeon's preference and echocardiographic criteria of TV. The DeVega repair was performed when the patient had minimal annular dilation and lower severity of pulmonary hypertension, while ring annuloplasty was performed in patients with severe tricuspid annular dilation and severe pulmonary hypertension. The DeVega repair was performed on a beating heart using pledget-supported two 4-0 polypropylene running parallel sutures. The MC3 ring annuloplasty was performed through right atriotomy using cardiopulmonary bypass and cardioplegic arrest. The ring size was determined after measurement of the length of the attachments of the tricuspid septal leaflet (the distance between the anteroseptal and septoposterior commissures) or the surface area of the anterior leaflet. The chosen ring was undersized by at least one size. The ring was implanted from the anteroseptal commissure to the middle of the septal leaflet. A series of 8 to10 mattress sutures with a 2-0 Ethibond multifilament suture were made on the tricuspid annulus starting from the center of the septal annulus to the anteroseptal commissure in the counter-clockwise direction, to avoid the atrioventricular conduction tissue. Thereafter, the sutures were placed through the sewing ring of the prosthesis (Fig. 1), followed by the lowering and securing of the ring to the annulus (Fig. 2).

The collected preoperative data included age, sex, New York Heart Association (NYHA) functional class, and the type of preoperative mitral valve disease. The primarily assessed postoperative outcome was residual TR (≥ moderate TR; ≥ grade + 2). Other assessed pre- and postoperative parameters included the NYHA functional class and echocardiographic data regarding the grade of TR, SPAP, tricuspid annulus (TA) diameter, tricuspid annular plane systolic excursion (TAPSE), left atrial diameter (LAD), left ventricular end-diastolic dimension (LVEDD), left ventricular end-systolic dimension (LVESD), and left ventricular ejection fraction (LVEF).

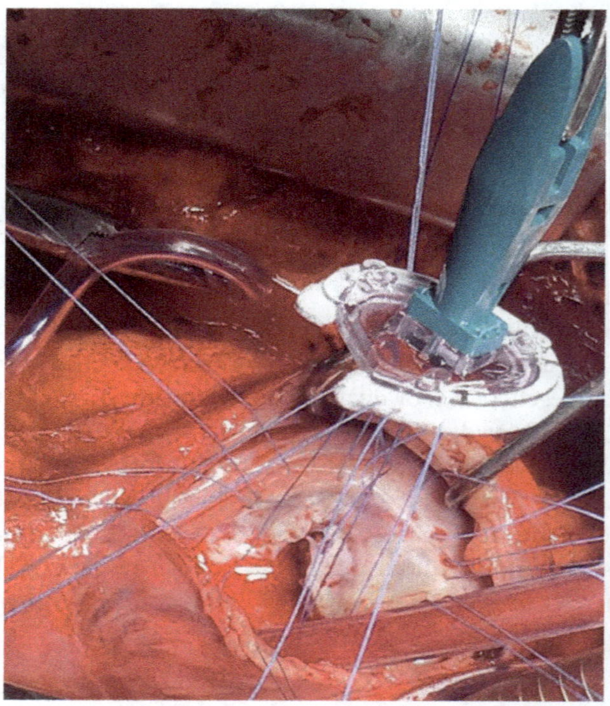

Fig. 1 Intra-operative view of the placement of the sutures through the sewing ring of the MC3 prosthesis

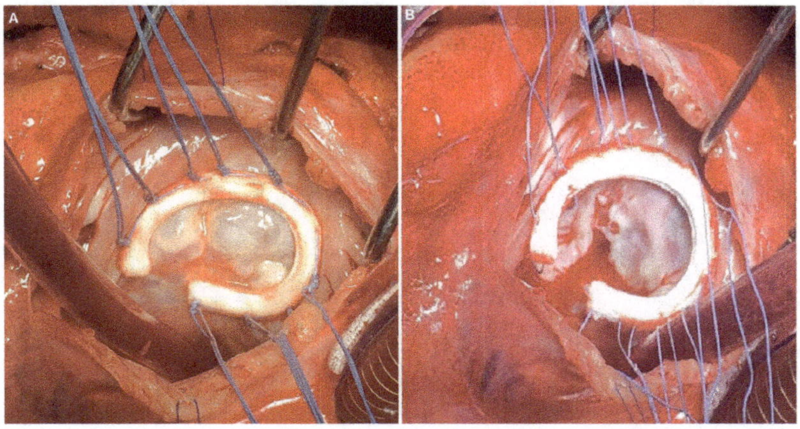

Fig. 2 Intra-operative view of lowering and securing of the MC3 ring to the tricuspid annulus. **a** During systole. **b** During diastole

Statistical analysis

The statistical analysis was performed using the SPSS software package (version 20.0; SPSS Inc., Chicago, IL, USA). The analyzed data were expressed as mean and standard deviation or as proportions. The studied groups were compared using the unpaired Student's *t* test for continuous independent variables and paired *t* test to compare related measurements. The categorical variables were compared using chi-squared test or Fisher's exact test if the expected frequency is less than 5. The Kaplan-Meier method was used to determine freedom from residual TR at the end of follow-up. *P* value < 0.05 was considered statistically significant.

Results

Preoperative demographic and clinical characteristics were similar between both groups (Table 1). There was a significant improvement in the preoperative grade of TR following surgery in each group (Fig. 3). There was no significant difference in the preoperative echocardiographic parameters between both groups of tricuspid annuloplasty regarding the grade of TR, SPAP, TA diameter, TAPSE, LAD, LVEDD, LVESD, and LVEF (Table 1).

Regarding comparisons of postoperative and baseline preoperative echocardiographic measurements in each group, there was a significant decrease in the mean of TR grade, SPAP, TA diameter, LAD, and LVESD in both groups, with a significant increase in the mean of LVEDD and LVEF. Moreover, there was a significant increase in the mean of postoperative TAPSE after MC3 ring annuloplasty (Table 2). Comparing the postoperative echocardiographic measurements between both groups revealed non-significant differences, except for the postoperative mean of TR in the MC3 group which was significantly lower than that in the DeVega repair group (0.17 ± 0.49 versus 0.77 ± 0.93, *P* = 0.004) (Table 3). The postoperative frequency of patients without TR (grade 0) in the MC3 group was significantly higher than that in the DeVega repair group (87% versus 51.2%, *P* = 0.002). The rate of TR recurrence (≥ 2+ TR) was significantly higher after MC3 ring annuloplasty (4.3% versus 23.1%, *P* = 0.03) (Table 4).

Regarding operative data and early postoperative outcomes (Table 5), the group of MC3 ring annuloplasty had significantly higher cardiopulmonary bypass (CPB) time (128.8 ± 24.7 min versus 141.9 ± 28.4 min, *P* = 0.03) and cross-clamp time (71.8 ± 23.7 min versus 84.3 ± 19.2

Table 1 Preoperative demographic, clinical, and echocardiographic data

Variables	DeVega (*n* = 82)	MC3 ring (*n* = 23)	*P* value
Age (years)	48 ± 11.8	46.2 ± 11.2	0.53
Female gender	53 (64.6%)	14 (60.9%)	0.74
NYHA class (III/IV)	52 (63.4%)	16 (69.6%)	0.58
Atrial fibrillation	45 (54.9%)	13 (56.6%)	0.88
Mitral valve disease			
Stenosis	18 (23.2%)	6 (26.1%)	0.68
Insufficiency	25 (30.5%)	4 (17.4%)	0.29
Stenosis and insufficiency	38 (46.3%)	13 (56.5%)	0.38
Preoperative TR grade	2.55 ± 0.61	2.39 ± 0.65	0.28
SPAP (mmHg)	47.87 ± 14.70	52.21 ± 15.43	0.21
TA diameter (mm)	34.62 ± 5.33	34.56 ± 5.56	0.96
TAPSE (mm)	18.23 ± 3.11	17.13 ± 2.76	0.12
LAD (mm)	42.97 ± 4.10	42.13 ± 4.33	0.39
LVEDD (mm)	42.34 ± 2.37	42.08 ± 2.87	0.66
LVESD (mm)	34.32 ± 1.79	34.21 ± 1.47	0.78
LVEF (%)	55.73 ± 8.93	55.13 ± 9.45	0.77

NYHA New York Heart Association, *TR* tricuspid regurgitation, *SPAP* systolic pulmonary artery pressure, *TA* tricuspid annulus, *TAPSE* tricuspid annular plane systolic excursion, *LAD* left atrial diameter, *LVEDD* left ventricular end-diastolic dimension, *LVESD* left ventricular end-systolic dimension, *LVEF* left ventricular ejection fraction

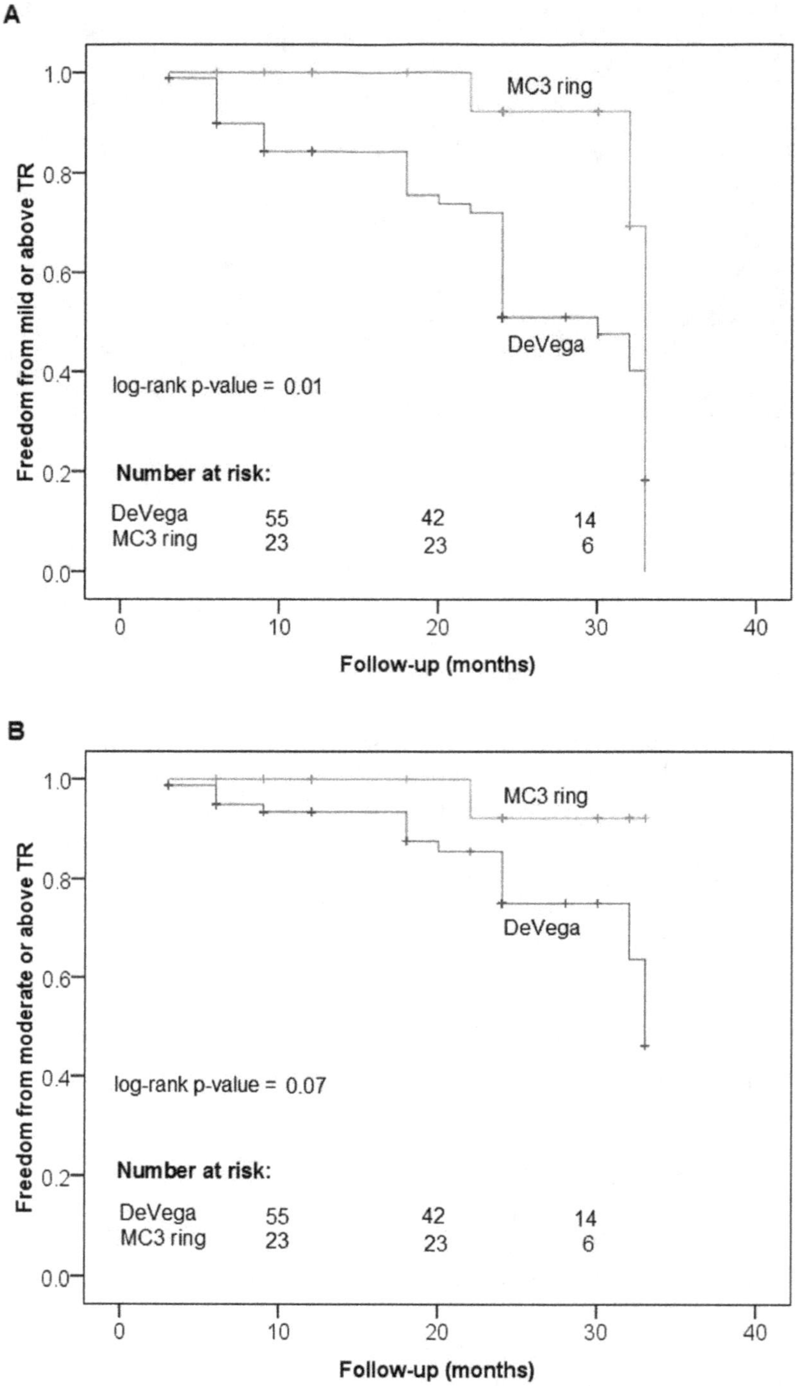

Fig. 3 **a** Freedom from ≥ mild tricuspid regurgitation (TR) after DeVega repair and MC3 ring annuloplasty. **b** Freedom from ≥ moderate tricuspid regurgitation (TR) after DeVega repair and MC3 ring annuloplasty

min, $P = 0.02$). There were no significant differences between both groups regarding the need for postoperative intraaortic balloon pump (IABP) support (2.4% versus 4.3%) and the incidence of heart block (1.2% versus 8.7%). During the follow-up period, freedom from mild TR was 30.5% in the DeVega group and 61% in the ring annuloplasty group ($P = 0.007$) (Fig. 3a). Freedom from residual TR was 76.8% in the DeVega group and 95.7% in the ring annuloplasty group ($P = 0.04$) (Fig. 3b).

Discussion

The repair of FTR in patients undergoing left heart valve surgery has a controversy among surgeons in terms of timing for intervention and technique of repair [10]. However, the persistence of moderate and severe TR after mitral valve surgery may lead to progressive heart failure or death [11].

The DeVega suture repair is the most commonly used technique of TV repair. However, high recurrence rates

Table 2 Mean difference between follow-up and preoperative echocardiographic data in relation to the type of tricuspid repair

Echocardiographic variables	DeVega ($n = 82$)		MC3 ring ($n = 23$)	
	Mean difference	*P* value	Mean difference	*P* value
TR grade	− 1.78	< 0.001*	− 2.22	< 0.001*
SPAP (mmHg)	− 15.35	< 0.001*	− 18.95	< 0.001*
TA diameter (mm)	− 4.20	< 0.001*	− 4.78	0.001*
TAPSE (mm)	+ 0.66	0.17	+ 1.87	0.02*
LAD (mm)	− 10.54	< 0.001*	− 8.96	< 0.001*
LVEDD (mm)	+ 0.16	0.001*	+ 2.22	0.002*
LVESD (mm)	− 1.28	< 0.001*	− 1.78	< 0.001*
LVEF (%)	+ 10.63	< 0.001*	+ 16.04	< 0.001*

TR tricuspid regurgitation, *SPAP* systolic pulmonary artery pressure, *TA* tricuspid annulus, *TAPSE* tricuspid annular plane systolic excursion, *LAD* left atrial diameter, *LVEDD* left ventricular end-diastolic dimension, *LVESD* left ventricular end-systolic dimension, *LVEF* left ventricular ejection fraction
*Significant difference between follow-up and preoperative values within the same group

have been reported with DeVega repair, particularly in patients with severe tricuspid annular dilation and/or pulmonary hypertension [12]. To overcome this issue, the search focused on the use of more anatomically relevant techniques for the management of FTR. For this purpose, ring annuloplasty has been used in the tricuspid position and achieved better results than suture repair [13–15]. The nonplanar, saddle-shaped, 3D structure, the tricuspid annulus favors the use of MC3 ring annuloplasty since its introduction in 2004 [16].

Table 3 Comparison of postoperative echocardiographic between types of tricuspid repair

Echocardiographic variables	DeVega ($n = 82$)	MC3 ring ($n = 23$)	*P* value
TR grade	0.77 ± 0.93	0.17 ± 0.49	0.004*
SPAP (mmHg)	32.52 ± 7.50	33.26 ± 8.83	0.69
TA diameter (mm)	30.42 ± 2.99	29.78 ± 3.20	0.37
TAPSE (mm)	18.89 ± 2.55	19 ± 2.81	0.85
LAD (mm)	32.43 ± 4.71	33.17 ± 5.22	0.52
LVEDD (mm)	43.50 ± 2.04	44.30 ± 1.22	0.07
LVESD (mm)	33.04 ± 1.46	32.43 ± 0.99	0.06
LVEF (%)	66.35 ± 2.07	66.73 ± 2.11	0.43

TR tricuspid regurgitation, *SPAP* systolic pulmonary artery pressure, *TA* tricuspid annulus, *TAPSE* tricuspid annular plane systolic excursion, *LAD* left atrial diameter, *LVEDD* left ventricular end-diastolic dimension, *LVESD* left ventricular end-systolic dimension, *LVEF* left ventricular ejection fraction
*Significant difference between follow-up and preoperative values within the same group

Our study compared early and midterm outcomes after MC3 ring annuloplasty in 23 patients with outcomes after DeVega repair in 82 patients, over an average follow-up period of 18.84 ± 9.90 months (range 3–33 months). We included patients with severe FTR or moderate TR with severe annular dilatation greater and/or pulmonary hypertension, and our primary outcome was residual TR (≥ moderate TR) during the follow-up period. The main findings in the present study are (1) the improvement of midterm echocardiographic parameters in both groups of tricuspid repair on comparison to preoperative values and (2) the superiority of MC3 ring annuloplasty in regards to lower postoperative grade of TR (0.17 ± 0.49 versus 0.77 ± 0.93, $P = 0.004$), lower recurrence rate of ≥ 2+ TR (4.3% versus 23.1%, $P = 0.03$), and higher midterm freedom from mild (61% versus 30.5%, $P = 0.007$) and moderate TR (95.7% versus 76.8%, $P = 0.04$). Additionally, we had acceptable incidences of heart block and postoperative use of IABP, beside the midterm absence of ring dehiscence, prosthetic ring endocarditis, and thromboembolic events.

Our favorable and superior outcomes after MC3 ring annuloplasty are comparable to other studies in literature [7–9, 16, 17]. The early study by Filsoufi et al. [7] included 75 patients with FTR with mean TR grade of 3.1 ± 0.9 and concomitant procedures of mitral valve repair, replacement, aortic valve replacement, coronary artery bypass grafting, and left atrial maze. The echocardiographic study demonstrated a stable significant decrease in TR (0.3 ± 0.5) after a median follow-up of 16 months (range 4–34), with no cases of ring dehiscence, prosthetic ring endocarditis, or thromboembolic events. The echocardiographic follow-up study by Fukuda et al. [16] of 136 patients with FTR confirmed the significant improvement in the severity of TR early after surgery and TR graded greater than moderate in 14% among patients followed more than 1 year. However, additional maneuvers to ensure valve competence were required in patients with extensive leaflet tethering. Jeong and Kim [8] investigated the clinical performance of MC3 rings in 103 patients with an average preoperative TR grade of 2.5 ± 0.8, during a mean follow-up of 26.7 ± 11.2 (range 0–52) months. The TR grade significantly decreased from 2.5 ± 0.8 preoperatively to 0.8 ± 0.8 before discharge ($P < 0.001$), which was stable through a median follow-up of 15 months. Additionally, there was a significant improvement in systolic pulmonary artery pressure. Moreover, comparing the outcomes of tricuspid annuloplasty with 3D-rigid versus flexible prosthetic ring for FTR in the study by Wang et al. [17] revealed that MC3 might be more effective for tricuspid ring annuloplasty in FTR in midterm postoperative periods regarding recurrence of TR in 30.3% of the rigid group versus 54.3% of the flexible group.

Table 4 Grades of tricuspid regurgitation at the last follow-up visit

Grades	DeVega ($n = 82$)		MC3 ring ($n = 23$)		P value
	N (%)	Mean follow-up (months)	N (%)	Mean follow-up (months)	
0	42 (51.2%)	23.5 ± 1.24	20 (87%)	20.5 ± 2	0.002*
1+	21 (25.6%)	28.3 ± 1	2 (8.7%)	32.7 ± 0.3	0.09
2+	16 (19.5%)	29.6 ± 0.92	1 (4.3%)	32.1 ± 0.18	0.11
3+	2 (2.4%)	32.7 ± 0.22	0 (0%)	–	1
4+	1 (1.2%)	32.6 ± 0.34	0 (0%)	–	1

SD standard deviation
*Significant difference

Overall, the midterm durability of MC3 rings and the superiority of the MC3 ring annuloplasty over the DeVega suture repair determined in our study and in other studies could be related to the superiority of the ring in remodeling of the TV annulus effectively compared to suture repair. Remodeling of the TV annulus could decrease the tension on suture lines, increase the leaflet coaptation, and prevent the recurrence of annular dilatation [18, 19].

Some authors investigated the predictors of midterm residual TR after MC3 ring annuloplasty [9, 20]. Little number of patients in our study was against multivariate regression analysis, but mentioning the results of these studies may be helpful for proper selection of patients for other surgical interventions with MC3 rings. Yoda et al. [9] investigated the midterm outcomes of MC3 ring in 136 patients with severe TR, or mild or moderate TR with pulmonary hypertension or TA dilatation. Although, the MC3 ring was effective for the correction of FTR, preoperative severe TR, left ventricular end-diastolic dimension > 70 mm, right ventricular dimension > 40 mm, dilated cardiomyopathy (DCM), and left ventriculoplasty associated with repair failure and residual TR. In the study by De Bonis et al. [20] tricuspid annuloplasty with the MC3 ring provided satisfactory early results in 135 patients which remain stable at mid-term follow-up of 22 ± 9.5 months (median 23 months). Those authors reported that the presence of other mechanisms besides annular dilatation (leaflet prolapse, pace-maker wires, and fibrotic leaflets' retraction) leads to residual TR after ring annuloplasty alone.

Interestingly, some authors developed certain methods in order to reduce the residual TR after MC3 ring annuloplasty, such as the placement of horizontal mattress sutures on the annulus beyond the anteroseptal commissure and away from the deemed atrioventricular node artery/vein [21], adjustment the point of fixation of the septal portion to the septal annulus [22], and septal plication technique [23]. These modifications are not the concern of our study, but its promising results encourage us to recommend its evaluation in the future studies.

In the present study, our finding of a significant increase in the postoperative TAPSE after MC3 ring annuloplasty in comparison to the preoperative values reflects more preservation of the global right ventricular function with MC3 rings. TAPSE is a parameter of global RV function which describes apex-to-base shortening. TAPSE correlates closely with the RVEF and has been found to be both highly specific and easy to measure [24].

Table 5 Operative data and early postoperative outcomes

Variables	DeVega ($n = 82$)	MC3 ring ($n = 23$)	P value
CBP time (min)	128.8 ± 24.7	141.9 ± 28.4	0.03*
Cross-clamp time (min)	71.8 ± 23.7	84.3 ± 19.2	0.02*
Postoperative IABP support	2 (2.4%)	1 (4.3%)	1
Heart block	1 (1.2%)	2 (8.7%)	0.11

CPB cardiopulmonary bypass, *IABP* intraaortic balloon pump
*Significant difference

Study limitations

This study is limited by being a single center experience, including a small number of patients. Moreover, the surgeon's preference directed the choice between DeVega repair and ring annuloplasty. Also, other types of annuloplasty rings were not available at our institution, and thus, it could not be compared to the 3D ring annuloplasty.

Conclusions

In conclusion, the low incidence of midterm residual TR and the preservation of the global right ventricular function after tricuspid annuloplasty using MC3 for FTR encourage its substitution to the traditional DeVega repair in patients with rheumatic mitral valve disease. However, there is a need to check its durability in long-term and randomized studies.

Abbreviations

AF: Atrial fibrillation; COPD: Chronic obstructive pulmonary disease; DM: Diabetes mellitus; FTR: Functional tricuspid regurgitation; LA: Left atrium; LAD: Left atrial diameter; LVEDD: Left ventricular end-diastolic dimension; LVEF: Left ventricular ejection fraction; LVEF: Left ventricular ejection fraction; LVESD: Left ventricular end-systolic dimension; NYHA: New York Heart Association; RHD: Rheumatic heart disease; SPAP: Systolic pulmonary artery pressure; TA: Tricuspid annulus; TAPSE: Tricuspid annular plane systolic excursion; TR: Tricuspid regurgitation; TV: Tricuspid valve

Acknowledgements

Not applicable

Authors' contributions

SEA conceived and planned the study and supervised the findings of the work. YSM conceived of the study, participated in its design and coordination, and helped to draft the manuscript. YAK participated in the design of the study, carried out the collection of the data and drafting the manuscript, and performed the statistical analysis. All authors cared for the patients. All authors read and approved the final manuscript.

References

1. Pozzoli A, Lapenna E, Vicentini L, Alfieri O, De Bonis M (2016) Surgical indication for functional tricuspid regurgitation at initial operation_ judging from long term outcomes. Gen Thorac Cardiovasc Surg 64(9):509
2. Shiran A, Sagie A (2009) Tricuspid regurgitation in mitral valve disease: incidence, prognostic implications, mechanism, and management. J Am Coll Cardiol 53(5):401–408
3. Nishimura RA, Otto CM, Bonow RO, Carabello BA, Erwin JP 3rd, Guyton RA et al (2014) AHA/ACC guideline for the management of patients with valvular heart disease: executive summary: a report of the American College of Cardiology/American Heart Association Task Force on Practice Guidelines. J Am Coll Cardiol 63(22):2438–2488
4. Belluschi I, Del Forno B, Lapenna E, Nisi T, Iaci G, Ferrara D et al (2018) Surgical techniques for tricuspid valve disease. Front Cardiovasc Med 5:118
5. Lee SI, Kim HJ, Kim JB, Jung SH, Choo SJ, Chung CH et al (2017) Medtronic Duran AnCore versus Edwards MC3 rings for tricuspid annuloplasty. Interact Cardiovasc Thorac Surg 24(6):848–854
6. Khorsandi M, Banerjee A, Singh H, Srivastava AR (2012) Is a tricuspid annuloplasty ring significantly better than a De Vega's annuloplasty stitch when repairing severe tricuspid regurgitation? Interact Cardiovasc Thorac Surg 15(1):129–135
7. Filsoufi F, Salzberg SP, Coutu M, Adams DH (2006) A three dimensional ring annuloplasty for the treatment of tricuspid regurgitation. Ann Thorac Surg 81:2273–2278
8. Jeong DS, Kim KH (2010) Tricuspid annuloplasty using the MC3 ring for functional tricuspid regurgitation. Circ J 74:278–283
9. Yoda M, Tanabe H, Kadoma Y, Suma H (2011) Mid-term results of tricuspid annuloplasty using the MC3 ring for secondary tricuspid valve regurgitation. Interact Cardiovasc Thorac Surg 13:7–10
10. Khallaf AN, Saleh HZ, Elnaggar AM, Rasekh FS (2016) Tricuspid valve repair by DeVega technique versus ring annuloplasty in patients with functional severe tricuspid regurge. J Egypt Soc Cardio Thorac Surg 24:131–134
11. Munasur M, Naidoo D (2016) Underlying rheumatic disease: an important determinant of outcome in tricuspid valve repair. J Heart Valve Dis 25(2): 203–210
12. Rivera R, Duran E, Ajuria M (1985) Carpentier's flexible ring versus De Vega's annuloplasty. A prospective randomized study. J Thorac Cardiovasc Surg 89: 196–203
13. Gatti G, Maffei G, Lusa AM, Pugliese P (2001) Tricuspid valve repair with the Cosgrove-Edwards annuloplasty system: early clinical an echocardiographic results. Ann Thorac Surg 72:764–767
14. Onoda K, Yasuda F, Takao M, Shimono T, Tanaka K, Shimpo H et al (2000) Long-term follow-up after Carpentier-Edwards ring annuloplasty for tricuspid regurgitation. Ann Thorac Surg 70:796–799
15. Tang GL, David TE, Singh SK, Maganti MD, Armstrong S, Borger MA (2006) Tricuspid valve repair with an annuloplasty ring results in improved long-term outcomes. Circulation 114(Suppl I):I-577–I-581
16. Fukuda S, Saracino G, Matsumura Y, Daimon M, Tran H, Greenberg NL et al (2006) Three-dimensional geometry of the tricuspid annulus in healthy subjects and in patients with functional tricuspid regurgitation: a real-time, 3-dimensional echocardiographic study. Circulation 114:1492–1498
17. Wang H, Liu X, Wang X, Lv Z, Liu X, Xu P (2016) Comparison of outcomes of tricuspid annuloplasty with 3D-rigid versus flexible prosthetic ring for functional tricuspid regurgitation secondary to rheumatic mitral valve disease. J Thorac Dis 8(11):3087–3095
18. Carpentier A, Deloche A, Dauptain J, Soyer R, Blondeau P, Piwnica A et al (1971) A new reconstructive operation for correction of mitral and tricuspid insufficiency. J Thorac Cardiovasc Surg 61:1–13
19. Guenther T, Mazzitelli D, Noebauer C, Hettich I, Tassani-Prell P, Voss B et al (2013) Tricuspid valve repair: is ring annuloplasty superior? Eur J Cardiothorac Surg 43:58 65
20. De Bonis M, Lapenna E, Taramasso M, Manca M, Calabrese MC, Buzzatti N et al (2012) Mid-term results of tricuspid annuloplasty with a three-dimensional remodelling ring. J Card Surg 27(3):288–294
21. Hata H, Fujita T, Shimahara Y, Sato S, Kobayashi J (2014) Early and mid-term outcomes of aggressive tricuspid annuloplasty with the MC3 ring. J Heart Valve Dis 23(5):601–608
22. Isomura T, Hirota M, Hoshino J, Fukada Y, Kondo T, Takahashi Y (2015) Tricuspid annuloplasty with the MC3 ring and septal plication technique. Asian Cardiovasc Thorac Ann 23(1):5–10
23. Kawaura H, Aoki A, Omoto T, Maruta K, Iizuka H (2015) Effect of the septal adjustment technique for tricuspid annuloplasty with an MC3 ring. Gen Thorac Cardiovasc Surg 63(5):273–278
24. Ueti OM, Camargo EE, Ueti Ade A, de Lima-Filho EC, Nogueira EA (2002) Assessment of right ventricular function with Doppler echocardiographic indices derived from tricuspid annular motion: comparison with radionuclide angiography. Heart 88(3):244–248

29

A case of needle embolism in a drug abuser, a diagnostic and therapeutic challenge

Valentina Scheggi[1*], Tiziano Mariani[2], Carlotta Mazzoni[2] and Pier Luigi Stefàno[3]

Abstract

Background: Needle embolism is a rare complication of intravenous habit. Clinical manifestations include recurrent pericarditis, tamponade, cardiac perforation, and infective endocarditis. We describe the case of needle embolization in a young intravenous opiate abuser.

Case presentation: We describe a rare complication of intravenous misuse in a 23-year-old patient. He presented at the emergency department with chest pain and shortness of breath. He complained of remittent fever ensued 6 months before. Echocardiographic and radiologic images revealed pericardial effusion and a needle fragment inside the pericardium. The needle was removed through left-anterior mini-thoracotomy, after CT-guided carbon tracking.

Conclusions: The presence of a foreign body within the heart resulted from the migration of a needle fragment from a peripheral vessel. It caused fever and recurrent pericarditis. In similar cases, surgical extraction is the therapy of choice.

Keywords: Cardiac tamponade, Embolism, Needle, Pericardial effusion, Drug abuse

Background

Needle embolism may be a rare complication of intravenous drug abusers, which has only been reported on rare occasions. Potential sequelae include cardiac perforation, tamponade, infective endocarditis, and recurrent pericarditis [1, 2].

A foreign body within the heart may result either from a direct injury to the heart or from embolization to the heart from distal sites, such as the migration of a needle fragment or a catheter from a peripheral vessel [1].

The embolism of fragments into the heart is favoured by reduced vascular turbulence and by the presence of hypotension, and it depends on the patient's position and the weight and shape of the foreign body; lower weight and smaller calibre facilitate embolization [2–4].

Foreign bodies can be trapped in the right cavities of the heart within the trabeculae of the endocardium with a fibrosis process, not causing clinical symptoms [5].

The most common symptomatic clinical manifestations are fever, pericarditis, and pericardial effusion, hemopericardium, arrhythmias, and also the formation of intracavitary thrombi. Fever is often the result of infection of the pericardium and/or endocardium by contaminated needle fragments [6].

Recurrent pericarditis and pericardial effusion, often due to an irritative stimulus given by the foreign body, are quite common in patients treated conservatively [7].

* Correspondence: scheggiv@aou-careggi.toscana.it; valentina.scheggi@gmail.com
All authors take responsibility for all aspects of the reliability of the data presented and their discussed interpretation.
[1]Division of Cardiovascular and Perioperative Medicine, Cardiothoracovascular Department, Azienda Ospedaliero-Universitaria Careggi and University of Florence, Largo Brambilla 3, 50133 Florence, Italy
Full list of author information is available at the end of the article

Case presentation

A 23-year-old heroin-addicted man was admitted to our department because of chest pain ensued 6 months before; the pain was sharp, was relieved by sitting up and leaning forward, and increased with coughing and swallowing. He also complained of fatigue and fever for 1 month before the presentation. His previous medical history was unremarkable. Echocardiography revealed non-haemodynamic pericardial effusion and right-sided pleural effusion, treated with thoracentesis. Three blood culture samples were negative. Cardiac biomarkers were negative. Human immunodeficiency virus (HIV), hepatitis B virus (HBV), and hepatitis C virus (HCV) serology were negative. He was treated with colchicine and ibuprofen and empiric antibiotic therapy with an initial improvement of symptoms. Echocardiography showed a progressive reduction of the effusion. The chest X-ray confirmed the pleural effusion resolution, with no other relevant findings. The diagnosis at discharge was idiopathic pericarditis. After 4 weeks from the discharge, the patient presented a recurrence of symptoms needing new access to the emergency care department. At admission, he was normotensive and apyretic; initial laboratory exams showed a white blood cell count of 15 K/μL and C-reactive protein of 105 mg/L.

An electrocardiogram showed widespread concave ST-segment elevation, and an echocardiogram revealed pericardial effusion relapse.

Chest radiography showed an unusual image near the right ventricle. The patient underwent computed tomography angiography that was able to localize a needle inside the pericardium (Fig. 1). A second echocardiogram confirmed the presence of the fragment in the pericardial cavity, beside the right ventricle (Fig. 2).

Before surgery, we performed a CT-guided carbon tracking of the needle.

The patient underwent left-anterior mini-thoracotomy, through the fifth intercostal space, with incision of the parietal pericardial layer and removal of 500 mL of haemorrhagic pericardial fluid.

The needle was easily found near the right ventricle, embedded in the thoracic wall, and was cautiously removed with a surgical needle driver (Fig. 3); it had an extremity inside the pericardial space, but without ventricular muscle laceration. After surgery, pericardial drainage was positioned; it was removed after 2 days because of the absence of fluid.

The patient's condition remained stable, and he was discharged home 1 week after surgery; echocardiography demonstrated the absence of pericardial effusion. Therapy at discharge included colchicine and ibuprofen. At the 2-month follow-up, he was asymptomatic, with a normal value of white blood cell and C-reactive protein and without pericardial effusion. In our case report, the foreign body penetrated the right cavities of the heart, embolizing through the venous bed.

Pericarditis resulted from the inflammation of the epicardium, due to the movement of the heart against the foreign body, which caused pericardial bleeding and local immune response; if untreated, this process may evolve in constrictive pericarditis [8].

The repeated use of intravenous drugs in numerous sites increases the likelihood of finding broken needle fragments. Given the location of the foreign body and the symptomatic presentation of the patient, we performed surgery to remove the foreign body [9].

An alternative therapeutic option for removal of foreign bodies from the heart is the percutaneous approach, with the use of a guidewire through the femoral vein and a magnet at its distal end. This is applicable only for small, intracavitary foreign bodies [10].

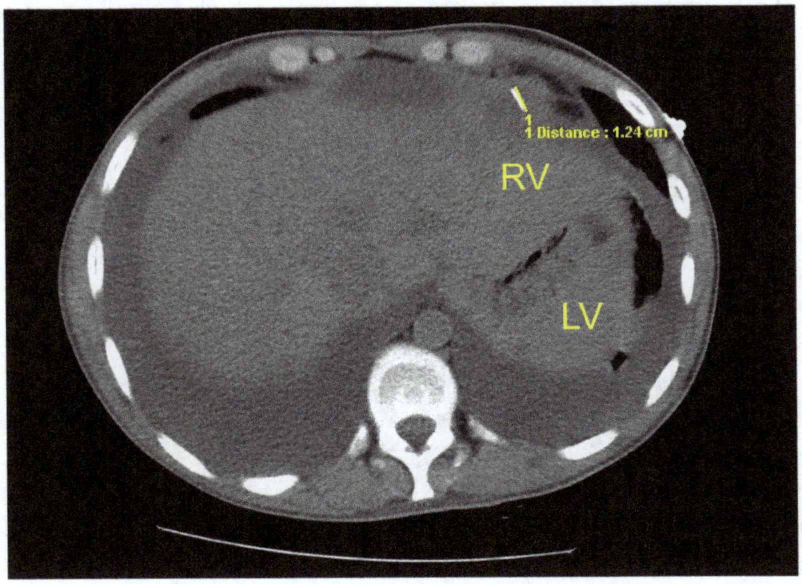

Fig. 1 Thoracic CT without contrast showing the needle beside the pericardium. RV, right ventricle; LV, left ventricle

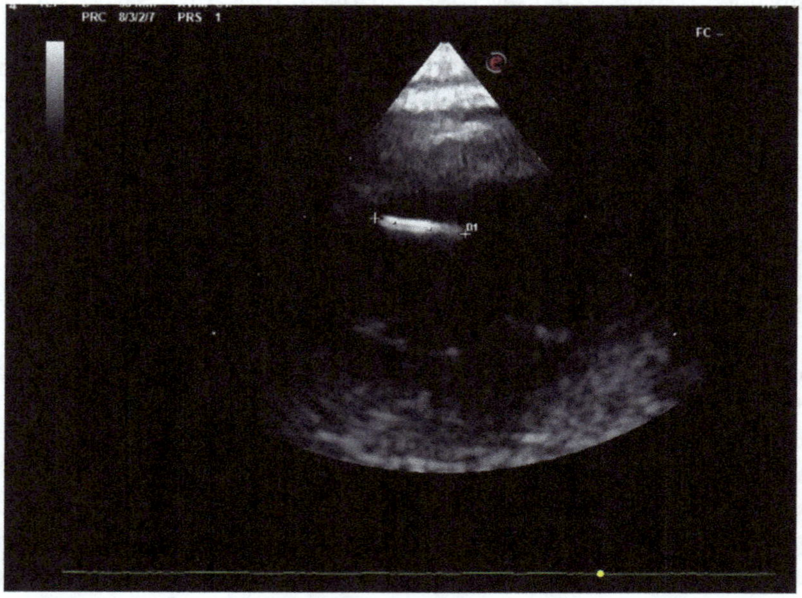

Fig. 2 Echographic image of the needle and the pericardial effusion

The management of foreign bodies in the heart should be individualized: (1) symptomatic foreign bodies should be removed, no matter their location; (2) asymptomatic foreign bodies diagnosed immediately after the injury with a high risk of infection, embolization, or erosions should be removed; (3) asymptomatic foreign bodies without associated risk factors or diagnosed late after the injury may be treated conservatively, particularly if they are completely embedded within the myocardium or the pericardium [5].

To our knowledge, only a few cases of needle embolization in pulmonary vasculature or inside the right heart are reported in the literature, most of them in drug abusers or after iatrogenic accidents [9–15].

Moreover, the literature describes different kinds of foreign bodies reaching the heart from peripheral sites, such as oral ingestion of safety pins causing cardiac injury or pericardial effusion, after migration through the lower oesophagus wall [16–18].

Other causes of foreign body embolization in the right heart and in the pulmonary artery are iatrogenic complications, such as embolization of inferior vena cava filter fragments [19, 20], or needle-like cement after percutaneous vertebroplasty [21], or embolization of subdermal contraceptive implants [22], all causing cardiac or pulmonary injury.

Conclusions

In drug abuse patients, we must consider the possibility of needle embolization. The medical history of these patients is sometimes difficult to acquire. In a drug abuse patient with recurrent pericardial disease, the hypothesis of a foreign body embolization, as in this case, should be part of the differential diagnosis.

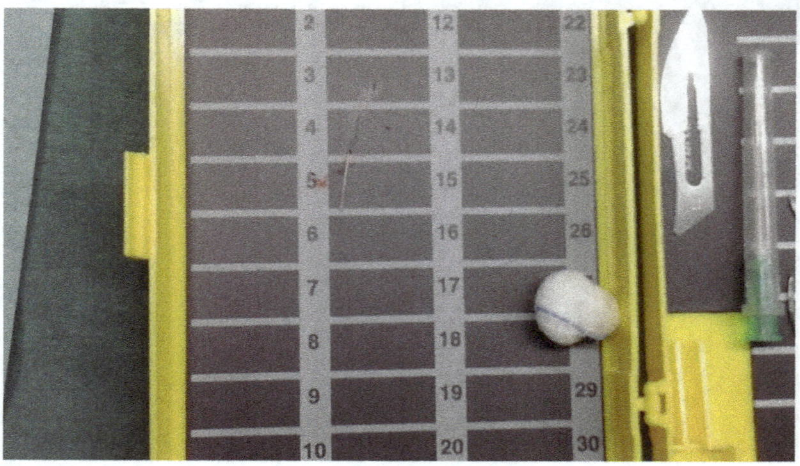

Fig. 3 The needle after surgical extraction

Abbreviations
HIV: Human immunodeficiency virus; HBV: Hepatitis B virus; HCV: Hepatitis C virus

Acknowledgements
Not applicable

Authors' contributions
VS made the diagnosis and followed the patient. VS and TM wrote the paper. CM revised the manuscript. PLS performed the surgical intervention. All authors read and approved the final manuscript.

Author details
[1]Division of Cardiovascular and Perioperative Medicine, Cardiothoracovascular Department, Azienda Ospedaliero-Universitaria Careggi and University of Florence, Largo Brambilla 3, 50133 Florence, Italy. [2]Division of General Cardiology, Cardiothoracovascular Department, Azienda Ospedaliero-Universitaria Careggi and University of Florence, Florence, Italy. [3]Division of Cardiac Surgery, Cardiothoracovascular Department, Azienda Ospedaliero-Universitaria Careggi and University of Florence, Florence, Italy.

References

1. Kim YJ, Kim JY, Choi BW, Nam JE, Kim TH, Choe KO (2006) Right ventricular acupuncture needle embolism detected on coronary computed tomography angiography. Circulation. 114:e623–e626
2. Wojda TR, Dingley SD, Wolfe S, Terzian WTH, Thomas PG, Vazquez D, Sweeney J, Stawicki SP (2017) Foreign intravascular object embolization and migration: bullets, catheters, wires, stents, filters, and more. https://doi.org/10.5772/68039
3. Gandhi SK, Marts BC, Mistry BM, Brown JW, Durham RM, Mazuski JE (1996) Selective management of embolized intracardiac missiles. Ann Thorac Surg 62:290–292
4. Shannon JJ, Vo NM, Stanton PE Jr, Dimler M (1987) Peripheral arterial missile embolization: a case report and 22-year literature review. J Vasc Surg 5:773–778
5. Actis Dato GM, Arslanian A, Di Marzio P, Filosso PL, Ruffini E (2003) Post traumatic and iatrogenic foreign bodies in the heart: report of fourteen cases and review of the literature. J Thorac Cardiovasc Surg 126:408–414
6. Roberts WC (2005) Pericardial heart disease: its morphologic features and its causes. Proc (Baylor Univ Med Cent) 18(1):38–55
7. Khandaker MH, Espinosa RE, Nishimura RA, Sinak LJ, Hayes SN, Melduni RM, Oh JK (2010) Pericardial disease: diagnosis and management. Mayo Clin Proc 85(6):572–593
8. LeMaire SA, Wall MJ Jr, Mattox KL (1998) Needle embolus causing cardiac puncture and chronic constrictive pericarditis. Ann Thorac Surg 65(6):1786–1787
9. Norfolk GA, Gray SF (2003) Intravenous drug users and broken needles–a hidden risk? Addiction 98:1163–1166
10. Bompotis G, Karkanis G, Chatziavramidis A (2016) Percutaneous removal of a tiny needle fracture from the right ventricle of the heart in a drug abuser. Vasc Endovasc Surg 50:575–578
11. Monroe EJ, Tailor TD, McNeeley MF, Lehnert BE (2012) Needle embolism in intravenous drug abuse. Radiology Case Reports 7:714
12. Yen AF, Homer CM, Mohapatra A, Langnas E, Gomez A, Hendrickson CM (2019) Embolic hypodermic needle causing traumatic cardiac tamponade: a case report. Crit Care Explor 1(8):e0038
13. Levy M, Hahn B, Aycock R (2019) Needle embolization: suspecting needle migration in intravenous drug abusers. J Emerg Med S0736-4679(19):30819-30814
14. Dell'Amore A, Ammari C, Campisi A, D'Andrea R (2016) Peripheral venous catheter fracture with embolism into the pulmonary artery. J Thorac Dis 8: E1581–E1584
15. Danek BA, Kuchynka P, Palecek T, Cerny V, Hlavacek K, Lambert L, Nemecek E, Podzimkova J, Linhart A (2016) Needle fragment embolism into the right ventricle: a rare cause of chest pain case report and literature review. Wien Klin Wochenschr 128(5-6):215–220
16. Sugunan S, Ajith Krishnan AS, Devakumar VK, Arif AK (2018) Safety-pin induced hemopericardium and cardiac tamponade in an infant. Indian Pediatr 55(6):521 522
17. Kalayci AG, Baysal K, Uysal S et al (2002) Hemopericardium caused by ingested safety pin. Endoscopy. 34:93
18. Choudhary S, Pujar Venkateshacharya S, Reddy C (2016) Sewing needle: a rare cause of intra-cardiac foreign body in a 3-year-old child. Cardiol Young 26:1425–1427
19. Shennib H, Bowles B, Hickle K (2014) Migration of a fractured inferior vena cava filter strut to the right ventricle of the heart: a case report. J Cardiothorac Surg 9:183
20. Kalavakunta JK, Thomas CS, Gupta V (2009) A needle through the heart: rare complication of inferior vena caval filters. J Invasive Cardiol 21:E221–E223
21. Kong M, Xu X, Shen J, Liu Q, Wang G (2019) Clinical characteristics and management of cardiac and/or pulmonary cement embolus after percutaneous vertebroplasty: a single center experience. Ann Transl Med 7(16):372
22. Hindy JR, Souaid T, Larus CT, Glanville J, Aboujaoude R (2020) Nexplanon migration into a subsegmental branch of the pulmonary artery: a case report and review of the literature. Medicine (Baltimore) 99(4):e18881

Pulmonary bullet embolism following cardiac gunshot wound: case report of a bullet that traversed the heart twice

Delan Ahmed Bakir[1], Yad N. Othman[1] and Abdulsalam Y. Taha[2*]

Abstract

Background: Cardiac gunshot wounds with bullet embolism (BE) into the pulmonary artery are rare. Most pulmonary BE follow injuries of peripheral veins without concomitant cardiac injury. Herein, we describe a case of cardiac gunshot injury in which the bullet migrated from right atrium through the inferior vena cava down to right internal iliac vein and back to the left pulmonary artery. Such bullet migration is too rare and unusual and to our knowledge not reported before.

Case presentation: On March 4, 2019, a man of 39 had a bullet injury during celebratory gunfire. He was clinically stable with entrance on right posterior chest but no exit. Chest CT scan showed a bullet in the right atrium. The next day, the bullet migrated to the right pelvis as shown by plain chest and pelvic radiographs. CT angiography 3 weeks afterwards displayed the bullet in the right internal iliac vein. Meanwhile, the patient was asymptomatic, thus discharged home. However, 3 months later, he was readmitted because of chest pain, dyspnea, and sweating. A repeat chest CT scan showed the bullet in the left lower lobe pulmonary artery. Hence, pulmonary BE was suspected and eventually a 0.36 bullet was removed via left thoracotomy.

Conclusions: This is a case of symptomatic venous BE with typical diagnostic criteria (a small low-velocity bullet with inlet but no exit located away from anticipated trajectory with migration proven by serial radiographs). Endovascular removal was preferred but was not available. BE of the heart is exceedingly rare. Hence, diagnosis requires a high degree of clinical awareness.

Keywords: Cardiac gunshot wound, Bullet, Pulmonary embolism, Inferior vena cava, Internal iliac vein, Case report

Background

To understand the effects of a bullet injury on the body, a range of factors should be considered. Besides the diameter of the bullet and its velocity, entrance profile and path of the bullet inside the body are important as well as the biological characteristics of the injured organ. Most high velocity bullets enter and leave the body in a straight trajectory while low velocity bullets may divert through bones or soft tissues and remain lodged, or may yet penetrate vessels, cardiac walls [1], or bowel [2] and behave as bullet emboli (BE) [3].

* Correspondence: abdulsalam.taha@univsul.edu.iq
[2]Department of surgery, Unit of Cardiovascular and Thoracic Surgery, School of Medicine, Faculty of Medical Sciences, University of Sulaimani, Sulaimaniyah, Kurdistan, Iraq
Full list of author information is available at the end of the article

The first instance of a traumatic projectile embolism was published by Thomas Davis in 1834, when he reported a case of a wooden fragment that embolized from the venous circulation to the right ventricle in a 10-year old boy [3–5]. Bullet embolus to the pulmonary artery was first reported by Moresten in 1903 (Moresten cited in [2]). Bullet embolism is a rare phenomenon in trauma [6], with only 300 cases published before 2011 [4]. A review of 7500 gunshot wounds during the Vietnam War demonstrated a 0.3% incidence of bullet embolism [5, 6]. In the Afghanistan and Iraq Wars, a 1.1% (4/346) incidence rate was reported. The true incidence in the civilian population is largely unknown. However, the rate may be higher given the prevalence of lower velocity weapons and lower kinetic energy [7].

Bullet emboli are either arterial (75%) or venous (20%). Very occasionally, BE may pass from veins to arteries (or vice versa) through a traumatic arteriovenous fistula (AVF) or an intra-cardiac communication [2, 4, 7]. Such (paradoxical) BE constituted 2.4% of emboli in Springer et al.'s review (Springer et al. cited in [4]) while they reached 5% in other reports [2, 7].The phrase "venous bullet emboli" refers to emboli to the right heart or pulmonary arteries [7].

Eighty percent of arterial BE produce early symptoms due to obstruction of distal arteries and hence require early endovascular or surgical removal. In regard to venous BE, 83% travel in the direction of venous blood flow into a bigger proximal vein, right heart, or pulmonary arteries while a minority (15%) are carried distally by gravity. Unlike arterial BE, symptoms of venous BE are usually late and confined to just one-third of cases. Consequently, treatment of venous BE has remained controversial [1, 4, 5].

Migration of bullets into the pulmonary artery is described most often with lesions of peripheral veins without concomitant cardiac involvement [8]. Gunshot wounds of the heart with migration of the bullet into the pulmonary artery are rare [2, 8]. Herein, we present a very rare case of bullet embolism from the right atrium (RA) to right internal iliac vein and back to right heart and left pulmonary artery in which the patient survived trans-thoracic extraction of the bullet from left lower pulmonary lobar artery. This work has been reported in line with the CARE criteria [9]. The management of bullet embolism in the literature is reviewed and discussed.

Case presentation

On March 4, 2019, a man of 39 received a low-velocity bullet injury. It was an accidental bullet falling from a height. After a CT scan of the chest revealing a bullet in RA and a moderate right-sided hemothorax, the patient was referred next day to our teaching hospital for further care.

Luckily, the patient on arrival to our hospital was clinically stable apart from mild shortness of breath (SOB) and slight hypotension. There was a 4-cm non-bleeding wound located in right 6th intercostal space 7-cm lateral to the spine. Air entry on right lower back was reduced. Heart sounds were muffled, abdomen was soft on palpation, and peripheral pulses were palpable. His vital signs were a Bp of 95/55 mmHg, pulse rate (PR) of 110 bpm, and O_2 saturation (PSO_2) of 91% that increased to 96% with O_2 supplementation via a mask.

Unfortunately, neither the CT scan films nor reports were brought with him. Therefore, a chest X-ray (CXR) was ordered. The hemothorax was evident but no bullet was seen in the region of the chest. A chest tube was placed and drained 400 cc of blood (Fig. 1a). To our surprise, the bullet had descended to the right pelvis as shown by a plain pelvic film (Fig. 1b). When the initial CT scan of the chest (Fig. 1c, d) was reviewed later, the

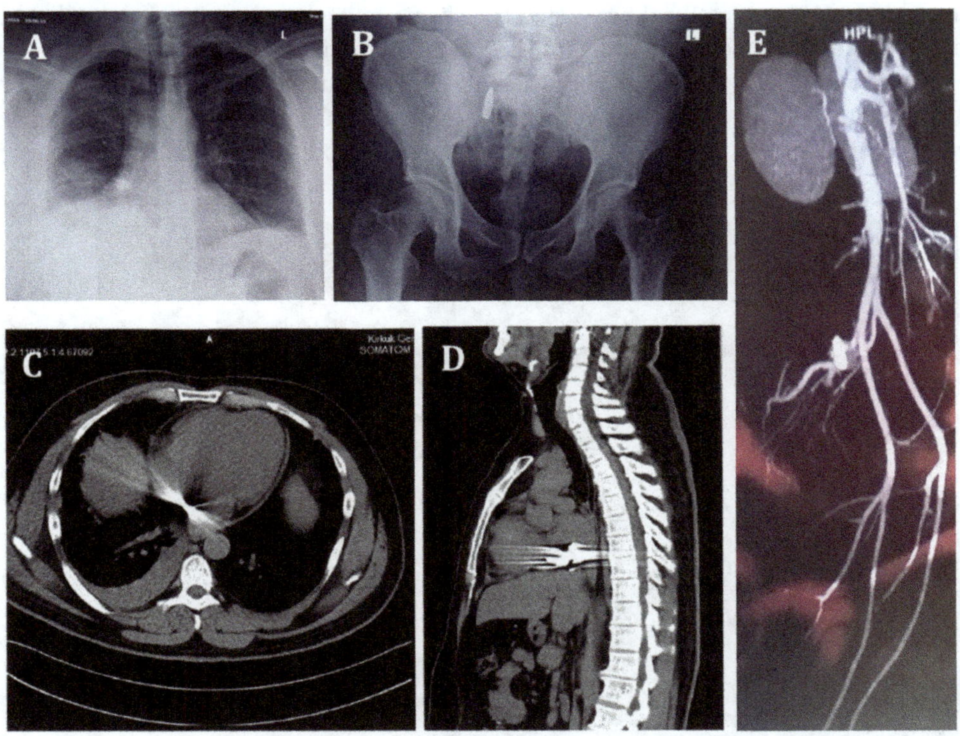

Fig. 1 **a** Right-sided hemothorax drained by closed tube thoracostomy. **b** Bullet migrated to right pelvis. **c**, **d** First day CT scan of the chest showing a bullet in the right atrium with moderate right sided hemothorax. **e** CT angiography showing the bullet adjacent to iliac artery mostly in the right internal iliac vein

bullet was seen in RA along with mild pericardial effusion, and hence, a migrating bullet was our provisional diagnosis. Doppler ultrasonography revealed normal abdominal vessels and failed to locate the bullet. CT angiography was arranged (Fig. 1e) and showed the bullet outside the arterial tree but adjacent to iliac arteries (most likely inside the right internal iliac vein). Meanwhile, the chest drainage ceased and chest tube was removed after 5 days.

Although our patient had no evidence of arterial or venous occlusion, we advised him for surgical exploration to extract the bullet and save him from potential complications of a bullet migrating in the major abdominal veins. Unfortunately, the patient refused surgery and left the hospital despite our warnings.

The dramatic change occurred 3 months later when the patient was re-admitted due to sudden onset of SOB, chest pain, and sweating which gradually worsened. On examination, he had a rapid pulse but normal blood pressure. CT scan of the chest (Fig. 2a) revealed a new surprise! The bullet was seen in left pulmonary artery. An urgent left thoracotomy was done and a 0.36 in caliber bullet (Fig. 2b) was extracted from a basal branch of left pulmonary artery. The patient had an uneventful recovery and left the hospital 4 days after surgery. He was in a stable condition when seen 2 months later. The path of bullet migration is displayed by Fig. 3.

Discussion

A bullet embolism occurs when a small-caliber, usually low-velocity bullet, penetrates a single vessel wall and remains within the circulation [4, 5]. Nearly all of the cases in literature involve bullets 0.38 in caliber and smaller, with only one recorded case of a 0.40 in caliber bullet embolism [4]. In our case, the bullet caliber was equivalent to 0.36 in with an inlet but no exit. An inconsistent number of entry and exit wounds may be indicative of a retained bullet or projectile [4, 5]. Moreover, bullet embolism should be suspected when a bullet lies outside the established trajectory, or a wandering bullet is demonstrated on radiographs [5]. A whole body radiography ± CT scan are often needed to make the diagnosis while angiography is usually reserved for supplementary diagnosis or may be used as therapeutic endovascular extraction procedure [1].

Venous BE may be complicated by pulmonary embolism, cardiac valve dysfunction, endocarditis, abscess formation, venous thrombosis, dysrhythmias, intraventricular communications, tissue erosion, hemorrhage, and cardiac ischemia. It is of interest to note that such complications may not occur immediately after the initial injury but may develop months, years, and even decades later [1, 4, 5].

In the presence of symptoms, venous BE undoubtedly warrant removal preferably with endovascular techniques. It has been proposed that objects > 5 mm in diameter, irregularly shaped, freely mobile, or only partially embedded within the myocardium should be considered for extraction [4, 5]. Hartzler reported percutaneous transvenous removal of a bullet from the right ventricle in 1980 (Hartzler cited in [4]). Six years later, Ruff et al. reported the removal of a bullet from the hepatic vein with a retrieval basket [3]. Currently, the endovascular techniques are increasingly employed for retrieval of venous, intracardiac, and pulmonary BE due to their increased success rates and safety [4, 5].

The situation is quite different when venous BE are asymptomatic. Existing evidence suggests that there is no significant outcome difference between patients managed

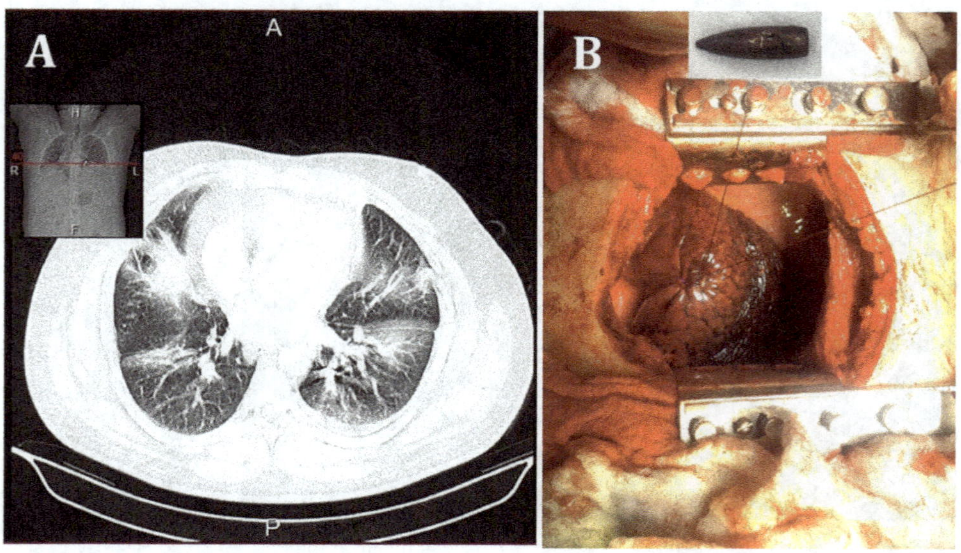

Fig. 2 a CT scan of chest (pulmonary window) showing the bullet in left lower pulmonary lobe. **b** Left thoracotomy for bullet extraction from left lower pulmonary lobe

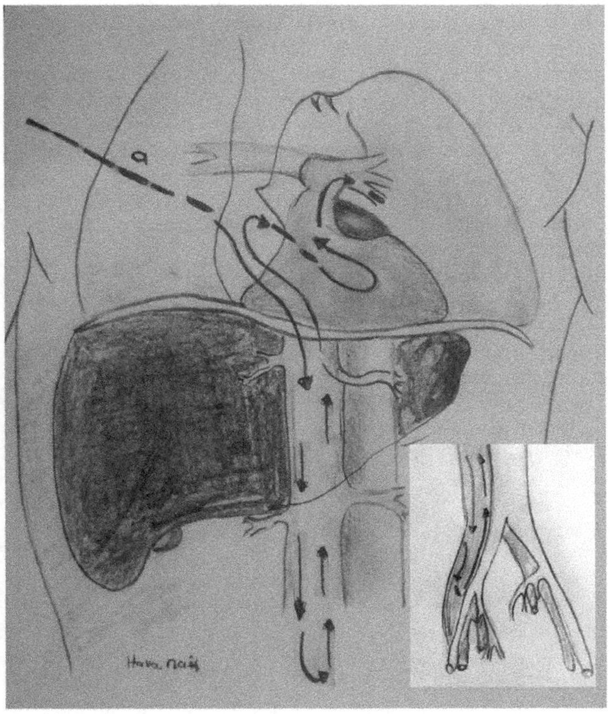

Fig. 3 Path of the bullet with an insert showing its distal-most location in right internal iliac vein

operatively versus non-operatively. Consequently, some authors recommend that retrieval of asymptomatic venous emboli should be considered only if an endovascular technique can be used, as the risks associated with invasive surgery may be too high to be considered on an elective basis [4].

Many authors reported cases of venous BE mostly managed by endovascular techniques [10–13] while others were managed by open surgery [14–20] or non-operatively [5, 21]. Open surgery was either used as a primary procedure or after failure of endovascular intervention. Likewise, non-operative approach was either chosen from the start or after failure of other techniques. The following are two patients' stories depicting endovascular, non-operative, and operative treatments.

Yamanari et al. from Brazil reported the case of a man of 30 with a venous BE from the left external iliac vein to the lingular segment of the left pulmonary artery. Diagnosis was made with whole-body radiography and computed tomography. Two attempts to extract the bullet at time of pulmonary arteriography were unsuccessful, thus the patient was managed conservatively [1].

Hassan et al. reported the case of 23-year-old farmer who sustained a gunshot wound to his left upper chest secondary to a hunter's errant shot. The projectile was impacted between cardiac apex and the diaphragm. The patient was treated conservatively and was discharged home but returned later on to the emergency department with chest pain. The projectile was then identified in the left inferior pulmonary vein. Operative management consisted of a median sternotomy, cardiopulmonary bypass, and a pulmonary venectomy [6].

In our country and many other countries with insufficient security, many people possess firearm weapons and may use them illegally contributing to an increase in civilian violence [22]. One common situation is shooting during social and national celebrations (celebratory gun fire) in which innocent persons may become injured or even killed. The case described herein was hit by a stray bullet falling from a height and therefore most likely it was of low velocity. "Bullets fired into the air usually fall back with terminal velocities much lower than their muzzle velocity when they leave the barrel of a firearm" [23].

The reported cases of pulmonary bullet embolism have mostly followed lesions of peripheral veins without concomitant cardiac involvement [8]. Cardiac gunshot wounds subsequently complicated by migration of bullets into the pulmonary arteries are reportedly rare [2, 8, 9]. Following trans-thoracic gunshot wound, the bullet in the index case penetrated the RA and made two migrations thereafter. First, it moved through the inferior vena cava (IVC) down to the right internal iliac vein. Such retrograde venous bullet migration is expected in the very large veins particularly in standing position and during coughing or a Valsalva maneuver [6]. Second, it returned back into the right heart to settle in the left lower pulmonary lobe artery. Such projectile pathway is very interesting and rare. We did not come through a similar case in the literature.

The patient was saved by surgical extraction of the bullet via left thoracotomy. However, one wonders what happened to the entrance wound of the bullet into the RA. Most likely this wound had sealed spontaneously after an initial bleed which produced the right hemothorax. The bullet could have caused an incomplete obstruction of the IVC or the iliac veins that is why there was no clinical evidence of venous occlusion.

Conclusions

We believe that radiographic confirmation of the location of an intravascular bullet is mandatory just prior to surgery as the bullet may suddenly change its location. The intraoperative use of fluoroscopy is also very helpful in such cases. Even without a Doppler ultrasonography, echo, and/or CT exam, if the plain radiographs show a change in position of bullet quickly from one body region to another, this should alert the physician to the possibility of intravascular bullet location.

Our case had the typical criteria of small-sized low-velocity bullet with inlet but no exit wounds and locations in body regions far from bullet trajectory. Due to symptoms and signs of pulmonary embolism, bullet extraction was indicated and was successfully accomplished by open surgery as our hospital lacked endovascular facilities. Two scenarios were involved in this case of pulmonary BE: a cardiac gunshot wound and migration of bullet through a peripheral vein.

Owing to their extreme rarity, no physician and no center had sufficient experience in management of intravascular migrating bullets. However, high clinical index along ancillary radiographic and imaging techniques may enable the physician in charge to make a timely diagnosis and initiate proper therapy.

Abbreviations

BE: Bullet emboli; Bp: Blood pressure; Bpm: Beat per minute; CXR: Chest X-ray; IVC: Inferior vena cava; PR: Pulse rate; PSO_2: Oxygen saturation; RA: Right atrium; SOB: Shortness of breath

Acknowledgments

We wish to thank Dr. Aram Baram (Assistant professor and consultant cardiothoracic and vascular surgeon) for providing surgical backup during surgery on this case. Our thanks are also extended to Dr. Rebaz J Abdul (consultant radiologist) for reviewing the images and Dr. Havana H Nadr for drawing Fig. 3.

Authors contribution

BDA and OYN collected the relevant patient data and wrote part of the manuscript draft. TAY reviewed the case, wrote the final manuscript, and reviewed the literature. All authors have read and approved the manuscript.

Author details

[1]Department of Thoracic and Cardiovascular Surgery, Shar Teaching Hospital, Sulaimaniyah, Kurdistan, Iraq. [2]Department of surgery, Unit of Cardiovascular and Thoracic Surgery, School of Medicine, Faculty of Medical Sciences, University of Sulaimani, Sulaimaniyah, Kurdistan, Iraq.

References

1. Yamanari MGI, Mansur MCD, Kay FU, Silverio PRB, Jayanthi SK, Funari MBG (2014) Bullet embolism of pulmonary artery: a case report. Radiol Bras 47(2):128–130
2. Bairagi A, Hardcastle TC, Muckart DJJ (2019) Left pulmonary artery bullet embolism following a penetrating cardiacgunshot injury.African. J Emerg Med 9:S61–S63
3. Ronsivalle J, Statler J, Venbrux AC, Arepally A (2005) Intravascular bullet migration: a report of two cases. Mil Med 170(12):1044–1047
4. Wojda TR, Dingley SD, Wolfe S, Terzian WT, Thomas PG, Vazquez D, Sweeney J, Stawicki SP (2017) Foreign intravascular object embolization and migration: bullets, catheters, wires, stents, filters and more. In: Embolic diseases: unusual therapies and challenges. IntechOpen
5. Fernandez-Ranvier GG, Mehta P, Zaid U, Singh K, Barry M, Mahmoud A (2013) Pulmonary artery bullet embolism—case report and review. Int J Surg Case Rep 4:521–523
6. Hassan AM, Cooley RS, Papadimos TJ, Fath JJ, Schwann TA, Elsamaloty H (2009) Pulmonary bullet embolism-a safe treatment strategy of a potentially fatal injury: a case report. Patient Saf Surg 3:12
7. Yoon B, Grasso S, Hofmann LJ (2018) Management of Bullet Emboli to the heart and great vessels. Mil Med 183:e307–e313
8. Imbert P-Y, Goin G, Goudard Y, De La Villeon B, Bonnet PM, Sockeel P, Pauleau G (2016) Pulmonary artery bullet embolism following cardiac gunshot wound. Ann Vasc Surg 36:290.e11–290.e14
9. Agha RA, Borrelli MR, Farwana R, Koshy K, Fowler A, Orgill DP, For the SCARE Group (2018) The SCARE 2018 statement: updating consensus surgical case REport (SCARE) guidelines. Int J Surg 60:132–136
10. Schroeder ME, Pryor HI, Chunk AK, Rahbar R, Arora S, Vasiri K (2011) Retrograde migration and endovascular retrieval of a venous bullet embolus. J Vasc Surg 53(4):1113–1115
11. Nolan T, Phan H, Hardy AH, Khanna P, Dong P (2012) Bullet embolization: multidisciplinary approach by interventional radiology and surgery. Semin InterventRadiol 29(03):192 196 New York: Thieme Medical Publishers
12. Miller KR, Benns MV, Sciarretta JD, Harbrecht BG, Ross CB, Franklin GA, Smith JW (2011) The evolving management of venous bullet emboli: a case series and literature review. Injury 42(5):441–446
13. Carter CO, Havens JM, Robinson WP, Menard MT, Gates JD (2012) Venous bullet embolism and subsequent endovascular retrieval—a case report and review of the literature. Int J Surg Case Rep 3(12):581–583
14. Yordanov Y, Pateron D, May A (2014) An unusual aetiology of abdominal pain: the forgotten bullet. BMJ Case Rep. https://doi.org/10.1136/bcr-2014-208268
15. Stallings LA, Newell MA, Toschlog EA, Thomas CC, Kypson AP (2013) Right ventricular bullet embolism: diagnostic and therapeutic decisions. Injury Extra 44(7):64–66
16. Pan GZ, Bastidas JG, Hasaniya NW, Floridia R Jr (2013) Bullet embolization from an aorto-caval fistula to the heart. Interact Cardiovasc Thorac Surg 16(5):710–711
17. Padula RT, Sandler SC, Camishion R (1969) Delayed bullet embolization to the heart following abdominal gunshot wound. Ann Surg 169(4):599
18. Manganas C, Iliopoulos J, Pang L, Grant PW (2003) Traumatic pulmonary arteriovenous malformation presenting with massive hemoptysis 30 years after penetrating chest injury. Ann Thorac Surg 76(3):942–944
19. Lu K, Sanjay G, Qureshi MA, Wright AS, Kantathut N, Noeller TP (2015) Approach to management of intravascular missile emboli: review of the literature and case report. Western J Emerg Med 16(4):489
20. Koirala B, Shrestha KR, Thapa B, Sayami P (2012) Migration of a piece of shrapnel: femoral vein to superior vena cava-azygous junction. Eur J Cardiothorac Surg 42(3):584–586
21. Duke E, Peterson AA, Erly WK (2014) Migrating bullet: a case of a bullet embolism to the pulmonary artery with secondary pulmonary infarction after gunshot wound to the left globe. J Emerg Trauma Shock 7(1):38–40
22. Taha AY (2005) Emergency thoracotomy for cardiac or great vessel injuries: a report of 5 cases. Basrah J Surg 11(1):100–109. https://doi.org/10.33762/bsurg.2005.55425
23. Celebratory Gunfire. In: Wikipedia. Available from https://en.wikipedia.org/wiki/Celebratory_gunfire. Accessed 15 Aug 2019.

Permissions

All chapters in this book were first published by Springer; hereby published with permission under the Creative Commons Attribution License or equivalent. Every chapter published in this book has been scrutinized by our experts. Their significance has been extensively debated. The topics covered herein carry significant findings which will fuel the growth of the discipline. They may even be implemented as practical applications or may be referred to as a beginning point for another development.

The contributors of this book come from diverse backgrounds, making this book a truly international effort. This book will bring forth new frontiers with its revolutionizing research information and detailed analysis of the nascent developments around the world.

We would like to thank all the contributing authors for lending their expertise to make the book truly unique. They have played a crucial role in the development of this book. Without their invaluable contributions this book wouldn't have been possible. They have made vital efforts to compile up to date information on the varied aspects of this subject to make this book a valuable addition to the collection of many professionals and students.

This book was conceptualized with the vision of imparting up-to-date information and advanced data in this field. To ensure the same, a matchless editorial board was set up. Every individual on the board went through rigorous rounds of assessment to prove their worth. After which they invested a large part of their time researching and compiling the most relevant data for our readers.

The editorial board has been involved in producing this book since its inception. They have spent rigorous hours researching and exploring the diverse topics which have resulted in the successful publishing of this book. They have passed on their knowledge of decades through this book. To expedite this challenging task, the publisher supported the team at every step. A small team of assistant editors was also appointed to further simplify the editing procedure and attain best results for the readers.

Apart from the editorial board, the designing team has also invested a significant amount of their time in understanding the subject and creating the most relevant covers. They scrutinized every image to scout for the most suitable representation of the subject and create an appropriate cover for the book.

The publishing team has been an ardent support to the editorial, designing and production team. Their endless efforts to recruit the best for this project, has resulted in the accomplishment of this book. They are a veteran in the field of academics and their pool of knowledge is as vast as their experience in printing. Their expertise and guidance has proved useful at every step. Their uncompromising quality standards have made this book an exceptional effort. Their encouragement from time to time has been an inspiration for everyone.

The publisher and the editorial board hope that this book will prove to be a valuable piece of knowledge for researchers, students, practitioners and scholars across the globe.

List of Contributors

Waleed Aty
Department of Cardiac Surgery, Liverpool Hospital, Level 1, New Clinical Building, Elizabeth St, Liverpool, Sydney, New South Wales, Australia
Department of Cardiac Surgery, Faculty of Medicine, Suez Canal University, Ismailia, Egypt

Eric Lo, Bruce French and Rebecca Verchin
Department of Cardiac Surgery, Liverpool Hospital, Level 1, New Clinical Building, Elizabeth St, Liverpool, Sydney, New South Wales, Australia

Wei Xuan
Sydney Southwest Clinical School, University of New South Wales, Liverpool, New South Wales, Australia

Rebecca J. Dignan
Department of Cardiac Surgery, Liverpool Hospital, Level 1, New Clinical Building, Elizabeth St, Liverpool, Sydney, New South Wales, Australia
Sydney Southwest Clinical School, University of New South Wales, Liverpool, New South Wales, Australia

Younes Moutakiallah, Abdelatif Boulahya, Aniss Seghrouchni, Reda Mounir, Noureddine Atmani, Youssef El Bekkali and Mahdi Aithoussa
Faculty of Medicine and Pharmacy, Mohammed V University, Rabat, Morocco
Cardiac Surgery Department, Mohammed V Teaching Military Hospital, Hay Riyad, PB 10100 Rabat, Morocco

Mohammed Drissi and El Ghadbane Abdedaim Hatim
Faculty of Medicine and Pharmacy, Mohammed V University, Rabat, Morocco
Intensive Care of Cardiac Surgery, Mohammed V Teaching Military Hospital, Rabat, Morocco

Zouhair Lakhal and Iliyasse Asfalou
Faculty of Medicine and Pharmacy, Mohammed V University, Rabat, Morocco
Cardiology Department, Mohammed V Teaching Military Hospital, Rabat, Morocco

Redouane Abouqal
Faculty of Medicine and Pharmacy, Mohammed V University, Rabat, Morocco
Laboratory of Biostatistics, Clinical and Epidemiological Research (LBRCE), Faculty of Medicine and Pharmacy, Mohammed V University, Rabat, Morocco

Mohamed Abdel Hafez Fouly
Cardiothoracic, Cairo University, Cairo, Egypt

Leena Moshref and Rana Moshref
Department of Surgery, King Abdulaziz University, Jeddah, Kingdom of Saudi Arabia

Mazen Faden
Department of Anesthesia and Critical Care, King Abdulaziz University, Jeddah, Kingdom of Saudi Arabia

Osman Al-Radi
Department of Surgery, King Abdulaziz University, Jeddah, Kingdom of Saudi Arabia
Cardiovascular Department, King Faisal Specialist Hospital & Research Center-General Organization, Jeddah, Kingdom of Saudi Arabia

Tamer Hamouda
Cardiovascular Department, King Faisal Specialist Hospital and Research Center, Jeddah, Saudi Arabia
Cardiothoracic Surgery Department, Faculty of Medicine, Benha University, Benha, Egypt

Mohamed Ismail
Cardiovascular Department, King Faisal Specialist Hospital and Research Center, Jeddah, Saudi Arabia
Cardiothoracic Surgery Department, Faculty of Medicine, Mansoura University, Mansoura, Egypt

Tamer Hamed Ibrahim
Department of Anaesthesia, Faculty of Medicine, Ain Shams University, Cairo, Egypt

Hesham Ewila
Department of Anaesthesia, Faculty of Medicine, Suez Canal University, Ismailia, Egypt

Ahmed Elmahrouk
Cardiovascular Department, King Faisal Specialist Hospital and Research Center, Jeddah, Saudi Arabia
Cardiothoracic Surgery Department, Faculty of Medicine, Tanta University, Tanta, Egypt

Osman O. Al-Radi
Department of Surgery, Faculty of Medicine, King Abdulaziz University, Jeddah 21589, Saudi Arabia
Cardiovascular Department, King Faisal Specialist Hospital and Research Center, Jeddah, Saudi Arabia

Abdelmonem Helal
Department of Paediatrics, Paediatric Cardiology Division, Faculty of Medicine, Cairo University, Giza, Egypt
Pediatric Cardiology Section, Department of Pediatrics, King Faisal Specialist Hospital & Research Center, Jeddah, Kingdom of Saudi Arabia

Mohammed Sanad
Department of Cardiothoracic Surgery, Faculty of Medicine, Mansoura University Hospitals, D17, F5. 60, El Gomhoria Street, Qism 2, Mansoura, Dakahlia 35516, Egypt
Department of Cardiothoracic Surgery, Egypt Ministry of Health and Population, Nasser Institute for Research and Treatment, Cairo, Egypt
Department of Cardiothoracic Surgery, Mansoura International Hospital, Egypt Ministry of Health and Population, Mansoura, Dakahlia, Egypt

Hatem Beshir
Department of Cardiothoracic Surgery, Faculty of Medicine, Mansoura University Hospitals, D17, F5. 60, El Gomhoria Street, Qism 2, Mansoura, Dakahlia 35516, Egypt
Department of Cardiothoracic Surgery, Egypt Ministry of Health and Population, Alexandria Directorate, Alexandria, Egypt

Aram Baram
Department of Surgery, School of Medicine, Faculty of Medical Sciences, University of Sulaimani, François Mitterrand Street, Sulaymaniyah 46001, Iraq
Department of Thoracic and Cardiovascular Surgery, Sulaimani Teaching Hospital, Al Sulaymaniyah, Kurdistan Region 46001, Iraq

Hiwa Sherzad
Kurdistan Board for Medical Specialization/ Cardiothoracic and Vascular Surgery, Sulaimani DOH, Al Sulaymaniyah, Kurdistan Region, Iraq

Ashraf A. H. El Midany and Ayman A. Doghish
Department of Cardiovascular & Thoracic Surgery, Faculty of Medicine, Ain Shams University Hospital, Cairo 11588, Egypt

Valentina Scheggi and Alterini Brunetto
Division of Cardiovascular and Perioperative Medicine, Cardiothoracovascular Department, Azienda Ospedaliero-Universitaria Careggi and University of Florence, Largo Brambilla 3, 50133 Florence, Italy

Iacopo Olivotto, Stefano Del Pace and Niccolò Marchionni
Division of General Cardiology, Cardiothoracovascular Department, Azienda Ospedaliero-Universitaria Careggi and University of Florence, Florence, Italy

Nicola Zoppetti
IFAC-CNR Institute of Applied Physics "Nello Carrara" of the National Research Council, Sesto Fiorentino, Florence, Italy

Alfredo Cerillo and Pier Luigi Stefàno
Division of Cardiac Surgery, Cardiothoracovascular Department, Azienda Ospedaliero-Universitaria Careggi and University of Florence, Florence, Italy

Ahmed F. Elmahrouk
Division of Cardiac Surgery, Cardiovascular Department, King Faisal Specialist Hospital and Research Center, MBC J-16, Jeddah 21499, Saudi Arabia
Cardiothoracic Surgery Department, Tanta University, Tanta, Egypt

Ahmed A. Jamjoom
Division of Cardiac Surgery, Cardiovascular Department, King Faisal Specialist Hospital and Research Center, MBC J-16, Jeddah 21499, Saudi Arabia

Jameel A. Al-Ata
Pediatric Cardiology Section, Department of Pediatrics, King Faisal Specialist Hospital & Research Center, Jeddah, Kingdom of Saudi Arabia
Section of Pediatric Cardiology, Department of Pediatrics, King Abdulaziz University, Jeddah, Saudi Arabia

Hysam Abdelmohty
Cardiothoracic Surgery Department, Faculty of Medicine, Mansoura University, Mansoura, Egypt

Mohamed A. Elanwar
Cardiothoracic Surgery Department, Faculty of Medicine, Cairo University, Cairo, Egypt

Basem M. Abdelgawad
Cardiothoracic Surgery Department, Faculty of Medicine, Benha University, 15 Hasan Muwafi St., Hi Elrawdah, New Benha, Qalyobia 13518, Egypt

Mohammed Ahmed El-Hag-Aly, Rafik Fekry Soliman, Mohamed Mordy Bakoush and Mohamed Gamal Hagag
Cardiothoracic Surgery Department, Faculty of Medicine, Menoufia University, Yassin Abdel Ghaffar Street, Shebin El-Kom, Menoufia, Egypt

Nehad Abdo Zaid and Mahmoud Said Eldesouky
Vascular Surgery Department, Faculty of Medicine, Menoufia University, Yassin Abdel Ghaffar Street, Shebin El-Kom, Menoufia, Egypt

Basem M. Abdelgawad and Mahmoud A. Elshafie
Cardiothoracic Surgery Department, Faculty of Medicine, Benha University, 15 Hasan Muwafi St., Hi Elrawdah, New Benha, Qalyobia 13518, Egypt

Suzan Bayoumy
Cardiology Department, Faculty of Medicine, Tanta University, Tanta, Egypt

Elatafy E. Elatafy
Cardiothoracic Surgery Department, Faculty of Medicine, Tanta University, Tanta, Egypt

Khaled D. Algarni
Department of Cardiac Sciences, College of Medicine, King Saud University, Riyadh 11472, Saudi Arabia
Department of Adult Cardiac Surgery, Prince Sultan Cardiac Center, Riyadh, Saudi Arabia

Amr A. Arafat
Cardiothoracic Surgery Department, Faculty of Medicine, Tanta University, Al-Geish Street, Tanta, Gharbyia 31529, Egypt

Mohamed Reda Zahran
Emergency Medicine, Faculty of Medicine, Tanta University, Mansoura, Egypt

Amr Abd El Monem Abd Elwahab
Cardiothoracic Surgery, Faculty of Medicine, Tanta University, Tanta, Egypt

Mohamed Mahmoud Abo El Nasr
Cardiothoracic Surgery, Faculty of Medicine, Tanta University, Tanta, Egypt

Mohamed Ahmed El Heniedy
Emergency Medicine Department, Faculty of Medicine, Tanta University, Tanta, Egypt

Mohammed Abd Al Jawad
Department of Cardiothoracic Surgery, Faculty of Medicine, Ain Shams University, Abbaseya Square, Cairo, Egypt

Abdallah Nosair and Hesham Alkady
Department of Cardiothoracic Surgery, Faculty of Medicine, Cairo University, Cairo, Egypt

Mohamed Elkahely
Department of Cardiothoracic Surgery, Faculty of Medicine for Girls, Al-Azhar University, Cairo, Egypt

Sherif Nasr
Department of Cardiothoracic Surgery, Faculty of Medicine, Fayoum University, Fayoum, Egypt

Walid Abu Arab and Abdel-maguid Ramadan
Cardiothoracic Surgery Department, Faculty of Medicine, University of Alexandria, Middan Al-Khartoum, Alexandria, Egypt

Mohamed Elshabrawy Saleh and Gehad Awad
Department of Cardiothoracic Surgery, Faculty of Medicine, Mansoura University, Mansoura, Egypt

Ahmed Deebis, Osama Saber, Kareem Elfakharany and Nezar Elnahal
Cardiothoracic Surgery Department, Faculty of Medicine, Zagazig University, Zagazig, Sharkia Governorate, Egypt

Hala Elattar
Anesthesia and Intensive Care Department, Zagazig University, Zagazig, Egypt

Mohamed Osman and Sameh Elameen
Cardiac Surgery Department, National Heart Institute, Cairo, Egypt

Reham Khalil
Radiology Department, Ain Shams University, Cairo, Egypt

Ahmed Hany Abdalla
Anaesthesia Department, National Heart Institute, Cairo, Egypt

Azza Katta
Cardiology Department, National Heart Institute, Cairo, Egypt

Samer Nashef
Cardiothoracic Surgery Department, Royal Papworth Hospital, Cambridge, UK

Mohammad Abdallah
Department of Cardiothoracic Surgery, National Heart Institute, Cairo, Egypt
Department of Cardiothoracic Surgery, Shebein Elkom Teaching Hospital, Shebein Elkom, Egypt

Shymaa Mamdouh, Abdel-Hady El-Gilany, Olfat Farag and Noha ElAdawy
Department of Public Health and Preventive Medicine, Faculty of Medicine, Mansoura University, Mansoura, Egypt

Wael Abdel-Aziz
Department of Cardiothoracic Surgery, Faculty of Medicine, Mansoura University, Mansoura, Egypt

Wael Abdel Aziz Abdel Hamid
Department of Cardiothoracic Surgery, Faculty of Medicine, Mansoura University, Mansoura, Dakahlia, Egypt
Department of Cardiothoracic Surgery, Nasser Institute for Research and Treatment, Egypt Ministry of Health and Population, Cairo, Egypt

Sherif Arafa
Department of Cardiology and Angiology, Faculty of Medicine, Mansoura University, Mansoura, Dakahlia, Egypt

Mohammed Adel Hegazy
Department of Anesthesia and Surgical intensive care, Faculty of Medicine, Mansoura University, Mansoura, Dakahlia, Egypt

Ahmed Hassouna, Mohamed El-Ghanam, Hasan Moftah, Khaled Samir and Khaled Refaat
Cardiothoracic Surgery Department, AinShams University, Cairo, Egypt

Shady Eid Al-Elwany, Yasser Shaban Mubarak and Yasser Ali Kamal
Department of Cardiothoracic Surgery, Faculty of Medicine, Minia University, El-Minya 61519, Egypt

Tiziano Mariani and Carlotta Mazzoni
Division of General Cardiology, Cardiothoracovascular Department, Azienda Ospedaliero-Universitaria Careggi and University of Florence, Florence, Italy

Delan Ahmed Bakir and Yad N. Othman
Department of Thoracic and Cardiovascular Surgery, Shar Teaching Hospital, Sulaimaniyah, Kurdistan, Iraq

Abdulsalam Y. Taha
Department of surgery, Unit of Cardiovascular and Thoracic Surgery, School of Medicine, Faculty of Medical Sciences, University of Sulaimani, Sulaimaniyah, Kurdistan, Iraq

Index

www.ingramcontent.com/pod-product-compliance
Lightning Source LLC
LaVergne TN
LVHW082227200926
848484LV00008B/2314